Emergency Orthopaedics and Trauma

Andrew Unwin BSc FRCS
Senior Registrar in Orthopaedics
Chelsea and Westminster Hospital

Kirsten Jones DA FRCS (A&E)
Accident and Emergency Department
Musgrove Park Hospital, Taunton

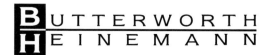
BUTTERWORTH
HEINEMANN

Butterworth-Heinemann Ltd
Linacre House, Jordan Hill, Oxford OX2 8DP

A member of the Reed Elsevier group

OXFORD LONDON BOSTON
MUNICH NEW DELHI SINGAPORE SYDNEY
TOKYO TORONTO WELLINGTON

First published 1995

British Library Cataloguing in Publication Data
A catalogue record for this book is available from the
British Library

ISBN 0 7506 2034 X

Library of Congress Cataloging in Publication Data
A catalogue record for this book is available from the
Library of Congress.

Typeset by Keyword Ltd, Wallington, Surrey
Printed in Great Britain

Emergency Orthopaedics and Trauma

To Diana and David

Contents

Foreword

Since one quarter of emergencies presenting in the accident and emergency department are the result of injury to the musculo-skeletal system, decisions on their management are critical. Without good diagnosis and treatment, lives can be lost or ruined. Senior and experienced orthopaedic surgeons cannot be present in the emergency department for twenty four hours every day so that an accurate and practical reference book is essential to avoid the many errors and pitfalls which, sadly, are not uncommonly encountered.

The authors of this book have achieved that elusive goal of a short and easily readable text with sufficient illustrations to guide the less experienced doctor safely through all the commonly encountered orthopaedic emergencies. The first part of the book, dealing with principles of diagnosis and mangement, is essential reading for orthopaedic and accident and emergency staff whilst the second part will surely become the definitive reference for specific injuries. Principles of applied anatomy, physiology, radiology, pharmacology and anaesthesia have all been concisely included in their relevant context. Practical procedures are clearly described when appropriate for the emergency setting but the strength of this book lies in the clear guidance on when a particular condition requires specialist referral. Providing the guidelines in the text are followed all the common errors will be avoided.

The authors are both young and closely involved with their subject which they clearly expound with an authority that derives from a thorough understanding. They and the publishers are to be congratulated for creating a much needed book which incorporates modern thinking in acute management of fractures and multiple injuries and will fill a gap in emergency text books. It should become an indispensable reference and guide for practitioners and students of Accident and Emergency Medicine and Orthopaedics.

A. J. Hall FRCS
Consultant Orthopaedic Surgeon
Charing Cross Hospital, London

There are many textbooks dealing with the immediate management of fractures and acute soft tissue injuries. The purpose of this text is to cover the field of trauma specifically for junior doctors working in Accident and Emergency departments with special emphasis on what should lie within their field of expertise, pointing out in clear terms when a junior doctor should be seeking early advice from a senior colleague.

A additional feature of this book (which I sure will become a well-thumbed practical reference manual) is the inclusion of the management of some of the common orthopaedic conditions not due to trauma which present to the emergency medicine service and which are less well covered in the undergraduate curriculum.

The authors draw heavily on their experience from the Advanced Trauma Life Support course in writing about major trauma and passing on the up-to-date basic tenets of trauma assessment and management.

The book, in especially covering hand injuries in detail, in indicating appropriate referral practice to fracture clinics and in dealing with the timing of referrals, fills a gap in the A/E reference library which will be welcomed by harassed casualty officers during the lonely hours of the night. The authors, being both currently senior registrars in orthopaedics and A/E respectively, are to be commended on their initiative and the clarity with which they present their ideas.

John Thurston MB FRCP FFAEM
*Honorary Registrar to the Faculty of
Accident and Emergency Medicine,
Queen Mary's Hospital, London*

Preface

This text is intended as an aid to all junior doctors who have to deal with the emergency presentation of musculo-skeletal disease. The book deals in detail with the initial management of the patient and specifically excludes details of in-patient care, for which there are many excellent texts. What is given is a reasoned account of the principles of patient management, including the conditions that require in-patient and out-patient referral.

What we believe to be a unique feature is the inclusion of not only fractures and soft tissue injuries but also some common non-trauma orthopaedic conditions that may present in the emergency setting. Many doctors find the latter difficult to manage, with little or no training in elective orthopaedic surgery. As an aid to this,

the basics of applied anatomy of the limbs and the spine are given.

The management of major trauma has changed radically in recent years, and the essentials of trauma assessment are explained. In addition, as head and chest injuries are common problems in the trauma patient, their assessment and management is given in detail.

Our aim is for the book to be both a comprehensive text and a manual for use in the Accident and Emergency Department. We hope it will be of use to Accident and Emergency staff, junior orthopaedic surgeons and medical students.

A.J.U.
K.E.J.

Acknowledgements

We would like to thank the following for their generous help and advice in addition to the use of their material incorporated into the text: Mr R. Allum, Dr A. Bremner-Smith, Mr M. Burwell, Miss G. Bryce, Mr M. Clancy, Mr C. Cutting, Dr. D. Hales, Mr A. Hall, Dr G. Hughes, Mr J. Jones, Mr C. McLauchlan, Dr S. Meek, Mr C. Oakland, Mr S. Palmer, Mr N. Rawlinson, Mr P. Salt, Mrs S. Sellars, Mr M. Thomas, Mr W. Williams, Ms C. Zank-McKelvey, and the Medical Illustration Departments of Bristol Royal Infirmary, Chelsea and Westminster Hospital, Frenchay Hospital, Taunton and Somerset Hospital and Wexham Park Hospital.

Part I
Management Principles

1

Orthopaedic diagnosis and referral

Orthopaedic diagnosis

Introduction

Emergency orthopaedics and trauma can, to some extent, be correctly assumed to cover injury to bones, joints and soft tissues. However, it must never be forgotten that these are part of a whole patient. The 'ankle in cubicle four' is also a patient; with a history of injury, a past medical history and, hopefully, other functioning parts of their body besides the musculo-skeletal system! If a blinkered approach to the examination is adopted, much valuable and important information may be missed. Whilst the examination will naturally focus upon the injured part, remembering that this belongs to a whole person will go a long way towards avoiding incorrect or incomplete diagnoses.

History

Taking a complete and appropriate history when one is often pressed for time requires experience and patience. Whilst it may be helpful to allow the patient to tell you what happened in their own words, most patients will need guidance through this if the salient facts are to be obtained.

If an injury has been sustained, you will need to know **what, how, when and where** it happened:

1. **What and how.** Ascertain exactly what the patient was doing at the time. Try to gain some idea of the degree of **force** involved and the direction and point of impact. This will give an indication of the extent of expected injury, and may also make you suspect other injuries. If a fracture has been sustained with the minimum of force, this may suggest a pathological fracture. Was the force direct or indirect? Again, this will suggest a pattern of injury.

2. **When** an injury happened is important, as it will give some idea as to the extent to which it has incapacitated the patient, the increased potential for infection if a wound is present, and the degree of shock that may exist in a multiply-injured patient.

3. **Where** the injury occurred is important if falls from heights are involved, or again, if a wound is present (a laceration to the leg sustained in a farmyard has a higher potential for infection than one sustained on the edge of a coffee table).

If the injury was sustained in a road traffic accident, important facts to elicit include:

1. Was the patient a car driver or passenger, a pedestrian, cyclist or motor cyclist?
2. The approximate speed involved.
3. If in a car:

- Where was the patient sitting, and were they wearing a seatbelt?
- Were they thrown from the car? This increases the chance of serious injury by 300%.

- What injuries have been sustained by the other occupants?
- Was the patient trapped, and for how long?
- What was the degree and position of damage to the car; this will reflect the damage to the patient.

4. If appropriate, was the patient wearing a helmet?
5. What treatment has been given by paramedics?

The most common and important complaint is of **pain**. The degree of pain experienced will depend upon the site of the injury, the instability of any fracture present, and the patient's response to their injury. Ask about factors that increase or decrease their pain, and whether it has changed since the time of injury. Discover what first aid measures have been employed. Try to assess the degree of functional impairment, but **remember some patients can have reasonable function even with a fracture**. This is especially so with impacted fractures of the humeral or femoral neck, fractures of the distal radius and greenstick fractures in children.

Enquire as to the presence of other symptoms such as loss of sensation or motor power, particularly distal to the site of the injury. It is also useful to ask if the patient is hurt anywhere other than their main complaint; this helps avoid overlooking other injuries.

It is important to discover the patient's occupation, and their dominant hand in the case of upper limb injuries. A brief past medical history, drug history, tetanus status and any allergies should also be elicited where relevant. **Always consider the possibility of an underlying medical condition that may have precipitated the injury**, e.g. syncope, epilepsy.

Examination

The examination can be easily divided into **look, feel, move**. All too often, insufficient time is spent on the inspection stage, where much important information can be learnt.

Look

Look at the whole patient, not just the affected limb. Look at their general state of health, for signs of systemic disease and their reaction to injury. Signs of systemic disease may give clues as to an underlying cause for the accident. Be aware of the possibility of other injuries.

It is important to inspect the whole limb. Look for old scars. Compare it with the other side, looking for asymmetry of both contour and posture. Is the limb bent, shortened or abnormally aligned? If swelling is present, determine if this is well localized or more diffuse. Remember that swelling may take up to 24 hours to develop. If a joint is injured, does the swelling confine itself to the joint or extend beyond it?

Look at the skin for abrasions and lacerations. If bruising is present, determine whether this is at the point of impact or has gravitated down the limb. Assess the general colour of the skin, particularly for signs of vascular impairment.

Finally, in patients with symptoms of more gradual onset or longer duration, inspect for signs of muscle wasting, particularly in the lower limbs.

Feel

This must be performed gently. Ask the patient to point to 'where it hurts'. Forcefully squeezing a fracture, whilst asking 'does this hurt?', will gain neither the confidence of the patient nor a great deal of information. Watch the patient's face; this will tell you if you are hurting them, even if they don't! Feel the skin, the soft tissues and the bone.

Feel the temperature of the **skin**. Increased temperature may suggest infection or an acute inflammatory process. A very cold extremity should raise suspicions of a vascular injury. Feel for a pulse distal to the site of the injury, and assess the capillary return of the skin. Assess whether the skin is unduly moist or dry, which may be due to an underlying nerve injury. It is vital to formally assess sensation in the dermatomes both around and distal to the site of injury.

Palpate the **soft tissues** for tenderness, swelling, surgical emphysema and the presence of underlying foreign bodies if appropriate. If a discrete swelling is present, palpate its size, shape, consistency and fluctuance. If tenderness is elicited, determine its extent by palpating from all directions.

Finally, gently palpate the **bones**. A fracture may be obvious at this stage. An important point to remember is that a fracture will be tender on palpation from every aspect. Soft tissue injury will usually only be tender on palpation directly over the site of injury. If a joint is involved, palpate for both the normal contours of the joint, which may suggest a dislocation or subluxation, and for the presence of an effusion.

Move

If, from the history and examination performed so far, a fracture is either obvious or highly suspected, **do not move the affected part to try to elicit crepitus or abnormal movement of the fractured bone**. This is will only increase the patient's pain and will not aid in your diagnosis. However this does not prevent you from assessing function at the joints above and below the site of a fracture.

In all other cases, active movement should be assessed before passive movement. When measuring the range of movement of a joint, it is often helpful to compare the injured side with the 'normal' uninjured side. When describing the range of movement, the normal anatomical position is usually regarded as 0 degrees, and measurements are taken from this point. If a loss of normal function exists, determine whether pain is the restricting factor, or whether weakness or a mechanical block is responsible. If weakness (secondary either to an acute nerve or tendon injury, or chronic muscle problem) is suspected, this can be confirmed by demonstrating an increased range of **passive** movement when compared with active movement.

At the same time as assessing movement, it is also necessary to assess strength. This is not only important in the more chronic problems with muscle wasting, but also in penetrating tendon injuries. Movement can be present in a tendon that is 90% lacerated, and **the injury will be overlooked unless power is also assessed**, which will be markedly reduced. Strength is assessed using the MRC (**Medical Research Council**) scale:

M5 – Normal power
M4 – Active movement against gravity and resistance
M3 – Active movement against gravity
M2 – Active movement but not against gravity
M1 – Flicker or trace of contraction.
M0 – No contraction

If a fracture of a bone is suspected, it is important to assess movement at adjacent joints, e.g. at the elbow and shoulder in a patient with a suspected Colles fracture. Movement at a joint should be assessed in all its possible directions, e.g. flexion, extension, adduction, abduction, internal and external rotation.

Finally, the presence of movement in an abnormal plane should be assessed. Injuries around particular joints can produce ligament injury and consequent instability, e.g. the ulnar collateral ligament of the thumb and the collateral ligaments of the knee. The joint should be stressed in the appropriate plane and abnormal movement detected. If necessary, compare with the normal side. This may be painful in the patient with an acute injury, and local or general anaesthesia may be required for a thorough assessment.

Radiography

By far the commonest imaging technique used in the emergency situation is radiography. If a thorough history and examination have been taken and performed, x-rays should be used to confirm the diagnosis and are mandatory in all cases of a suspected fracture. However, they should never be used as a substitute for clinical assessment. **A patient should not be sent to x-ray before being examined**. This may be dangerous; the management of serious injuries requiring resuscitation, manipulation or analgesia may be delayed. This practice may also lead to the wrong area being x-rayed, e.g. the ankle rather than the 5th metatarsal. It should also be remembered that requesting an x-ray is the same as prescribing a dose of radiation for the patient, and therefore radiography should not be used indiscriminately.

Why x-ray?

Failure to diagnose a fracture is an important matter for both the patient and the doctor from a medico-legal point of view. The x-ray allows the exact site and nature of the injury to be determined, including the number of fragments, degree and direction of displacement and angulation of a fracture, and gives evidence of pre-existing disease. It may also reveal signs such as air in the soft tissues suggestive of a penetrating injury. Radiography allows future management decisions about the patient's care to be made. The risk of missing a fracture can be minimized if the following guidelines are adhered to.

The x-ray request

The correct x-ray cannot be requested until the patient has been formally assessed. The request form should include brief clinical details and the particular area of the bone or joint suspected of being injured, e.g. *'inversion injury; swollen/ tender lateral malleolus, unable to weight-bear. X-ray left ankle please'*.

If this doctrine is not followed, fractures will be missed; the classic example is the fractured scaphoid bone missed when ordinary views of the wrist are requested. Similar examples are the missed fracture of the base of the fifth metatarsal on ankle views, and the fractured calcaneum on ordinary foot views.

If hairline or stress fractures are suspected, request a 'coned down' view over the specific area of maximum tenderness. When looking for foreign bodies, e.g. glass, the request form should specify this, as the radiographer will take the film using a different exposure to look at the soft tissues, and place a marker at the site of the wound. X-rays of children, especially joints such as the elbow, are often very difficult to interpret, and it is acceptable to request views of the uninjured side as a comparison.

However, this should only be done once the films of the injured limb have been scrutinized.

The x-ray itself

There are certain minimum standards expected of an adequate radiograph. It should be taken in **at least two planes**, usually anteroposterior and lateral. If only a single projection is taken, an injury such as a posterior dislocation of the shoulder may be missed, with serious consequences for both the doctor and the patient. Furthermore, an apparently minor fracture can appear alarmingly displaced on a second view. Specific areas may require other views, such as oblique projections for suspected scaphoid fractures. The whole length of the bone must be visualized, **including the joint above and below.** This avoids missing pitfalls such as the Monteggia and Galeazzi fractures.

Examination of the x-ray

Check that the x-rays you are viewing **belong to your patient**, and **check in the x-ray packet.** It can be guaranteed that the only film that demonstrates the fracture is the one that has been left in the bottom of the packet.

Before scrutinizing the film at close quarters, stand back and assess the x-ray as a whole. This may reveal useful information such as the size, shape and quality of the bones, and their alignment. This applies also to chest x-rays; a pneumothorax is usually much easier to see from 2 feet rather than 2 inches!

It is then important to adopt a methodical approach to your assessment. Examine the **soft tissue shadows** for swelling, foreign bodies and signs of joint effusion, e.g. the anterior 'fat pad sign' at the elbow. In patients with major trauma, look for subcutaneous air on the chest film.

Assess the bones by carefully tracing round their contours, looking for deformity or breaks in the cortex. Assess the joint spaces, and look particularly for bony fragments lying within them. Finally, assess the alignment of the bones, and their relationship with neighbouring bones.

If you find a fracture, decide whether you think the injury is traumatic, stress-related or pathological. Is the injury new or old? Finally, and importantly, **look for the second fracture**. It is all too easy to stand back satisfied once you have identified an injury, and miss a second one.

The referral

The referral for admission

This referral will usually take place over the telephone. Prior to this, ensure that you have all the information about the patient to hand, and be clear in your mind **why** you are making the referral. It is polite to know both the name and grade of the doctor you are telephoning, and be sure that it is someone of the appropriate seniority. Whilst hospitals differ as to which grade referrals are made to, it would be wholly inappropriate to refer a patient with a partial amputation of the lower leg to the House Officer.

Once contact has been made, clearly introduce yourself and establish who you are speaking to. There is nothing more frustrating than pouring out a long complicated story, only to find that at the end of this you are speaking to the theatre orderly, who has answered the Registrar's bleep as he is operating.

State at the outset that you are making a referral. i.e. 'I would like to refer you a 19-year-old . . . '. Give the sex, age, occupation and hand dominance (if appropriate) of the patient, with any relevant past medical history. Give a concise account of the history, stating precisely when the injury occurred and the relevant examination and x-ray findings. Describe the injury in precise accepted terms. For example, when describing a fracture, indicate whether it is closed or open, comminuted, displaced, rotated or angulated. If appropriate, give details of any other injuries, e.g. a head injury, and a general status of the patient.

Relate any treatment that has been given in the Accident Department, including splintage, manipulation, dressings, analgesia, antibiotics and tetanus prophylaxis.

If the patient is expected to require a general anaesthetic, know when they last ate or drank **anything.**

Finally, give the reason for your referral. This may be blatantly obvious, as in the partially amputated leg, but otherwise state whether you are referring because, for example, the patient requires fracture manipulation or open reduction, wound debridement, admission for pain relief, neurological observation following a head injury etc.

It is always polite to thank your colleague for accepting the referral – this goes a long way towards establishing harmonious working relationships.

The referral for advice

Whilst the information given in this situation will, on the whole, be the same as that for a referral for admission, it is important to state at the outset that you are telephoning for **advice**. Also, make it clear whether you are requesting telephone advice only, or for your colleague to come and see the patient personally.

Telephone advice alone, without personal review of the patient, is potentially dangerous. It should not be sought for all but the most simple advice. If telephone advice alone is given, it is **essential** to record this in the medical notes, together with the name and grade of the doctor giving it. If this is not done, the potential for medico-legal problems should the patient develop future complications, is considerable. Remember, however, good advice can only be given if you pass on accurate information.

When advice has been given, ensure that you clearly understand all the facts; it is often worth repeating them back to your colleague. Also, clearly establish what follow-up arrangements are required, and when. Again, thank your colleague for their time and advice.

Referral to the fracture clinic

Many orthopaedic departments have clear guidelines regarding what are appropriate fracture clinic referrals, and what would be better seen in a routine orthopaedic clinic or by the General Practitioner. The majority of orthopaedic injuries not admitted to hospital will require fracture clinic follow-up. Problems that are **not** suitable for fracture clinic referral include chronic mechanical back pain, aggravation of long-standing degenerative change, tenosynovitis or other 'elective' chronic conditions.

The information that the fracture clinic will require is essentially that recorded in a clear, comprehensive and legible set of A & E notes. The time and mechanism of injury, time of presentation and complaint of the patient should be recorded. Relevant positive and negative examination findings, together with results of investigations, are required. If x-rays are taken, their findings should be clearly recorded.

The details of treatment must include manipulations, wound dressings, splintage, antibiotic therapy, analgesia and tetanus prophylaxis administered. If a manipulation has been performed, record also the findings of the post-manipulation x-ray; **this is essential**.

Finally, record any advice given to the patient, e.g. rest, elevation, to remain non weight-bearing etc.

Whether the patient is referred to the next days' clinic, or in a few days' time, will depend largely on hospital policy. Injuries that must be reviewed in the next available clinic include all children's fractures and all fractures that have been manipulated.

2
Orthopaedic conditions

Osteoarthritis

Osteoarthritis is characterized by a **degenerative disease** of joints. There is a destruction of the articular cartilage with secondary destruction of bone. Two major forms exist:

1. **Primary osteoarthritis** – no obvious cause.
2. **Secondary osteoarthritis** – degenerative change within a joint as a consequence of an underlying pathology, e.g. malunion of intra-articular and peri-articular fractures, avascular necrosis, inflammatory arthropathies and many other joint problems.

The **radiological features** of osteoarthritis are:

1. Narrowing of the joint space.
2. Subchondral sclerosis.
3. Osteophytes.
4. The formation of pseudocysts around the joint.

Patients rarely present as an emergency with osteoarthritis but you should be able to differentiate the radiological changes from acute trauma.

The inflammatory arthropathies

Rheumatoid arthritis

Rheumatoid arthritis is the commonest of the inflammatory arthropathies. The primary pathology is one of synovial inflammation which may spread to destroy the surrounding cartilage, bone, ligaments and tendons by the **pannus** that is formed. Although many cases of established rheumatoid are easy to diagnose, remember that the disease may present itself as a monoarticular arthropathy to your Accident and Emergency Department!

The disease process usually starts in the small joints of the hand. Rheumatoid arthritis is usually a symmetrical polyarthropathy although it may involve only one joint initially. Extra-articular manifestations are common; tiredness, myalgia and fever are often found at presentation.

Radiological features at the outset are often unremarkable, merely showing a joint effusion. Intermediate signs are erosions but later a destructive arthritis occurs. Markers for the condition, although sometimes unreliable, are a raised erythrocyte sedimentation rate (ESR), C-reactive protein (CRP) and rheumatoid factor (but 30–40% of rheumatoids have a normal serology).

Psoriatic arthropathy

Psoriasis may be complicated by an inflammatory arthropathy primarily affecting the distal joints of the hands and feet. Monoarticular arthropathies may also occur.

Crystal arthropathies

If crystals accumulate within a joint an intense inflammatory reaction may result. The two most common types are urate crystals causing **gout** and pyrophosphate crystals causing **pseudogout**.

Gout and pseudogout may present as an acute inflammatory arthropathy of one or more joints. The condition can resemble a septic arthritis and is therefore an important condition to diagnose. The acute attacks may subside and chronic disease may result with a destructive arthropathy.

The diagnosis is confirmed by aspiration of joint fluid that demonstrates crystals under polarized light. The serum urate may be raised in classic gout. Treatment in the acute stage is with anti-inflammatories (allopurinol should not be given in the acute stage as it may worsen the symptoms).

Infective arthropathy

Some organisms may result in antigenic stimulation of synovium and other structures and the condition is termed a **reactive arthropathy**. The commonest form of reactive arthropathy is **Reiter's syndrome** whereby the patient presents with arthropathy associated with conjunctivitis and urethritis. The condition usually affects the smaller joints of the hand but it may also result in monoarticular swelling. Treatment should be directed at the primary treatment of the infective organism (if appropriate) as well as symptomatic relief with anti-inflammatory drugs.

Ankylosing spondylitis

Ankylosing spondylitis is an auto-immune disorder that results in an inflammatory arthropathy, most commonly of the back and sacroiliac joints. The end result in untreated cases is a stiff and rigid spine. The most common abnormal investigation is a raised ESR. Suspect the disease in a young adult patient presenting with low back pain with any features of an inflammatory arthropathy. Referral to a rheumatologist should be arranged if the disease is suspected.

Causes of a monoarticular arthropathy

The patient with a non-traumatic monoarticular arthropathy (i.e. pain and swelling in only one joint) is a frequent reason for presentation to Accident and Emergency. Common causes include:

1. Synovial pathology, e.g. rheumatoid arthritis, ankylosing spondylitis.
2. Structural derangement within the joint, e.g. meniscal tears (remember that meniscal tears may not have a definite recent history of trauma).
3. Crystal arthropathy – gout and pseudogout (pyrophosphate arthropathy).
4. Reactive arthropathy, e.g. Reiter's syndrome.
5. Psoriatic arthropathy.
6. Septic arthritis – **always exclude this in any case of monoarticular swelling**.
7. Osteoarthritis.
8. Miscellaneous, e.g. loose bodies, synovial chondromatosis, osteochondritis dissecans.

Diseases of abnormal bone quality

Osteoporosis

Osteoporosis is a condition characterized by a decreased amount of bone per unit volume. Most cases occur without any underlying disorder but osteoporosis may be associated with immobilization (e.g. within a plaster cast), drugs (e.g. steroids), metabolic conditions (e.g. Cushing's syndrome, thyrotoxicosis) and malignancy (e.g. multiple myeloma).

Most cases do not present until the bone involved undergoes structural failure, e.g. fracture or collapse. The most common sites affected are metaphyseal regions, e.g. the distal radius, the proximal femur and the spine. Many fractures seen in the Accident and Emergency Department will have osteoporosis as an underlying cause.

Osteomalacia and rickets

These conditions represent **decreased mineralization of bone**. Rickets is the form encountered in childhood whilst osteomalacia is seen in adults. The commonest cause is vitamin D deficiency, although other causes are renal failure, gastrointestinal malabsorbtion and other metabolic disorders.

Rickets may present with systemic problems (e.g. tetany associated with hypocalcaemia) or structural bone changes, which include bowing of long bones and prominent epiphyses. X-rays usually demonstrate widened epiphyses as well as the structural consequences of the condition.

Osteomalacia most commonly has an insidious presentation (e.g. backache) but may also present with a fracture. On radiography the appearances are very similar to osteoporosis but in addition stress fractures called **Looser's zones** may be seen. Investigation may reveal a raised alkaline phosphatase; the serum calcium is usually in the normal range but may be decreased.

Paget's disease

Paget's disease, or **osteitis deformans,** is a disease of unknown cause characterized by inappropriately increased bone turnover. There is both increased osteoblastic and osteoclastic activity, the proportions of which vary at different stages in the natural history of the condition.

The disease is commonly asymptomatic. Most cases present with fracture or other structural bone failure. Some may have bone pain or other complications such as nerve entrapment (e.g. of the VIIIth cranial nerve resulting in deafness), heart failure (due to the increased bone vascularity) or spinal stenosis. A small number may develop an **osteosarcoma** and this should always be borne in mind in any patient with Paget's disease who presents with new symptoms.

The treatment of Paget's disease lies outside the scope of this book but includes simple analgesics, calcitonin and biphosponates.

Osteomyelitis and septic arthritis

Acute osteomyelitis

Active recent infection of bone is termed acute osteomyelitis. It is most commonly seen in children although occasional cases occur in adults.

The infection is usually haematogenous and nearly always starts in the metaphyseal region of a long bone. A recent upper respiratory tract infection is a common finding. Bone infection is an extremely serious condition as very rapidly the patient becomes systemically unwell with fever etc. Untreated the condition may lead to death via septicaemia and multiple organ failure.

An early presentation of acute osteomyelitis is a child with a painful hot limb who is unwell and with a fever. If untreated the condition may present as:

1. Breakthrough of the infection through the bone into the surrounding tissues and ultimately the skin – this is the forerunner of chronic osteomyelitis.
2. The infection may be partially walled-off by the patient's immune system, resulting in an intra-osseous abscess termed a **Brodie's abscess**.

Any child who presents with the clinical suspicion of acute osteomyelitis **must** be admitted. **The x-rays are initially normal.** Do **not** give any antibiotics until adequate specimens have been taken from the bone, by biopsy or trephine if necessary. The child may be dehydrated and intravenous fluids are often necessary. The ESR, CRP and white cell count (WCC) should be measured and blood cultures taken. Most cases of acute osteomyelitis are due to one of two organisms – *Staphylococcus aureus* and *Haemophilus influenzae*.

Once admitted and appropriate specimens are taken, the child should be given the appropriate intravenous antibiotic. If there is any evidence of pus or abscess formation, or of a deterioration in the clinical condition of the child, the involved area of bone should be trephined.

The risk of septic arthritis following acute osteomyelitis

The differences between acute osteomyelitis and septic arthritis should be clearly understood. Whilst acute osteomyelitis is a serious condition, septic arthritis is calamitous and unless effectively treated will result in permanent and significant deformity.

Certain metaphyseal regions are intracapsular; hence if osteomyelitis is present within the metaphysis, there is a likelihood of spread of infection to within the joint, resulting in septic arthritis. This is the case in the **hip, shoulder, knee, elbow and wrist.**

Chronic osteomyelitis

Chronic osteomyelitis is the almost inevitable result of untreated acute osteomyelitis. Be aware that a patient may present acutely with an exacerbation of the problem.

The bone in chronic osteomyelitis is infected. Attempts are made at new bone formation which surrounds the old infected dead bone. The dead bone is termed **sequestrum** and the new bone **involucrum**. A **sinus** exists from the site of the sequestrum through to the skin. The sinus episodically discharges pus and/or dead bone. The chronic osteomyelitis may become acute and require antibiotic treatment, which will temporarily help the situation but not cure the condition.

A patient with chronic osteomyelitis should be referred to the next available clinic for further assessment. It is probably best not to give any antibiotics until appropriate specimens have been taken. Occasionally the patient may need to be admitted for intravenous therapy and elevation etc.

The patient with chronic osteomyelitis may present with one of the complications of the disease, for example:

structural deformity
amyloidosis (secondary to the chronic infective process)
malignant change at the site of the sinus.

Septic arthritis

Septic arthritis is a **surgical emergency** and needs to be managed expertly and quickly to prevent serious morbidity and possible mortality. Pus within a joint results in its rapid destruction. If the condition is suspected rapid action is required in terms of surgical drainage and antibiotic therapy.

Septic arthritis may occur as a result of:

1. Osteomyelitis where the metaphysis is intracapsular (see above).
2. Haematogenous spread (there is often a history of recent upper respiratory tract infection or instrumentation at a distant site such as umbilical catheterization).
3. Local direct infection from wounds etc.

The patient with septic arthritis, often a child, presents with a painful swollen joint with fever and systemic upset. There is a joint effusion (**pyarthrosis**). The outstanding feature of the condition is that **the joint cannot be moved at all without causing extreme pain**. Take care, however, in the patient on steroids or in the diabetic – such patients may not present with a florid clinical picture and thus may have more significant pathology at presentation.

If the condition is at all suspected, **refer the patient immediately**. Give intravenous fluids to prevent dehydration. Relevant investigations are a WCC, ESR and CRP. Blood cultures should be taken. The x-rays are usually normal initially although an effusion may be seen. **Do not give any antibiotics at this stage**. The patient should be taken as soon as possible to the operating theatre for washout and lavage of the joint under general anaesthesia. A broad spectrum antibiotic can then be given and the choice modified from the results of the washout specimens.

3
Fractures and other musculo-skeletal injuries

Introduction

Although it is easy to think of a 'fracture' purely in terms of the bony injury, for a bone to fracture there is often significant damage to the surrounding structures, i.e. skin, muscle, nerves, arteries etc. If there is a fracture within a limb, always think of all the structures rather than simply the bone. Similarly, remember that bones may break as a result of many different mechanisms and forces. It is very helpful to have some indication of the forces involved in trauma; for example an ankle fracture caused by a high velocity road traffic accident is likely to be more severe than that caused by a slip on the pavement.

Fractures may occur as a result of **direct** forces, e.g. the direct blow to the shin in soccer resulting in a tibial fracture, or by **indirect** forces, e.g. a skiing injury whereby twisting forces are applied to the tibia (Fig. 3.1). In general terms, direct forces result in a greater degree of soft tissue injury.

Always remember that a fracture does not belong to an x-ray but to a patient! You cannot diagnose or treat a fracture properly without taking a history and examination. The injury may be worse than the x-ray suggests in that

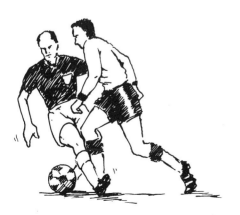
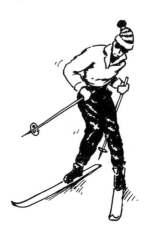

Figure 3.1 - Direct and indirect forces

the forces applied to the patient may have resulted in more deformity at the time of impact than the x-ray indicates. Remember the rest of the patient – other injuries are possible, and the mechanism of injury may give you clues as to what they may be.

Diagnosis of musculo-skeletal injuries

History

This can be very helpful, not only in diagnosis but also in treatment; a good principle in fracture reduction is to apply force in the opposite direction to the deforming forces. Important information to obtain is the mechanism of injury, the magnitude of the force involved and any prior reduction and treatment by paramedical personnel. It is necessary to realize that an underlying medical precipitant, e.g. epilepsy or myocardial infarction, may have resulted in the fall that led to the injury.

Examination

This should include both a general examination of the patient as well as a local evaluation of the injured part. The general examination will reveal any evidence of hypovolaemic shock, precipitating medical condition and other injuries. Local examination should proceed **with great care not to hurt the patient,** but sufficient to exclude any concomitant pathology, e.g. arterial injury. It should include the following elements.

- **Inspection** The skin should be carefully inspected to ensure that the fracture is not open. Any asymmetry of the limb may suggest an injury (Fig. 3.2). Bruising and skin shadowing may be present.
- **Palpation** A fracture is usually tender on palpation and this should be **carefully** carried out without undue distress for the patient. Other areas of a limb need to be palpated to exclude an associated injury, e.g. in medial malleolar fractures the fibula throughout its length needs to be palpated (Fig. 3.3). It is **mandatory** to examine the limb distal to a fracture to assess the neurovascular status. The examination should be repeated

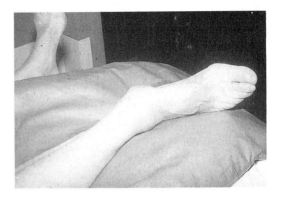

Figure 3.2 – Deformity can be obvious

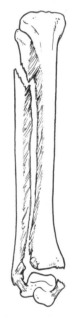

Figure 3.3 – Medial malleolar fractures may be associated with high fibular fractures. If they are, the interosseous membrane between them has torn, rendering the relationship between the two bones unstable.

with time. The signs of a compartment syndrome should be carefully excluded (see below, Complications of Fractures and Dislocations).
- **Movements** The elicitation of crepitus at a fracture site is both unnecessary and distressing and should **not** routinely be performed. The movement of surrounding joints, exclusion of distal neurological problems and tendon function is helpful however.

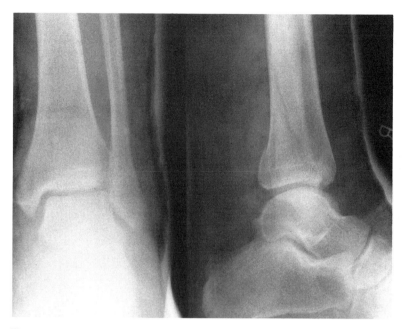

Figure 3.4 – Two views are always needed – this fibular fracture is only apparent on one view

Radiography

If a fracture is suspected, an x-ray is mandatory (unless your unit has a protocol for clinical diagnosis of certain injuries, e.g. toe fractures). Some important principles are:

1. Always obtain two views of the area (e.g. anteroposterior and lateral) as one view may not show the injury (Fig. 3.4).
2. In long bone injuries, always radiograph the whole of the bone and the joints above and below it. For example, a Monteggia frac-ture of the forearm (fracture of the ulna with associated radial head dislocation at the elbow) may be missed if the elbow is not seen on x-ray (Fig. 3.5).
3. Always be specific about the views you wish the radiographer to take. For example, with suspected scaphoid bone fractures, it is necessary to obtain not only AP and lateral views but also oblique films (Fig. 3.6).
4. In children, if you are not sure if a fracture is present on a film (e.g. at the elbow with multiple epiphyseal growth plates, Fig. 3.7), x-ray the uninjured limb to compare. In addition, a fracture tends to hurt, which is a useful diagnostic tool!

Commonly missed fractures

It is only too easy to miss a fracture or dislocation, but this risk is minimized by thorough history and examination skills and appropriate radiography.

Commonly missed injuries are:

1. Impacted fractures of the neck of the femur – the lateral view is the most helpful (Fig. 3.8).

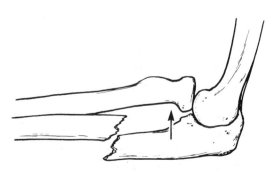

Figure 3.5 – Monteggia fracture – fracture of the ulna associated with dislocation of the radial head

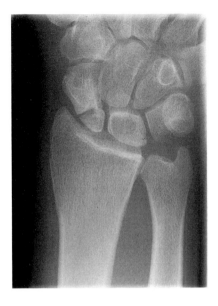

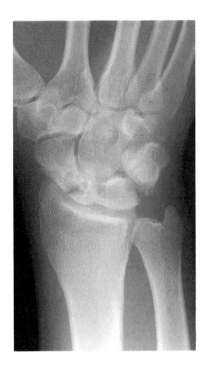

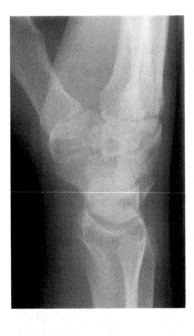

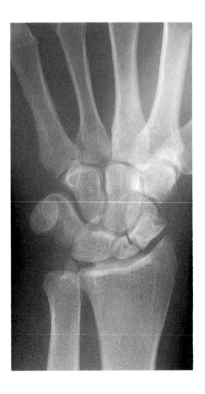

Figure 3.6 – Scaphoid views – to adequately visualize the scaphoid, in addition to AP and lateral views, it is mandatory to obtain oblique projections.

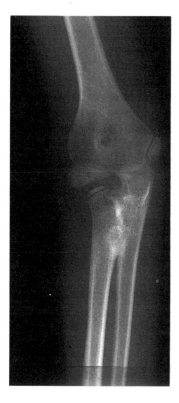

Figure 3.7 – Epiphyseal lines at the elbow – do not confuse them for fractures!

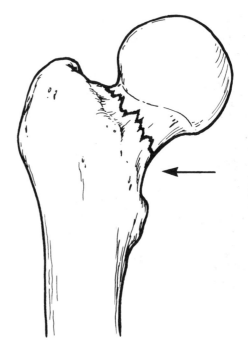

Figure 3.8 – Impacted fractures of the neck of the femur are notoriously easy to miss – the lateral view is usually helpful

2. Pubic ramic fractures, especially when looking for femoral neck fractures!

3. Patellar fractures – some are not evident on the lateral view. Suspect patellar fractures in dashboard injuries (also associated with femoral shaft fractures and hip dislocations).

4. Posterior dislocation of the shoulder – 'the AP view may look reassuringly normal (Fig. 3.9)! Always obtain an axillary view. Suspect the injury in patients with epilepsy.

5. Calcaneal fractures – commonly caused by a fall from a height. If there is a calcaneal fracture on one side there is a high chance of an injury on the contralateral limb. Remember to look for associated femoral fractures, hip dislocations and thoraco-lumbar injuries.

6. Fifth metatarsal fractures in 'ankle injuries' – standard ankle x-rays do not include the base of the fifth metatarsal (Fig. 3.10), and so if this area is not examined, you will miss the fracture!

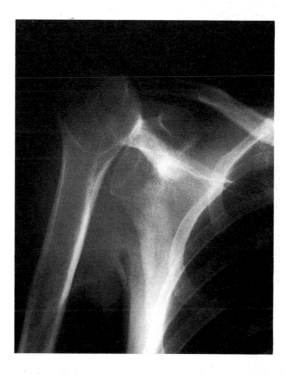

Figure 3.9 – Posterior dislocation of the shoulder

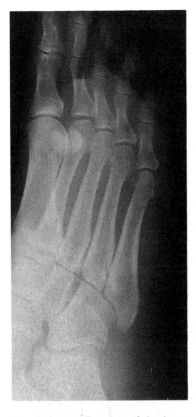

Figure 3.10 – Fracture of the base of the fifth metatarsal

7. Cervical spine fractures in head-injured patients. **All unconscious trauma patients must have adequate views of the cervical spine, maintaining the neck immobile until this is done.** Remember that all seven cervical vertebrae and the C7/T1 interspace must be visualized (Fig. 3.11).

8. Fractures of the radial head.

9. Avulsion fractures of the base of the proximal phalanx of the thumb as part of ulnar collateral ligament injuries (gamekeeper's or skier's thumb).

10. Scaphoid fractures – oblique views as well as standard AP and lateral views are necessary. If a scaphoid injury is clinically suspected and the initial x-rays are normal, it is standard practice to immobilize the wrist and bring the patient back for reassessment in 10–14 days.

11. Galleazi and Monteggia fracture-dislocations of the forearm – missed if the whole forearm including the wrist and elbow joints are not examined and radiographed (Fig. 3.12).

12. Impacted fractures of the neck of the humerus.

13. Stress fractures – easily missed up until the time of periosteal callus formation. e.g. The 'march' fracture of the second metatarsal shaft or neck (Fig. 3.13).

14. Skull fractures – vault fractures can be easily missed. The diagnosis of a basal skull fracture is a clinical one as the x-ray is usually unremarkable (see Chapter 7)

15. Maxillary fractures in head-injured patients.

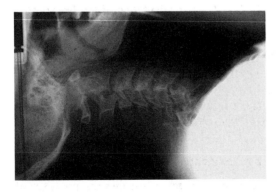
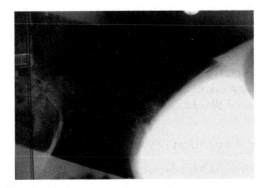

Figure 3.11 – An inadequate lateral cervical spine x-ray can be dangerous. The film on the left appears normal, but it does not demonstrate the C7/T1 interspace. When the shoulders are depressed to produce the film on the right, the injury is obvious.

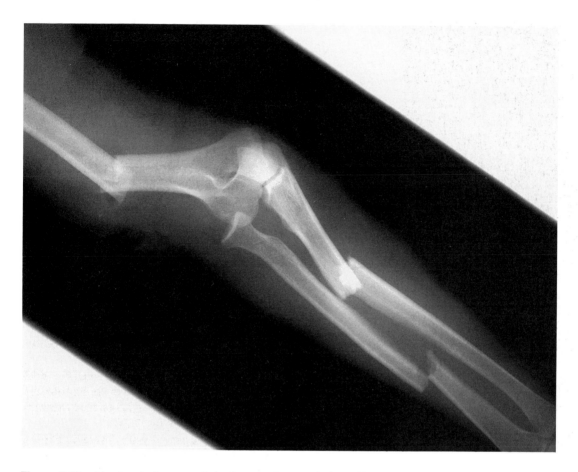

Figure 3.12 – Monteggia fracture of the forearm in association with a mid-shaft radial fracture and a humeral fracture.

How to describe a fracture

A **fracture** is a loss of continuity of the margins of a bone.

A **subluxation** of a joint is a partial shift of the surfaces of a joint but where some contact remains.

A **dislocation** of a joint is a complete separation of the surfaces of a joint (Fig. 3.14).

How can a fracture be described?

When documenting an injury or communicating with colleagues, it is vital to be able to satisfactorily and accurately describe a fracture pattern. This may be done by answering the following questions:

1. Is the fracture **open** or **closed?**
2. **Where** is the fracture?
3. What is the **orientation** of the fracture?
4. What is the **nature** of the fracture?
5. What is the **mechanism of injury** of the fracture?
6. Have the fracture fragments **moved**?

If you can adequately answer these questions, appropriate advice on treatment can be given.

Is the fracture open or closed?

A fracture is **closed** when there is no external communication via the skin with the fracture site. An **open** fracture is one where there is a communication between the fracture site and a

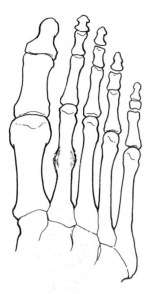

Figure 3.13 – March fracture of the second metatarsal shaft – note the periosteal callus formation

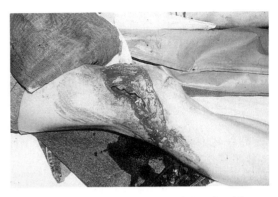

Figure 3.15 – An open fracture of the distal femur

wound (Fig. 3.15). (Closed and open fractures were formerly referred to as simple and compound fractures – these terms were misleading and have now been discarded.)

An open fracture is a **surgical emergency**. Throughout this book, it should be appreciated that all open fractures must be urgently managed. Open fractures carry with them the risk of infection and usually imply a larger causative energy force than in a similar closed fracture. The management of open fractures has radically changed in recent years – formerly it was said that all forms of internal fixation should be avoided for open fractures.

Some authorities would now advocate that many open fractures demand aggressive debridement and internal fixation **as soon as the patient comes into hospital.** The management of open fractures is discussed more fully later in this chapter.

It is therefore important to inform a senior colleague immediately that the injury is open as this will often drastically alter the management plan of the fracture. The soft tissue severity can be graded and this can be useful both in planning treatment and in prognosis. The most commonly used grading system is that of Gustilo and Anderson.

Type 1 Open fractures with a clean wound less than 1 cm long.

Type 2 Open fractures with a clean wound more than 1 cm long but without extensive soft tissue damage or skin loss.

Type 3a Open fractures with extensive soft tissue damage but where the bone is adequately covered with soft tissue.

or Any segmental or severely comminuted fractures regardless of the size of the skin laceration.

Type 3b Open fractures with extensive soft tissue loss **and** bone exposure.

Type 3c Open fractures with an arterial injury that requires repair.

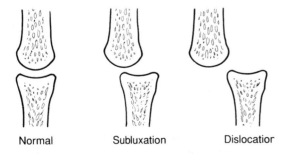

Normal   Subluxation   Dislocatior

Figure 3.14 – Subluxation and dislocation of joints

Where is the fracture?

You should be able to describe the anatomical location of a fracture. There are a number of classification systems available to do this, but these are largely unhelpful except to the specialist. The simplest plan is as follows:

1. State which bone is broken, e.g. radius, tibia, calcaneum.
2. If the bone has an anatomically named part, then state it as such, e.g. radial head, tibial plateau, intertrochanteric region of femur etc.
3. For long bones, state whether the fracture is within the diaphysis (mid-shaft), metaphysis or epiphysis (Fig. 3.16).
4. State if the fracture is **intra-articular** (Fig. 3.17) – fractures into joints usually demand an accurate reduction to restore joint function and prevent later degenerative change.

What is the orientation of the fracture (Fig. 3.18)?

The orientation of a fracture may be:

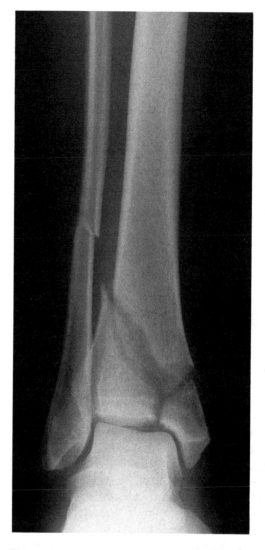

Figure 3.17 – An intra-articular fracture of the distal tibia

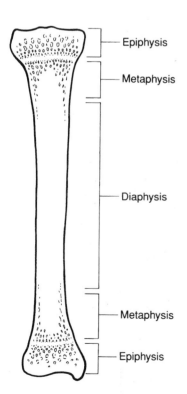

Figure 3.16 – Diaphysis, metaphysis and epiphysis

1. **Transverse** These fractures may be the result of both direct and indirect forces. The injuries tend to be relatively stable but can take longer to unite than spiral fractures.
2. **Spiral or oblique** These fractures are usually the result of indirect forces. These fractures can be unstable but tend to unite more quickly than transverse fractures.
3. **Segmental** Where a long bone is broken in two sites, a central fragment of bone is left unattached to the rest of the skeleton and

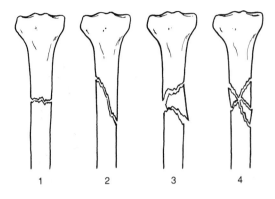

Figure 3.18 – Orientation of a fracture pattern; 1 transverse, 2 oblique, 3 segmental, 4 comminuted

this is termed a segmental fragment. Segmental fractures tend to be high energy injuries and usually require operative stabilization as there is a high risk of non-union at one of the fracture sites.

4. **Comminuted** Direct forces applied to a bone may result in a fracture configuration of more than two fragments, and this is termed a comminuted fracture. In some cases the fragments may be very small and defy surgical reconstruction. Bone loss may be appreciable.

5. **Avulsion** Avulsion fractures are a special form of injury whereby a musculo-ligamentous unit pulls a segment of bone from the main skeleton, e.g. avulsion fractures of the olecranon (by triceps) and the calcaneum (by the achilles tendon).

6. **Crush fractures** These are fractures of cancellous bone where compressive forces crush the bone, e.g. the vertebral body, tibial plateau, calcaneum. Bone loss may be extensive.

7. **Greenstick fractures** These fractures occur in the immature skeleton. Rather than both cortices of a bone breaking, the less brittle bone of the child deforms rather than breaks. The cortex on one side of the bone is buckled whilst the other side remains intact. Nevertheless deformity may be considerable, especially angulation of the radius and ulna in the forearm.

What is the nature of the fracture?

Most fractures occur in normal bone and are a result of an appropriately large force required to break bone. However, fractures may occur within abnormal bone and may be the result of much smaller forces. Such fractures are termed **pathological fractures** (Fig. 3.19). Although they may be suspected from the bone quality and appearance on x-ray, a thorough history and examination may suggest a pathological fracture, e.g. in women with fractures of the mid-shaft of the humerus with a history of carcinoma of the breast. Some causes of pathological fractures are:

1. **Osteoporosis** By far the commonest cause of pathological bone.
2. **Osteomalacia and rickets**
3. **Benign bone cysts and tumours**

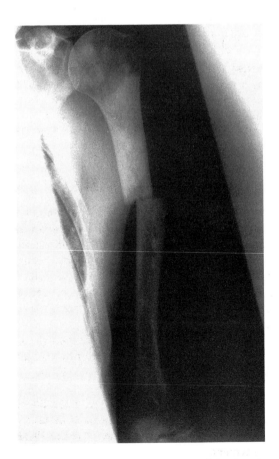

Figure 3.19 – Pathological fracture of the humerus

4. **Malignant primary and secondary bone tumours** Primary bone tumours are relatively rare. Secondary deposits are common; metastasis from almost any primary site is known but the common tumours that metastasize to bone are lung, breast, prostate, thyroid and kidney tumours.
5. **Paget's disease**
6. **Infections** Acute and chronic (including tuberculosis).
7. **Congenital,** e.g. osteogenesis imperfecta.

What is the mechanism of injury?

A fracture may be caused by:

1. **Direct** forces, e.g. a direct blow to the ulna in self-defence.
2. **Indirect** forces, e.g. rotational forces to the tibia and fibula in skiing injuries.

Other mechanisms may be responsible however, such as:

Stress fractures (fatigue fractures) Fracture as a result of repeated cyclical stressing of a portion of bone, e.g. the 'march' fracture of the second metatarsal shaft.
Pathological fractures Trivial force through pathological bone.

Have the fracture fragments moved?

In an **undisplaced** fracture the bone ends have not moved appreciably and are in near-correct anatomical position. A form of undisplaced fracture is the **impacted fracture** – this occurs in cancellous bone due to compressive forces. Impacted fractures are easy to miss on radiography but generally show sclerotic bone margins.
If the bone ends of a fracture have moved, then it is said to be **displaced**. A fracture may displace in three different ways (Fig. 3.20):

1. The bone ends may **shift** with respect to one another. The displacement is described in terms of the displacement of the distal fragment.
2. The bone may **angulate**

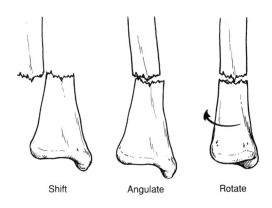

| Shift | Angulate | Rotate |

Figure 3.20 – A bone may displace in three ways – shift, angulate or rotate

3. The long axes of long bones may **rotate** – this is the most important displacement to detect and correct, especially in the forearm and the lower leg.

Fracture pathophysiology

The phases of fracture healing

The phases of fracture healing can be divided into:

1. **Inflammatory phase** A blood clot forms between the bone ends as a result of bleeding from the marrow cavity. This clot is gradually invaded by granulation tissue with cells that transform into osteoblasts, the bone-forming cells.
2. **Repair phase** Fibrous tissue forms between the bone ends, so that the fracture, although mobile, becomes 'sticky'. Bone-precursor material, termed **callus**, starts to form. If the bone ends are not rigidly fixed (as is the case in plaster immobilization) external bridging callus forms around the bone ends in a fusiform pattern. Rigidly fixed bones (e.g. those internally fixed with plates) do not form this external callus and unite with internal callus at a much slower rate. **Woven bone** is formed from this callus.
3. **Remodelling phase** This process begins 2–3 weeks after the repair phase commences

and can take several years to complete. The woven bone is remodelled into **lamellar bone**, chiefly due to the forces applied to the bone.

Times to bone union

Cancellous bone unites more quickly than cortical bone, usually within 6 weeks. Cortical bone, in general terms, unites within 6–8 weeks. This figure is halved in children and takes twice as long in the lower limb. Thus a tibial shaft fracture routinely takes 12–16 weeks to unite whilst a forearm fracture in a 4-year-old unites within 3-4 weeks.

Complications of fractures and dislocations

The complications of fractures and dislocations can be categorized as:

> **Systemic complications**
> **Local complications**
>   early
>   intermediate
>   late

Systemic complications of fractures and dislocations

Haemorrhage and hypovolaemic shock

Bleeding from fractures can be profuse and devastating (Fig. 3.21). Blood may be lost from the fracture site itself (more in open fractures) but in addition the obligate soft tissue swelling around fracture sites decreases the intravascular volume. Prompt recognition of **hypovolaemic shock** is mandatory (see Chapter 4) in the trauma victim. Average blood losses in closed fractures are: tibia – 2 units; femur – 4 units; pelvis – at least 8 units.

The metabolic response to trauma

The body metabolism reacts to trauma by a number of compensatory mechanisms, and these can be dramatic in major trauma. Major

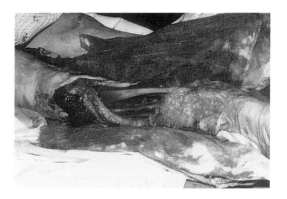

Figure 3.21 – Traumatic amputation of the leg – the potential for haemorrhage is great

complications as a result of these changes include the following.

1. The **adult respiratory distress syndrome (ARDS)** – this may be a reflection of severe trauma but may be precipitated by aspiration of gastric contents, fluid depletion or overload and poor fracture management. It is characterized by diffuse pulmonary vascular hyper-permeability manifested clinically by pulmonary oedema and hypoxia. Prompt stabilization of long bone fractures in multiply-injured patients has been shown to decrease its incidence and severity.

2. The **fat embolism syndrome** – this is a part of the spectrum of ARDS that follows long bone fractures. It was formerly thought to be due to microvascular embolization of fat globules to the lungs, but is probably a disorder of lipid metabolism. The condition presents within 2–3 days of injury with hypoxia, tachypnea and tachycardia. Multiple petechiae may be present. Clotting abnormalities are common. As with ARDS, prompt long bone stabilization is beneficial.

3. **Other manifestations of 'stress'** – for example, disseminated intravascular coagulation (DIC), peptic ulceration, paralytic ileus with spinal fractures.

The complications of prolonged immobility

These are a very important group of complications that contribute greatly to the morbidity and mortality of trauma, especially in the elderly age group. They include:

1. Thrombo-embolic disease – deep venous thrombosis (DVT) and pulmonary embolism (PE).
2. Pressure sores (decubitus ulcers).
3. Respiratory tract infections.
4. Urinary tract infections.

The complications of surgery and anaesthesia

Any operative procedure carries a risk proportionate to the general health of the patient. Errors in surgical treatment also occur!

Early complications local to the injury

Arterial obstruction in association with a fracture

It is mandatory to examine the limb distal to a fracture to ensure that there is no interruption of the blood supply. **The clinical symptoms and signs of an ischaemic limb are extreme pain, cold skin, a poor capillary return, absence of distal pulses, paraesthesiae and ultimately paralysis.** Causes of obstruction include kinking of the vessel around a fracture site, intimal stripping, thrombosis and spasm. If obstruction is noted the fracture or dislocation should be immediately reduced. If this does not improve the clinical state, prompt surgical intervention is necessary. Be aware that the cause of an ischaemic limb may be a compartment syndrome (see below).

Acute neurological disturbance

This is uncommon in closed injuries and when present is almost always due to a neurapraxia rather than nerve division. Examples include the sciatic nerve in hip dislocations, the common peroneal nerve in knee injuries, the axillary nerve in shoulder dislocations and the ulnar nerve in elbow dislocations. If recognized, the fracture or dislocation should be promptly reduced. Open injuries with nerve deficit should be explored by an experienced surgeon, prefer-

ably within a week of injury. They should *not* be explored in the Accident and Emergency Department!

Skin and soft tissue damage

Remember that an injury resulting in a fracture does not only involve an injury to bone. The skin, muscle and vital structures are also damaged. This is dealt with more fully in the following section. Be careful not to overlook **degloving injuries** whereby the skin is separated from the underlying tissues by shearing forces (Fig. 3.22).

Compartment syndrome

This is a potentially devastating **surgical emergency**. If diagnosis or treatment are delayed, permanent and severe disability will result.

A compartment refers to any closed tissue space. Increased pressure within this compartment will compromise capillary blood flow to muscles and nerves. The normal pressure within a compartment is normally less than 10 mmHg; if this rises to more than 20 mmHg, capillary blood flow will be compromised. At pressures of over 30–40 mmHg, ischaemic necrosis of muscles and nerves occurs. It is important to note that at these pressures flow through arteries and arterioles remains virtually normal, that is, **significant muscle necrosis can occur whilst a pulse remains palpable.**

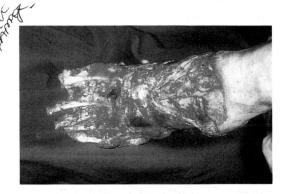

Figure 3.22 – Degloving injury of the foot

Increased compartmental pressure can be caused by either **compression**, e.g. burn eschar, constrictive dressings or casts, or by a **volume increase** in the compartment due to haemorrhage or oedema. Direct trauma, either soft tissue or bony injury, with consequent bleeding and oedema is the commonest cause. Prolonged immobilization with limb compression as a result of alcohol or overdose is another frequent cause. Almost any muscle mass within a fascial envelope can develop compartment syndrome. The anterior compartment of the lower leg is most commonly affected. The anterior compartment of the forearm may also be affected.

The typical features of a compartment syndrome are:

1. **Pain** – there is unremitting pain, not relieved by strong analgesia.
2. Pain on **passive extension of the muscles within the compartment**, e.g. for the anterior forearm compartment, pain on passive extension of the fingers.
3. **Paraesthesiae** – nerve function can be affected by raised compartmental pressures.
4. Cool skin distally.
5. Muscle paralysis and eventual contracture.

Not all these features need be present; the first two are by far the most important. **Note that the distal pulses are nearly always present in a compartment syndrome – their presence should not be reassuring!**

If a compartment syndrome is suspected, **call immediately for senior advice.** If the diagnosis is confirmed, a **decompressive fasciotomy** will be required as an emergency.

Infection

Infection in closed injuries is very uncommon. In open injuries, however, there is a very real risk of infection, and the early management of such patients is crucial in minimizing this risk. (See discussion of open fractures below.)

Remember : never primarily close the wound of an open fracture, no matter how tempting!

Intermediate complications local to the injury

Abnormalities of bone union

Bone union may be abnormal in a number of ways:

1. **Malunion**   The fracture does not unite in a near-anatomical position.
2. **Delayed union**   The fracture takes longer than normal to unite but will eventually do so.
3. **Non-union**   The fracture does not unite at any stage. Non-unions demand surgical intervention in most cases. There are two major types:

   (a) **Hypertrophic non-union**, in which the bone ends make an attempt at union and there is an abundance of callus around the bone ends. Such cases are aided by open reduction and internal fixation.
   (b) **Atrophic non-union**, in which the bone ends make little attempt at union or callus formation. Bone grafting is usually necessary.

4. **Cross-union**   Two adjacent bones that are fractured may join together, e.g. the radius and ulna. Such an union may restrict movement, particularly rotation.

Joint stiffness

This is a great problem in fracture management. There is little point in obtaining an attractive x-ray if clinically the patient has no movement. All fractures to some extent result in stiffness, usually temporarily. However, intra-articular fractures are very prone to stiffness that may be permanent. Stiffness may be minimized by early mobilization, accurate intra-articular fracture reduction and aggressive movement of all non-immobilized joints in an injured limb.

Reflex sympathetic dystrophy

This is a baffling condition that may follow any injury. It is also known as Sudek's atrophy or post-traumatic oligodystrophy. An abnormality of the sympathetic nervous system is probably responsible. The patient complains of a painful limb, which is swollen, tender and stiff. X-rays show profuse decalcification. This distressing condition usually resolves but may take up to 2 years to do so. In the interim period the joints must be mobilized so as to prevent permanent deformity.

Late complications local to the injury

Post-traumatic osteoarthritis

This occurs not only with intra-articular fractures but also in malunited fractures that place abnormal loads on surrounding joints, e.g. varus malunion of the tibia may result in premature degenerative change of the ankle joint.

Avascular necrosis

Certain peri-articular bones receive their blood supply exclusively via one route, which if interrupted may result in the death (necrosis) of that portion. This is termed **avascular necrosis**. Examples include:

1. The femoral head in subcapital fractures of the proximal femur.
2. The proximal pole of the scaphoid bone in scaphoid wrist fractures (Fig. 3.23).
3. The head of the talus in talar neck fractures.

Avascular necrosis inevitably results in collapse of the bone, which may demand surgical intervention.

Myositis ossificans

Ectopic bone may form around injured joints. This is especially common in head-injured patients.

Soft tissue injuries associated with fractures

Remember that all injuries include a soft tissue component. Do not neglect management of the

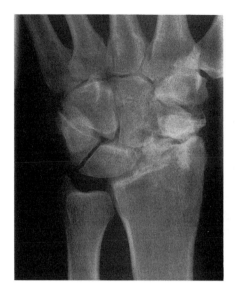

Figure 3.23 – Avascular necrosis with secondary degenerative change.

muscles, nerves, arteries etc. when dealing with fractures. Management of the skin is a difficult problem but certain principles need to be emphasized.

1. **Never** primarily close the wound over an open fracture, no matter how tempting this may seem. This almost inevitably leads to infection of the underlying tissues and carries with it the risk of osteomyelitis, which is very difficult to eradicate.
2. Remember that all open fractures are **surgical emergencies**. It has clearly been shown that early operative debridement of the wound with appropriate fixation increases the chances of union without infection. In this context 'early' is ideally within **6 hours** of the accident.
3. Do not be fooled by the innocent 'Grade 1' open fracture said to be 'from within out'. These fractures have a definite potential to become infected and should be aggressively treated. Remember that the limb may have been deformed to a much greater extent at the time of injury than it looks once in your department.

4. Be able to categorize open fractures according to the Gustilo and Anderson grading (see above) as this aids communication with colleagues.

The management of open fractures

1. An open fracture is a **surgical emergency.** There should be no avoidable delay in the management of open fractures and appropriately senior personnel should be summoned immediately.

2. If there is extreme deformity of the limb, this should be corrected as soon as possible with appropriate analgesia. This is especially important if other intact areas of skin are under tension by bone fragments.

3. A polaroid photograph of the injured part should be taken. This not only serves as a permanent record of the state of the limb on admission but also allows other personnel to assess the injury without further tampering with the wound.

4. A swab of the wound should be taken and sent for microbiological analysis.

5. The wound should be covered with an antiseptic-soaked swab and a splint applied. The wound should not need further inspection until the time of formal debridement.

6. Intravenous broad spectrum antibiotics should be given routinely. Your hospital may have an antibiotic policy as to which should be given. Remember to provide anaerobic cover if there is any contamination from soil etc.

7. Antitetanus toxoid should be given according to the patient's immunization record (see below).

8. Appropriate analgesia should be given.

9. The patient should be taken to the operating theatre as soon as possible, and certainly within 6 hours of injury, for debridement at a minimum, and in most cases for stabilization of the fracture. Debridement involves the thorough decontamination and lavage of the soft tissues – this should always be done under a general anaesthetic and there is no place for this to be done under local anaesthetic in the Accident and Emergency Department.

10. This book does not deal with the surgical strategy for stabilization of open fractures. Note, however, the recent shift to aggressive stabilization of the fracture on **day 1** in combination with lavage, with early soft tissue procedures if required. Infected non-stabilized fractures are a disaster and must be avoided if at all possible. It is worth repeating that **the open wound must never be primarily sutured – the wound should be left open to granulate or sutured as a delayed procedure.**

General principles of closure of skin wounds

Skin wounds without an underlying fracture are a common problem in the Accident and Emergency Department. The wound should only be primarily sutured if caused by a clean mechanism (e.g. a sharp knife) with no skin loss; the skin edges should be able to come together with no skin tension.

A crushed or contaminated wound should **not** be primarily closed as this will inevitably become infected. In such cases the wound should be cleaned, dressed and arrangements made for delayed suture. Although in some cases skin and soft tissues are beneficially excised, consult senior personnel before you do this as such excision may compromise later wound closure.

Degloving injuries

Take great care to recognize degloving injuries, which are shear injuries of the skin from the underlying soft tissues with consequent loss of its blood supply (Fig. 3.24). The mechanism of injury is a great clue, e.g. running over a limb with a vehicle tyre or a ring shearing the tissues of a finger. The skin may be completely devitalized and require extensive plastic surgical procedures to provide soft tissue cover and avoid sloughing of the skin. **The skin may initially seem reassuringly normal** but look for evidence of imprints and devitalization.

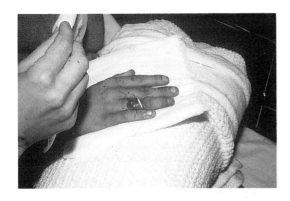

Figure 3.24 – Degloving injury of the finger

Gunshot wounds

These are fortunately rare in the UK. Distinguish between three major types of gunshot injury:

1. Low velocity guns – these generally propel a large bullet but do not cause significant soft tissue damage.
2. High velocity guns – these are very destructive in that the bullet's energy creates a cavitation effect within the soft tissues.
3. Shotgun injuries – multiple small pellets are embedded in the tissues and it is rarely practicable for them all to be removed.

Never primarily close a gunshot wound. They need to be treated as contaminated wounds, with appropriate cleaning, soft tissue debridement and delayed closure. In any significant injury this needs to be performed under a general anaesthetic.

Tetanus prophylaxis

There were 116 cases of tetanus reported in England and Wales between 1984 and 1991. The elderly are the population at greatest risk, particularly females over the age of 65 years. Whilst great emphasis is placed upon immunization, the equal importance of thorough surgical toilet and careful debridement should not be forgotten. Although classically tetanus develops from deep, soiled and necrotic wounds, it can also arise from any breach of the body surface,

including burns, ear-piercing, corneal abrasions and intramuscular injections. In the United States, the disease is reported with surprising frequency in intravenous drug abusers.

Recommendations on tetanus prophylaxis are based upon:

1. The condition of the wound.
2. The patient's immunization history.

Condition of the wound

Wounds with these features are considered to be tetanus prone:

- More than 6 hours old.
- Significant degree of devitalized tissue.
- Puncture type wounds (> 1 cm).
- In contact with soil, manure or faeces (Fig. 3.25).
- Clinical evidence of sepsis.

All other wounds should be considered as not tetanus prone.

Immunization status (see Table 3.1)

1. Complete course of vaccine or booster within the past 10 years
   – check wound status and give **A** if necessary.
2. Complete course of vaccine or booster > 10 years ago
   – check wound status and give **B** if necessary.

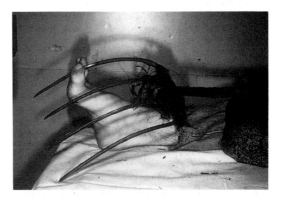

Figure 3.25 – There is a high potential for tetanus inoculation with this injury

Table 3.1   Schedule for immunization

	Tetanus prone	*Not tetatnus prone*
A	No action unless very high risk of infection 1 dose of vaccine	No action required
B	1 dose of vaccine **plus** human tetanus Ig – 1 dose	1 dose of vaccine
C	Complete vaccine course **plus** human tetanus Ig – 1 dose	Complete vaccine course
D	Complete vaccine course **plus** human tetanus Ig – 1 dose	Start vaccine course

Ig, immunoglobulin. **The tetanus vaccine should be given in a different limb from the immunoglobulin.**

3. Has not had a complete course of vaccine
   – check wound status and give **C** if necessary.
4. Immunization status unknown
   – check wound status and give **D** if necessary.

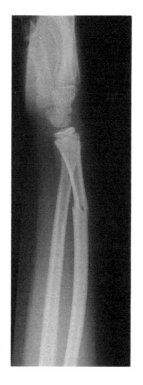

Figure 3.26 – Greenstick fracture of the distal radius

Fractures within the immature skeleton

Children differ from adults in many ways in terms of musculo-skeletal injury.

1. Children's bones are more malleable than those of adults. This can result in the following:

(a) **Greenstick fractures**   Incomplete fracture of the bone with the cortex and periosteum on one side remaining intact (Fig. 3.26).

(b) **Torus fractures**   An impaction injury in the metaphyseal region of a long bone may result in buckling of the bone rather than fracturing (Fig. 3.27).

(c) **Bowing of long bones**   Because the bones are more malleable, a child's bone may bow under force rather than fracture.

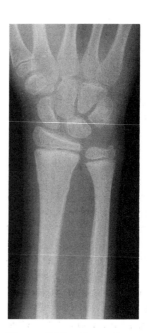

Figure 3.27 – Torus fracture of the distal radius

2. The pattern of injury differs from adults, e.g. the child falling on the outstretched hand is more likely to sustain a greenstick fracture of the distal radius, a supracondylar fracture of the humerus or a fracture of the clavicle than the adult with a similar mechanism of injury.

3. There is a far greater power of remodelling in childhood injuries, although angulation remains a problem, as in the adult.

4. Fractures in young children unite more quickly than in adults.

5. Epiphyseal injuries may occur (see below).

Epiphyseal injuries

The immature skeleton may undergo damage within the epiphyseal region. These injuries must be very carefully analysed as the potential for growth disturbance can be significant.

The most useful and common classification of epiphyseal injuries is that by **Salter and Harris** (Fig. 3.28).

Type 1 Complete separation of epiphysis from metaphysis. Traumatic cases tend to have a good prognosis if accurately reduced.

Type 2 Fracture of the epiphysis with a triangular portion of metaphysis. This is by far the most common epiphyseal injury and if accurately reduced has an excellent prognosis.

Type 3 Intra-articular fracture of a portion of the epiphysis. Accurate reduction is essential if growth disturbance is to be avoided. Most cases demand operative stabilization.

Type 4 Vertical split of the epiphysis and a triangular portion of the metaphysis. Again accurate reduction and stabilization is necessary to avoid growth disturbance. The prognosis of these fractures is intermediate.

Type 5 Crush fracture of the epiphysis. This is a very rare injury, which may be difficult to diagnose as the epiphysis is largely cartilagenous and therefore does not show on x-ray. There is a high incidence of growth disturbance or arrest with this injury.

Type 6 This is a recent addition to the classification and is characterized by a crush

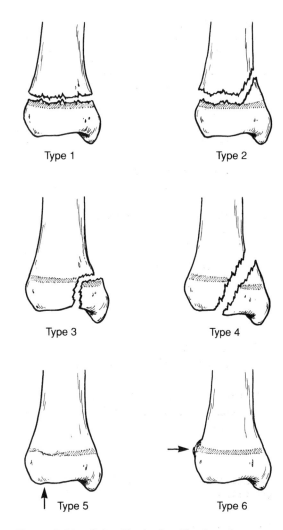

Figure 3.28 – Salter-Harris classification of epiphyseal injuries (arrows denote point of impact)

injury (as in type 5) with in addition an injury to the periosteum at the periphery of the epiphysis. Again, growth disturbance is common.

The principles of fracture management

The primary aim of fracture management is to allow union of bones in the correct position whilst providing adequate analgesia for the patient. There are numerous ways of achieving this but the outcome should be achieved by the simplest means and with the minimum of complications.

In fracture management there are three main phases:

1. **Reduction** (if necessary) of the fracture.
2. **Maintenance** of the reduction
3. **Mobilization** once the fracture is sufficiently united.

For the admitting doctor dealing with a fracture, the initial stages of management can be thought of as:

1. What is the diagnosis of this fracture?
2. Does this fracture need reduction?
3. If the fracture requires reduction, how do I achieve this?
4. Once I have achieved this reduction, how do I maintain the position?
5. Does the patient require to be admitted?
6. If not admitted, what form and urgency of outpatient follow-up is required?

What is the diagnosis of this fracture?

Before any attempt can be made at treating an injury, an accurate diagnosis must be made. If not the wrong treatment may be carried out to the detriment of both the fracture and the patient, e.g. to treat a Smith's fracture as a Colles fracture would not provide adequate reduction or maintenance of position. Remember that a diagnosis includes:

- Is it an open or closed injury?
- Where is the fracture?
- What is the orientation of the fracture (e.g. oblique, transverse etc.)?
- What is the nature of the fracture (e.g. traumatic, pathological)?
- What is the mechanism of injury?
- Have the fracture fragments moved and if, so, in what direction?

Does this fracture need reduction?

This is a question that many doctors find difficult to answer. Undisplaced fractures clearly do not require reduction.

Grossly displaced fractures in most cases demand reduction (Fig. 3.29). Minimally displaced fractures may require reduction depending upon the location of the fracture and the physiological age of the patient. All epiphyseal and most intra-articular injuries should be accurately reduced. Moderately displaced fractures in the elderly may not necessarily require reduction. Some knowledge of the natural history of fractures is useful in determining the need for reduction.

If the fracture requires reduction, how do I achieve this?

The best and simplest way of working out how to reduce a fracture is via the mechanism of injury. In general terms, the fracture is reduced by the opposite forces that caused the injury.

However, the next question to ask yourself is whether you have the necessary **ability, experience, personnel and equipment** to provide an adequate reduction. For example, an intra-articular fracture of the distal humerus will require accurate open reduction and internal fixation whilst an extra-articular fracture of the distal radius in many cases can be adequately reduced by manipulation. Before you attempt to reduce a fracture you must work out a **reduction plan**, practising it if necessary prior to the procedure itself.

Reduction can be achieved by:

1. Traction and manipulation – for most fractures, e.g. Colles fractures.

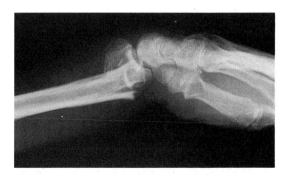

Figure 3.29 – A grossly displaced distal radial fracture – reduction is clearly required

2. Continuous traction – for many long bone fractures, e.g. distal tibial fractures, femoral shaft fractures, and also for the cervical spine.

3. Open reduction with or without internal fixation.

4. External fixation.

Once I have achieved reduction, how do I maintain this position?

Nearly all fractures that have been reduced will require some form of maintenance device to hold the position achieved. The methods available are:

1. Gravity, e.g. application of a collar and cuff to a humeral shaft fracture.

2. Casts – mostly plaster of paris but also synthetic materials. Cast braces can also be used in selected cases, usually after a period of time has passed and the fracture has become 'sticky'.

3. Continuous traction.

4. Internal fixation.

5. External fixation.

Undisplaced fractures also require some form of 'maintenance device' – this is not to maintain a reduction but to prevent pain and to protect the fracture from the patient.

Does the patient require to be admitted?

Admission is needed if:

1. The planned treatment should be as an in-patient, for example:
   open reduction;
   continuous traction of a long bone fracture.

2. The patient requires nursing care as a result of the injury, for example:
   pelvic fracture.

3. The fracture, although treated, requires monitoring of the circulation for a short period, for example:
   supracondylar fractures of the humerus.

4. Other injuries require admission to hospital.

5. The patient will not be able to cope at home without further support, for example:
   elderly patients with lower limb plasters.

If not admitted, what form and urgency of out-patient follow-up?

This is a very important aspect of fracture management that is often badly thought out. The patient should not be inappropriately brought up to a busy fracture clinic but the patient with a serious injury should not be neglected for a long period.

The fracture clinic functions to confirm the diagnosis and provide follow-up care of all fractures. As many patients must pass through the clinic, it is inappropriate in most instances to refer elective or semi-elective orthopaedic problems to the clinic. The clinic should be regarded as an emergency clinic.

Your hospital may have a protocol for the referral of injuries to the fracture clinic, but all fractures should routinely be seen at least once by experienced orthopaedic personnel.

You must then ask **when** that patient should be seen in the fracture clinic. For a clinically suspected scaphoid fracture with no radiological evidence of injury, for example, it would be inappropriate to send the patient to the clinic the next day. The patient should be seen approximately 10 days after injury so that the standard reassessment can be made. On the other hand, any fractures that have a potential for redisplacement should be seen as soon as possible in the fracture clinic.

It is the opinion of most orthopaedic units that referral of mechanical back pain to a fracture clinic is wholly inappropriate.

The closed treatment of fractures

The soft tissue hinge in closed fracture reduction

One of the most important principles underlying successful closed fracture reduction is that of the **soft tissue hinge**, present in most fractures

(Fig. 3.30). Unless the fracture is grossly displaced the soft tissues are intact along one side of the fracture. The hinge:

1. Allows an easier reduction of the fracture by realigning the soft tissues under the correct tension.
2. Makes over-reduction almost impossible unless large forces are applied that destroy the hinge.

Hence, when attempting a closed fracture reduction, try to work out where this hinge exists on the plain radiographs. This applies particularly to angulated greenstick fractures. The theory that the intact periosteum should be broken by overdistraction of the fracture should be regarded with great caution as this is a sure way of converting a stable fracture into an unstable pattern.

Closed fracture reduction

As noted previously, there are a number of phases involved in successful fracture union:

1. Reduction (if necessary) of the fracture.
2. Maintenance of the reduction.
3. Mobilization once the fracture is sufficiently united.

Once reduced, the fracture position may be maintained by a number of methods:

1. Gravity or other forms of functional splintage.
2. Casts.
3. Continuous traction.
4. Internal fixation.
5. External fixation.

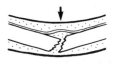 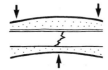

Figure 3.30 – The soft tissue hinge in closed reduction of fractures

Slings

Slings may be used to provide support for injuries of the upper limb. The main devices available are:

1. **Collar and cuff** This should be applied to the distal forearm so that it does not support the elbow, thereby allowing the arm to become dependent. It is useful in fractures of the humerus where gravity aids reduction of the fracture.
2. **Broad arm sling** These triangular bandages are applied so that they support the elbow and thereby support the arm. It is useful for fractures of the clavicle.
3. **High sling** These are used in hand injuries for elevation.

Reduction of fractures with maintenance of position with a cast

When reducing any fracture to be immobilized within a cast, three phases should be performed:

1. Practise reduction without any plaster.
2. Plastering of the fracture.
3. Reduction and moulding of the fracture within the plaster.

You should satisfy yourself that the fracture can be reduced to a satisfactory position prior to the application of any plaster. The reduction is most easily effected by forces applied in the opposite direction to those causing the fracture. For example, in the forearm the initial force is traction in the longitudinal axis which leads to disimpaction and partial reduction of the fracture. Any residual deformity is then corrected by the appropriate force worked out from the mechanism of injury.

Ideally all fractures should be reduced under image intensifier control so as to provide radiological confirmation of an adequate reduction. However in many units this facility is not available and plain films only can be obtained. If the latter is the case, it is impractical to take plain films without the limb in plaster. Good clinical features of an adequate reduction are a straight minimally deformed limb (there is usually some swelling which may obscure the view) without telescoping of the fracture.

Once you are satisfied that you can obtain a satisfactory reduction, plaster of paris may be applied to the limb so as to hold this position. It is usually impracticable to hold the reduction **effectively** whilst applying a plaster, although maintenance of a traction force is useful. The plaster should be **quickly** applied (whether it be a partial slab or a complete cast). Once applied the fracture should again be reduced by the same mechanism as your practice reduction. The plaster should be **moulded** so that the fracture is not allowed the freedom to redisplace. Remember the axiom 'a straight plaster ensures a bent limb' – the plaster must be locally moulded to prevent later displacement. You will find that if the plaster is immersed in hot water it then dries much more quickly and leaves little time for reduction and moulding. Therefore use cold water instead.

Application of plaster of paris

Most doctors find this a difficult skill to master. A book cannot give you this experience. Go to your plaster technician and ask him or her to show you how to apply a plaster cast and other synthetic materials. Start with 'easy' plasters (e.g. for undisplaced fractures) so that when you need to apply moulded plasters you have some experience.

The safest form of plaster to apply is a 'lightly padded plaster'. Unpadded plasters (i.e., plaster directly on to skin) are rarely used nowadays although they do offer excellent moulding properties. Heavily padded plasters, however, have a very high risk of allowing redisplacement; the fracture may be allowed to move as the swelling of the injury settles because of air contained within the padding. A lightly padded plaster is best – the padding should be enough to cover any bony pressure areas but should otherwise be applied very sparingly. When applying a plaster bear in mind the following points:

1. Use tepid or cold but not hot water.
2. Apply the padding layer evenly and sparingly but with adequate covering over bony pressure points.

3. If a plaster slab is to be used make sure that the gauze used to wrap around the plaster is wet or else it will shrink once applied and overly compress the soft tissues.
4. If a complete plaster is applied, apply it **without tension**. Any tension should be within the padding layer and not the plaster. If the fracture has been reduced apply only one portion at a time, and later add a second component. For example, in an above-elbow plaster for a forearm fracture, apply the below-elbow portion first and later complete the plaster with the above-elbow component.
5. Make sure that the edges of the plaster are smooth and applied in the correct position. Allow movement of all joints that are supposed to be free!
6. **If a complete plaster is applied to a new fracture or one that has been manipulated it is mandatory to split the plaster throughout its length.** The cast should be split **down to the skin** as the padding itself may have compressive properties. Many medico-legal authorities consider it negligent to send a patient home with an unsplit plaster after a recent fracture.
7. Make sure that there is no obstruction to the circulation as a result of the plaster cast. Give the patient clear instructions for when at home regarding what to do should the circulation become impaired. All injured distal extremities should be elevated. If a limb has the signs of circulatory insufficiency, the plaster should be removed. Remember the possibility of a compartment syndrome!
8. Once a fracture is within a cast it should not be unduly painful. If pain persists consider a compartment syndrome, a plaster that is too tight or localized pressure within the plaster. A 'window' can be removed if the latter is the case, which must subsequently be replaced (or the soft tissues may try to 'escape' through the window).

Plaster slab or complete plaster?

The idea behind a plaster slab is to surround the fracture by plaster whilst allowing some of the soft tissues room to expand. Although the slabs can be useful in this respect they are not as effective as a complete plaster in holding the fracture. Both slabs and complete plasters will require 'completion' after a few days as **all complete plasters must be split down to the skin**.

Many units have their own policies as to when to apply plaster slabs. If in doubt apply a slab rather than a complete cast. Examples of plaster slabs commonly used are the radial slab (not a 'backslab') for Colles fractures, the volar radial slab for Smith's fractures and the ankle backslab. Note the correct method of application of an ankle backslab – both a dorsal slab **and** a U-slab must be applied **with the foot in full dorsiflexion**, unless otherwise indicated.

Continuous traction

Some fractures require continuous traction, either to aid reduction of the fracture or to maintain its position. Two major forms are:

1. **Skeletal traction**   A metal pin is inserted through bone by which traction may be applied. Common sites are the calcaneum, proximal tibia and distal femur. They are the form needed for long-term traction in adults.

2. **Skin traction**   This is useful in children and for short-term traction in adults. However, heavy weights cannot be used and problems can occur including skin sloughing and allergic reactions to the tape used.

4

The management of major trauma

Introduction

It is the responsibility of every doctor working in the Accident and Emergency Department to have a good working knowledge of the principles of major trauma management. Some units receive many multiply-injured patients as part of their workload whereas others may only see one or two cases per year. Nevertheless all doctors should be trained in basic patient resuscitation.

Following major trauma, there are three temporal peaks of death:

1. The **first peak** occurs at the scene of the accident within minutes and is due to injuries for which little effective treatment could be offered in appropriate time, e.g. massive head injuries, high spinal cord and aortic transections.
2. The **second peak** of deaths occurs within the first few hours after an accident. Examples of causes include pneumothorax, haemothorax, abdominal bleeding, hypovolaemic shock and secondary brain damage.
3. The **third peak** of deaths occurs from several days to weeks following trauma and is generally due to the metabolic effects of trauma, e.g. 'shock lung', renal failure and systemic infection.

It has been realized that effective initial trauma management can reduce the number of deaths, not only in the second peak where timely intervention can literally save the life of a patient, but also in the third peak. **Advanced Trauma Life Support courses** are now common throughout the world and effectively teach the management of multiply-injured patients. Attendance on one is highly recommended.

This text cannot go in detail into the management of the trauma victim, but the basic management pathway is presented.

Overview of trauma management

The principles of trauma management are similar for all patients whatever the injuries. Remember:

1. **If a patient has one major injury, there is a high probability that other serious injuries are also present.** Never satisfy yourself that you have 'found the injury' and stop there.
2. **Constant re-evaluation** of the trauma patient is essential. Many injuries may present themselves at some time after your initial assessment.
3. To treat any **life-threatening injuries** as soon as you recognize them, e.g. if a tension pneumothorax is recognized, decompress it immediately – do not wait for an x-ray to confirm the diagnosis!
4. **Trauma management can be very difficult and demands experience** – summon senior colleagues as soon as possible.

The stages of trauma management

1. **Pre-hospital treatment** Before you see the patient in the Accident and Emergency Department, the paramedical team will have attended the victim. Depending on protocols the patient may have been simply 'picked up and rushed to hospital' or may have been more thoroughly assessed and given primary treatment such as intravenous lines, intubation and application of a cervical collar. **Remember to gain every piece of information about the accident, the mechanism of injury, the initial treatment and other details from the paramedical crew** (Fig 4.1).

2. **Primary survey** Examine the patient for evidence of treatable life-threatening injury.

3. **Immediate resuscitation** This depends in large part on the findings of the primary survey but includes certain 'standards', e.g. the insertion of wide-bore intravenous cannulae.

4. **Secondary survey** A thorough examination of the entire patient to detect the presence of all injuries.

5. **Re-evaluation of the patient.**

6. **Appropriate finalized care,** e.g. fixation of fractures, plastic surgical procedures etc.

The primary survey and resuscitation

The aim of the primary survey is to detect life-threatening injuries as soon as possible and **to treat them appropriately and immediately.** Hypoxia must be prevented at all costs.

Airway and cervical spine control

This is rightly the first priority in that a patient without a patent airway will die no matter what other injuries are treated. **Concurrent with airway management is mandatory cervical spine protection** (Fig. 4.2).

The airway must be confirmed clear and without obstruction. All foreign debris must be removed and suction should be available. Gargling sounds or abnormal breath sounds may indicate airway obstruction. Facial fractures may predispose to both intrinsic and

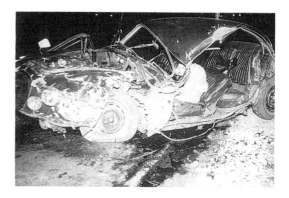

Figure 4.1 – The information the paramedical team give about the accident may help you in the mechanism and severity of injury

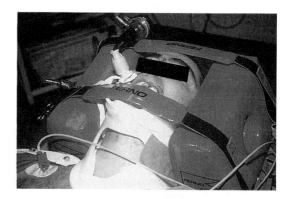

Figure 4.2– The cervical spine must be protected with a cervical collar, sandbags and tape

extrinsic airway obstruction. A talking cooperative patient does not have an airway problem **at that time.**

In the conscious patient, a simple manoeuvre to establish airway patency is to lift the chin anteriorly, and this should not hyperextend the neck. For this to be maintained in a conscious patient a nasopharyngeal airway may be inserted; oropharyngeal airways should only be used in unconscious patients without a gag reflex.

If the patient requires ventilatory support or if an airway cannot be easily maintained and protected, an endotracheal tube will need to be passed. If this cannot be done effectively, a surgical airway should be established (a cricothyroidotomy preceded by jet insufflation through the cricothyroid membrane if required).

One hundred per cent oxygen must be administered as soon as possible.

Throughout airway management the cervical spine must be protected. This can be done either by **manual in-line immobilization** or by the application of a rigid **cervical collar** supplemented by sandbags taped to the side of the patient's head. The immobilization should not be removed until the neck is cleared from injury both clinically and radiologically.

Breathing (ventilation)

As well as requiring a patent airway, the trauma patient requires an adequate ventilation mechanism if hypoxia is to be avoided. There are several life-threatening conditions that may be found in the trauma victim. These include tension pneumothorax, flail chest, open pneumothorax, massive haemothorax, cardiac tamponade and intimal rupture of the arch of the thoracic aorta.

Inspect the respiratory rate and note any chest wounds and flail segments. **Palpate** any rib fractures that may be present. **Percuss** the lung fields – hyper-resonance suggests a pneumothorax whilst dullness suggests the accumulation of blood. **Auscultate** for air entry.

It is of vital importance to realize that many of the life-threatening thoracic conditions **may be diagnosed without a chest x-ray** – the patient may die whilst an x-ray is being taken. This applies especially to the following.

1. **Tension pneumothorax**   Due to a one-way valvular mechanism, air builds up between pleura and chest wall with resultant mediastinal shift. This is a **clinical diagnosis** with a shocked patient, tachypnoea, tracheal shift, hyper-resonance and decreased air entry on one side of the thorax. **There is no place for x-ray in the presence of the above signs.** The tension pneumothorax should be immediately decompressed with a cannula (in the mid-clavicular line of the second intercostal space) with subsequent chest drain placement.
2. **Open pneumothorax**   This should be treated by the placement of a sterile dressing over the defect in the chest wall (preferably taped on three sides and left open on one side) with additional chest tube placement.
3. **Massive haemothorax**   This can be drained with a chest drain. Large amounts of blood may be released and it is therefore necessary to have intravenous access with fluid replacement prior to decompression.
4. **Cardiac tamponade**   The management of this condition lies outside the scope of this text but realize that it is a cause of a shocked patient. Treatment is by aspiration of the pericardial collection of blood through the subxiphoid approach.

As with all airway/breathing problems, ensure adequate **oxygen** delivery to the patient and appropriate **ventilation**.

Circulation

Once the airway and ventilation of the patient has been managed, the next step is to ensure that the patient is not in shock. Shock may be defined as **inadequate organ perfusion and tissue oxygenation**. By far the most common cause of shock in the trauma patient is **hypovolaemic shock,** but other causes also exist such as tension pneumothorax, cardiac tamponade and neurogenic shock.

Shock can only be diagnosed clinically. No investigations or x-rays will help you. The features of hypovolaemic shock are:

1. **Early shock** With blood loss of up to 750 ml (0–15% of blood volume) there is a mild tachycardia.
2. **Intermediate shock** With blood loss of up to 1.5 litres (up to 30% of blood volume), there is a tachycardia, tachypnoea and a decreased pulse pressure. (The pulse pressure is the difference between the systolic and diastolic blood pressures.) **Note that 30% of the blood volume may be lost before the systolic blood pressure begins to fall.** The pulse pressure decreases due to a rise in the diastolic pressure secondary to an increase in the total peripheral resistance of blood vessels which vasoconstrict.
3. **Late shock** With blood loss of up to 2 litres (40% of blood volume) the patient

begins to become very ill with tachycardia, tachypnoea, cool extremities, narrow pulse pressure, **fall in systolic blood pressure** and a change in mental status.

4. **Catastrophic shock**   Blood loss of over 2 litres (40% of blood volume) is a situation in which the patient will die unless immediately resuscitated. The limbs are very cold, the patient begins to lose consciousness, tachycardia and hypotension coexist with tachypnoea and an absent urinary output.

All trauma patients should have the following management of their circulatory status.

1. The insertion of **two** intravenous cannulae which are of a **large calibre**. These should be placed in a peripheral vein. If a peripheral vein cannot be cannulated because the patient is 'shut-down' then cut-downs are necessary, optimally at the long saphenous vein (ankle) or the median basilic vein (elbow). Central lines should be avoided in the acute setting for the purposes of intravenous access.

2. In children under the age of six, **intraosseous access** (best in the proximal tibia) may be used if a vein cannot be cannulated.

3. ECG monitoring is essential.

4. An initial fluid replacement bolus should be given, e.g. 2 litres of crystalloid or colloid. If there is no cardiovascular response or your assessment of the shock status indicates high blood loss, blood must be given **but in addition thought must be given as to whether bleeding needs to be controlled.** This may be due to:

(a) **External haemorrhage** – pressure dressings should be placed over any external arterial bleeding (Fig. 4.3).

(b) **Abdominal bleeding** – if it is clear that there is an abdominal injury in a shocked patient **then the patient should undergo laparotomy immediately. This should be at this stage, even before x-rays etc. have been taken.** Of course the patient should be stabilized on spine boards etc. with cervical spine protection until a later stage when further investigations can take place. **Note that there is no place for peritoneal lavage in the primary survey** – this should take place in the secondary survey if there is a question of whether the patient is bleeding.

(c) **Pelvic fracture** – very large quantities of blood may be lost in pelvic fractures. The pelvis should always be radiographed in major trauma as the injury may not always be clinically obvious (Fig. 4.4). Application of an external fixator, in selected cases, may tamponade the blood loss – this should only be performed by experienced orthopaedic personnel.

(d) **Limb fractures** – blood may be lost in limb fractures, especially if they are open. Reduction of the fracture may decrease this but blood replacement is needed in this situation.

(e) **Other** – other injuries may cause blood loss, e.g. massive haemothorax. **Remember that a head injury does not cause hypotension or shock** (except in very rare circumstances).

5. In some circumstances the stomach may dilate and actually cause 'shock' or aggravate it. It is usually beneficial to decompress the stomach with a nasogastric tube as long as there is no contraindication (e.g. a facial fracture).

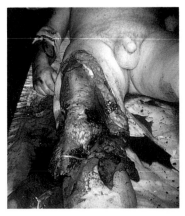

Figure 4.3 – Injuries such as this may lose large quantities of blood. Simple pressure dressings nearly always control the haemorrhage

6. Similarly a urinary catheter should be passed (but remember that urethral catheterization is dangerous in the presence of a pelvic fracture).

Neurological injury

As part of the primary survey, a brief assessment of the neurological status should be made. This is best done by the **Glasgow Coma Scale** (see Chapter 7). This is useful not only in establishing a baseline for later reference but also in determining whether the patient needs further detailed neurological assessment to prevent catastrophic brain damage, e.g. a rapidly expanding extradural haematoma. It must be borne in mind, however, that the patient's **airway, breathing and circulation** are normalized before an adequate assessment can be made, e.g. a shocked patient may well be unconscious because the blood supply to the brain is inadequate rather than secondary to cerebral pathology.

Exposure

Remember to fully expose and, at some stage, to log-roll the patient to examine the back. Maintain spinal immobilization until spinal injury has been excluded both clinically and radiologically.

Radiography

Certain x-rays should be taken at the end of the primary survey. These are:

1. **A lateral cervical spine film**
2. **A chest x-ray.**
3. **An AP film of the pelvis.**

No other x-rays are essential at this time. Furthermore no x-ray should interfere with the resuscitation of the patient during the primary survey.

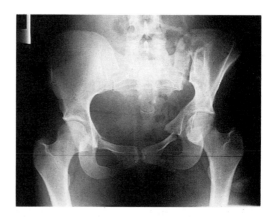

Figure 4.4 – Pelvic fracture

Note that the lateral cervical spine film should include the C7/T1 interspace, and that it does not exclude all cervical spine injuries.

Review

At the end of the primary survey the patient should be stable. If this is not the case, **re-evaluate** from the start, i.e., airway first etc. Re-evaluation is of crucial importance. Also consider at this stage whether the patient requires transfer to a more specialist centre. **Never transfer an unstabilized patient – it is a recipe for disaster!**

The secondary survey

Once the patient is stabilized, a full examination should be made, and at this time a history should also be fully evaluated. Remember that all limb fractures, unless with catastrophic arterial bleeding requiring external pressure, should not be assessed until this stage. Once all the injuries are evaluated, appropriate definitive treatment may commence.

5

Analgesia, sedation and local anaesthesia

It is important to distinguish between **analgesia** and **sedation**. Although possibly decreasing the pain threshold, no amount of sedation will allow a patient comfortably to undergo a painful procedure. Similarly, analgesics are not ideal for sedation. In the emergency setting, both methods may be required. Patients with musculo-skeletal injuries should not be allowed to remain in pain. The underuse of analgesia is well documented. This is particularly so in children; they are often unable to express their pain, and the doctor is often hesitant in prescribing for a patient group with which he is unfamiliar.

Non-pharmacological methods

The importance of simple non-pharmacological methods should not be forgotten. Significant pain relief and reassurance can be achieved through correct splintage, elevation of a limb, early manipulation and a calm and reassuring manner. In patients undergoing brief, painful procedures such as manipulation of dislocations, systemic analgesia and/or sedation may be required.

Systemic analgesia

Nitrous oxide

Nitrous oxide is usually delivered in a 50:50 mixture with oxygen, known by the trade name of **Entonox**. It is a useful way of provid-

ing analgesia and a state of conscious sedation, with feelings of euphoria. It can be used alone or as an adjunct to local anaesthetics. It is usually given via a self-administered demand valve system; the patient must inhale through a mouthpiece or mask to receive the gas (Fig. 5.1). Advantages of the method are its rapid uptake and excretion, with minimal cardiovascular or respiratory effects. Disadvantages include a degree of patient cooperation and understanding. **Its use is contraindicated in patients with suspected pneumothorax or altered mental status.**

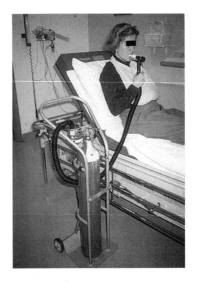

Figure 5.1 – Patient using inhalational anaesthesia

Intravenous analgesia

The use of intravenous analgesia has much to commend it in the emergency setting. It allows the dose of drug to be titrated to the patient response, and further doses to be given later without the need for repeated injections. Patients with very painful injuries often have a degree of vasoconstriction secondary to increased sympathetic output. The absorption of drugs delivered via an intramuscular route is therefore unpredictable and erratic, with the risk of repeated doses being administered just as the first dose is reaching its peak plasma level. This problem is avoided by the intravenous route.

When choosing an intravenous analgesic, important considerations include the nature of the injury or procedure, the desired onset and duration of action and the general health of the patient. It is vital that the doctor not only calculates the safe maximum dose, but also considers the patient's state of health. Remember that the elderly have a very slow circulation time. The drug should be administered slowly, waiting sufficient time for effect.

Opiates are the most commonly administered intravenous analgesic. If they are used, the doctor must have oxygen, suction equipment, oral airways, bag and mask and intubation equipment readily available, **and know how to use them**. It is wise also to have naloxone, an opiate antagonist, readily available.

If opiates are being administered for long lasting analgesia, morphine remains the gold standard. However, when performing brief, painful procedures, opiates with a shorter speed of onset and duration of action should be used. Fentanyl and alfentanyl are very useful drugs in this context. They **must be administered slowly** to avoid respiratory depression. It is important to stress that opiates are only recommended for analgesia, **not** for sedation. If sedation is required, a specific sedative drug should be used.

Non-steroidal anti-inflammatory drugs (NSAIDs)

These are commonly used drugs for orthopaedic injuries, via oral, rectal or intramuscular routes. Severe pain, however, will require an opiate. NSAIDs should be avoided in patients with active gastrointestinal ulceration, and with a history of asthma precipitated by NSAIDs.

Intravenous sedation

If intravenous sedation is used for performing brief, painful procedures, the following rules must **always** be obeyed.

1. Full resuscitation facilities must be available **in the same room**, not down the corridor (Fig. 5.2).
2. The doctor must be fully familiar with all the resuscitation equipment, and its use.
3. This equipment must be checked prior to **every** reduction, it is too late to discover the battery in the laryngoscope is flat when it is needed in an emergency.
4. Reduction under intravenous sedation is a **two**-doctor technique, one doctor must always be available to look after the airway if necessary.
5. The outdated cocktail of long-acting drugs such as pethidine and diazepam should **not** be administered; this is an unsafe technique that cannot be recommended.
6. Short-acting drugs, e.g. midazolam should be used, and the doctor familiar with their dosage on a milligram per kilogram basis.

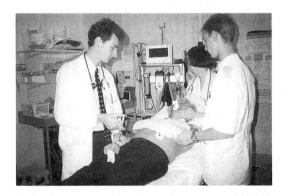

Figure 5.2 – Intravenous sedation is a two-doctor technique, with full resuscitation facilities available

7. Intravenous drugs should be administered slowly, titrating to effect. Remember that the elderly have a slower circulation time.

Midazolam

This is a short-acting benzodiazepine with a duration of action of 30–40 minutes. Children require a higher dose on a milligram per kilogram basis than do adults. As well as causing sedation, it is also an excellent amnesic. Flumazenil is a benzodiazepine antagonist. Whilst it is useful to have this drug at hand, overdose of midazolam should be avoided by slow, careful titration against effect.

Local anaesthesia

Local anaesthesia is the commonest form of anaesthesia used in the Accident and Emergency Department. **Remember that local anaesthetics are useful for providing analgesia as well as anaesthesia.** Local anaesthetic agents can be used for infiltration, nerve blocks and intravenous regional anaesthesia (Bier's block). Infiltration is the most commonly used technique.

The advantages of local anaesthesia are that it is simple, cheap, relatively safe in competent hands and can be used in the unstarved patient, or the patient with poor general health. Disadvantages include the need for full patient cooperation; the patient may dislike either being awake or aware during the procedure, or being able to still sense pressure at the operation site. The use of a local anaesthetic is also limited by the maximum safe dose for a particular patient. Absolute contraindications to their use are patient refusal, known allergy to local anaesthetics, anticoagulant therapy, bleeding diatheses and infiltration into areas of established infection.

The choice of anaesthetic is governed by the severity of pain on injection, the speed of onset and duration of anaesthetic activity, dose limitation and local toxic manifestations. The amide local anaesthetics have far fewer allergic and sensitivity reactions than the esters, and therefore are the agents of choice. The most commonly used amides are lignocaine, bupivacaine and prilocaine. Some of their properties are described in Table 5.1.

When calculating the maximum safe dose, remember that 1 ml of a 1% solution contains 10 mg, 1 ml of a 2% solution contains 20 mg etc. A useful formula for calculating the weight of a child is **(age in years + 4) × 2** (kg).

Lignocaine is the usual drug of choice for infiltration and nerve blocks. Bupivacaine, with a longer duration of action than lignocaine, is a useful alternative when a longer period of anaesthesia is required. However, remember that in certain areas, e.g. fingertips and mouths, prolonged anaesthesia may be undesirable. Prilocaine, with a higher maximum dosage, is the drug of choice for intravenous regional anaesthesia.

Adrenaline can be added to local anaesthetics (in pre-prepared ampoules), usually in a concentration of 1:200 000. Its vasoconstrictive activity means that it decreases local bleeding by creating an ischaemic field. This vasoconstriction also decreases absorption, allowing a larger dose of the anaesthetic to be used. Local anaesthetic with adrenaline must **NEVER** be used in areas with end arteries, e.g. fingers, toes, the nose, the ear and the penis. Always check the ampoule **yourself** before use. Ideally local anaesthetic with adrenaline should be kept locked away separately from plain local anaesthetic. Adrenaline should be avoided in patients with cardiac disease or taking tricyclic or related antidepressants, because of the risk of hypertension and dysrhythmias. It should be used with caution around heavily contaminated

Table 5.1 Properties of the amide local anaesthetics

Agent	Speed of onset	Duration	Dose (mg/kg)	+ Adrenaline (mg/kg)
Lignocaine	Fast	Moderate	3	7
Prilocaine	Fast	Moderate	4	8
Bupivacaine	Moderate	Long	2	2

wounds, as the resultant local ischaemia can limit white blood cell function, therefore decreasing defence against infection.

Side-effects and complications of local anaesthetics

These can be categorized as allergic reactions or systemic toxicity.

True allergic reactions to the amide group of local anaesthetics are rare, as these are thought to be incapable of stimulating antibody formation. Patients believed to be allergic to these agents are actually allergic to the added preservatives or stabilizers; it may be difficult to identify a true allergic reaction as the symptoms are similar to those of systemic toxicity.

Systemic toxicity is usually due to either intravenous injection of the agent, injection into a highly vascularized bed or administration of an excessive dose. Adverse effects primarily involve the central nervous system (CNS) and the cardiovascular system (CVS), and can be divided into four stages.

1. Premonitory symptoms include dizziness, tinnitus, periorbital tingling and nystagmus. These are treated by discontinuation of the drug, airway maintenance and administration of high flow oxygen.
2. Convulsions may follow, which are usually self-limiting, but can be treated with intravenous diazepam if persistent.
3. The next stage is CNS depression which may cause respiratory depression requiring ventilatory assistance. Finally CVS collapse can ensue requiring intravenous fluids and occasionally inotropic support.

The best treatment for toxicity is prevention. Always check the maximum safe dose and administer the drug slowly, aspirating first to avoid intravenous injection. If the patient has a convincing history of allergy to amide local anaesthetics, an alternative technique is the injection of an antihistamine around the wound. This provides anaesthesia for about 30 minutes by an unknown mechanism.

Local anaesthetic techniques

Infiltration

This is the simplest and most commonly used technique for anaesthetizing an area. The subcutaneous branches of the sensory nerves are anaesthetized. Inject the agent through the skin. Injection through the wound, although less painful, can disseminate bacteria throughout uninvolved tissue. Injection in the deep dermal tissues rather than the superficial dermis decreases the pain experienced. Advance a 23–25 gauge needle subcutaneously, aspirate to confirm you are not in a vessel, and inject slowly as the needle is withdrawn. Injection will also be less painful if performed slowly, e.g. over 10 rather than 2 seconds. Care needs to be taken to avoid injection of large volumes of anaesthetic as this can lead to localized oedema causing distortion of wound edges and tissue hypoxia.

Nerve blocks

These can be extremely useful techniques for both pain relief and performing minor procedures, e.g. fracture manipulation, wound exploration and repair. In wound management blocks have the advantage that they do not distort the wound edges. In some circumstances they are less painful than infiltration of anaesthetic around the wound, e.g. the sole of the foot or the palm.

Always formally assess nerve integrity before performing the block. As when injecting local anaesthetic at any site, **always** aspirate first to ensure the needle tip is not lying in a vessel. All the blocks described below can be performed safely with adequate initial supervision and training in their use. The risk of complications is minimized by exercising care in the performance of each block.

Femoral nerve block (Fig. 5.3)

This is a useful block in the emergency setting; for pain relief with a fractured femoral shaft or a fractured patella, to decrease quadriceps spasm or when applying skin traction.

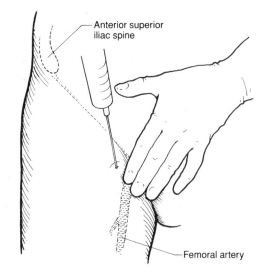

Figure 5.3 – Femoral nerve block

The femoral nerve (L2,3,4) arises from the lumbar plexus, and enters the thigh beneath the inguinal ligament. At this point it lies 2–3 cm lateral to the femoral artery. To perform the block, place the index finger of your non-dominant hand over the femoral artery and anaesthetize the skin just lateral to your finger, approximately 1 cm below the inguinal ligament. Inject 10–15 ml of solution in a fan-like distribution lateral to the artery perpendicular to the skin. Aspirate at regular intervals. Suitable agents are 1–2% lignocaine, with or without adrenaline, or bupivacaine 0.375–0.5%. Wait approximately 10 minutes for the block to take effect.

Ankle block

This block is very useful when performing procedures on the sole of the foot, an extremely painful area to infiltrate with local anaesthetic. The details are beyond the scope of this book, but ask senior colleagues to demonstrate this useful technique.

Wrist blocks

These blocks can be used alone or in combination with each other. They are very useful for procedures such as manipulating metacarpal fractures, management of wounds on the palm, or pain relief for severe injuries to one or more fingers.

They are performed at the level of the proximal volar skin crease, using a 23 or 25 gauge needle. The tendon landmarks are often more easily identified if the wrist is flexed against resistance. Wait 5–10 minutes for the full effect of the block.

Median nerve block (Fig. 5.4)

This should not be performed if there is a history of carpal tunnel syndrome. The solution (4–5 ml) is injected perpendicular to the skin between flexor carpi radialis and palmaris longus. The anaesthetic is injected in a fan at right-angles to the axis of the forearm.

Ulnar nerve block (Fig. 5.5)

In this technique, 4–5 ml of anaesthetic is injected perpendicular to the skin between flexor carpi ulnaris and the ulnar artery, again in a fan-like direction. **Remember** to aspirate first.

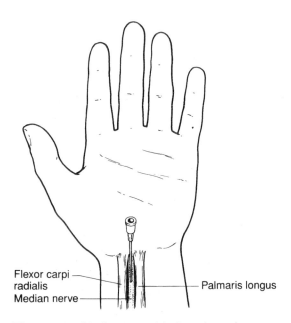

Figure 5.4 – Median nerve block at the wrist

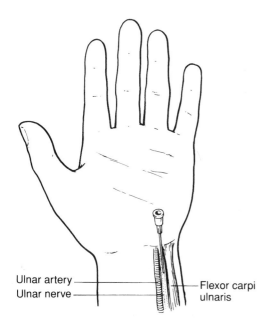

Figure 5.5 – Ulnar nerve block at the wrist

Radial nerve block (Fig. 5.6)

A subcutaneous ring is raised around the radial border of the wrist using 5–10 ml of solution.

Digital nerve block (Fig. 5.7)

These are often incorrectly known as ring blocks, which implies circumferential injection of anaesthesia. The block involves injection of agent either side of the finger (radial and ulnar sides), proximal to the interdigital web, to anaesthetize the digital nerves. Always assess sensation carefully first. Use approximately 2 ml of solution on each side of the finger. Use of more than 4 ml risks impeding blood flow by oedema. Plain lignocaine 1 or 2% is suitable. **Never** use adrenaline. Introduce the needle perpendicular to the skin on the dorsal aspect and advance until the skin on the volar aspect blanches. Try not to pierce the volar skin, this is very painful. Inject whilst slowly withdrawing the needle, and repeat on the other side. Wait 2–5 min for the block to take effect.

Similar blocks can be used for the toes, but for the big toe the block is modified slightly. Having injected on both sides of the toe, also inject 1ml across the dorsal aspect of the toe, introducing the needle through anaesthetized skin.

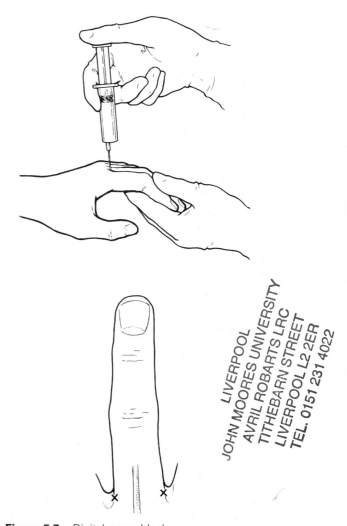

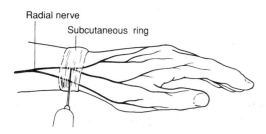

Figure 5.6 – Radial nerve block at the wrist

Figure 5.7 – Digital nerve block

Part II
The Axial Skeleton

6
Chest injuries

Pathophysiology of chest injuries

Thoracic trauma is the primary cause of mortality in approximately 25% of fatal trauma cases, and also contributes towards 50% of other trauma deaths. Unfortunately, many of these deaths could be avoided by early, aggressive and relatively simple management. As many as 85% of patients with major chest injuries can be managed with oxygen therapy, intravenous fluids and appropriate placement of intercostal chest drains.

Thoracic trauma must be excluded in the multiply-injured. It should be suspected in any patient, but particularly in those with signs of respiratory distress. These signs include tachypnoea, paradoxical movements of the chest and abdomen, use of accessory muscles, altered level of consciousness, pallor and sweating. **Cyanosis is a late sign of respiratory distress.**

In all serious chest injuries, the pathophysiological events that occur culminate in **hypoxia**. The following changes can occur, either alone or more commonly in combination.

1. **Hypovolaemia** may result from lacerations to the lungs, intercostal or internal mammary vessels, or to the great vessels.
2. **Ventilation–perfusion mismatch** results from ventilation of non-perfused areas of lung. The commonest cause of this mismatch is lung contusion, and it also occurs as a result of severe pain or flail chest.
3. **Mechanical obstruction**, secondary to either tension pneumothorax, cardiac tamponade or mediastinal haematoma will cause hypoxia due to decreased cardiac output by preventing adequate cardiac filling.

General management of chest injuries

Injuries to the chest are often under-estimated. All available pre-hospital information about the mechanism of injury must be obtained from paramedics before they leave the resuscitation room. As described in Chapter 4, care of the multiply-injured patient involves the **simultaneous identification and management** of problems detected in the primary survey. This assessment follows the established ABC order of priorities (**A**irway with cervical spine control, **B**reathing and **C**irculation).

Nothing takes priority over care of the airway and cervical spine. It is no use treating chest injuries before ensuring a patent airway exists via which to ventilate the lungs. Look, listen and feel at the mouth for obvious obstruction and the movement of breath. A talking patient has a patent airway. If a patent airway is not being maintained, simple measures include suction and/or forceps removal of debris, chin lift and jaw thrust (Fig. 6.1) to open the airway, and insertion of an oral or nasal airway. All patients must receive 100% inspired oxygen.

A patent airway is no guarantee of adequate ventilation. Causes of inadequate ventilation include:

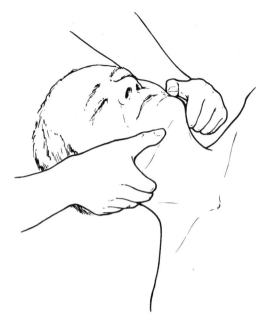

Figure 6.1 – Jaw thrust manoeuvre to open the airway (cervical immobilization is not shown to aid clarity)

1. Airway obstruction
   Any level
   Any cause
2. Central nervous system dysfunction
   Brain injury – primary, or secondary to hypoxia or hypotension
   Drugs/alcohol
3. Chest wall injuries
   Flail segment
   Sucking chest wounds
   Pain secondary to rib fractures
4. Pleural collections
   Haemothorax
   Pneumothorax (Fig. 6.2)
5. Diaphragmatic injuries
6. Lung tissue injuries

Whilst chest x-rays are important, excessive reliance upon them may lead to delays in performing life-saving procedures.

Symptoms

Symptoms of thoracic injury include chest pain, shortness of breath and tachypnoea greater than 20 per minute.

Examination

Expose the whole chest.

1. **Inspect**

(a) The chest – for contusions and patterns of bruising. Look for asymmetry of chest wall movement, flail segments and sucking chest wounds.
(b) The neck – for (1) the presence of distended neck veins, but remember that this sign of intrathoracic circulatory obstruction may be absent in hypovolaemia, and (2) for subcutaneous emphysema and swelling, which may indicate major airway injury.

2. **Palpate**

(a) The trachea – for any deviation from the normal midline position.
(b) The chest wall – for tenderness, crepitation at fracture sites and subcutaneous emphysema. Abnormal movement, especially of the sternum, may be better detected by palpation rather than inspection.

3. **Percuss** the chest in all areas, especially for the dullness of haemothorax at the bases, and the hyper-resonance of pneumothorax at the apices.

4. **Auscultate** in a symmetrical fashion, listening for the absence of breath sounds or the presence of abnormal sounds such as wheeze.

By following this step-by-step approach, the clinical signs of life-threatening thoracic injuries should be detected. **Many of the signs detected may be very subtle, and the importance of the history cannot be stressed too highly.**

Life-threatening chest injuries

The following conditions are potentially life-threatening thoracic injuries:

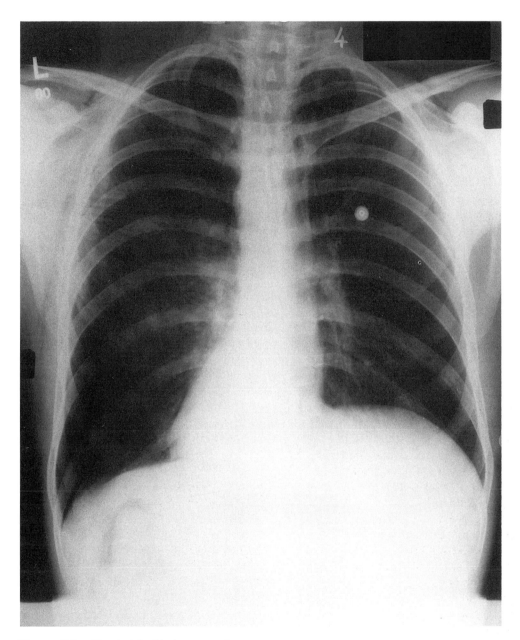

Figure 6.2 – Simple left-sided pneumothorax

1. Flail segment
2. Tension pneumothorax
3. Open pneumothorax
4. Massive haemothorax
5. Cardiac tamponade
6. Pulmonary contusion
7. Myocardial contusion
8. Diaphragmatic rupture

Flail segment

A flail segment is a serious chest wall derangement in which a section or segment of the chest wall does not have bony continuity with the rest of the thoracic cage. The flail segment usually results from a crush injury; for example, that sustained by a car driver when the chest makes contact with the steering wheel at high speed. The most severe injuries are those in which multiple bilateral rib fractures and fractures of the sternum coexist. A flail segment can also arise when two or more fractures exist in the same rib. Anterior flail segments are likely to cause more functional disturbance than posterior injuries.

The flail segment disrupts normal chest wall movement. It moves inwards on inspiration and outwards on expiration; this paradoxical movement alone however does not cause hypoxia (Fig. 6.3). The main problems associated with a flail segment arise from the associated trauma to the underlying lung. Management is therefore directed towards maintaining adequate respiratory function.

A flail segment may initially be difficult to diagnose because of splinting of the chest wall. Asymmetrical, uncoordinated or poor movements of the chest wall are suggestive findings on examination. The abnormal chest wall expansion may be detected on palpation, together with the crepitus of fractures. The multiple rib fractures and possible laceration of underlying lung may lead to considerable blood loss. The possibility of a coexistent haemothorax or pneumothorax must always be remembered.

Management of a flail segment can be difficult, and depends upon a number of factors. The patient who presents in extremis should immediately be intubated and ventilated. This should be followed by the insertion of an intercostal drain to the injured side (and bilaterally if bilateral flail segments exist) because of the risk of a tension pneumothorax developing when positive pressure ventilation is applied to the injured lung.

Most patients, however, lie along a spectrum of severity less than this, and their management depends upon assessment of their respiratory function, degree of pain, age and presence of associated injuries. A flail segment alone is not an indication for ventilation. All patients should receive high flow oxygen, humidified if possible, and intravenous fluids must be administered carefully to avoid overhydration of the sensitive injured lung.

Pain is an important factor in the patient with a flail segment because it is often severe and causes decreased movement of the chest wall, poor ventilation of the lung bases, inhibition of coughing and exhaustion. Therefore adequate analgesia is essential, and intercostal blocks or a thoracic epidural can be extremely useful. The patient may often be successfully managed without ventilation if adequate analgesia is used. If ventilation remains inadequate despite pain relief as judged by arterial blood gases ($Pa_{CO_2} > 45$ mmHg or $Pa_{O_2} < 50$ mmHg), or the patient is becoming exhausted, artificial ventilation must be considered, i.e. the decision is made upon the functional rather than anatomical consequences of the injury.

Tension pneumothorax

A tension pneumothorax develops when 'air leaks' through a defect in either the lung or chest wall that acts as a 'one-way valve'. With each breath, more air is forced into the thoracic cavity without means of escape (Fig. 6.4). The lung on the same side collapses and the mediastinum and trachea are displaced to the other side. This disrupts both venous return to the heart and ventilation of the other lung, which will also collapse if the situation is allowed to continue.

In the trauma victim the commonest causes of a tension pneumothorax are blunt trauma (causing parenchymal lung injury that does not then seal), or penetrating injuries to the chest wall. Iatrogenic causes include mechanical ventilation with PEEP (positive end expiratory pressure) and insertion of central lines via the subclavian route.

A tension pneumothorax must be diagnosed clinically, not radiographically. The immediate

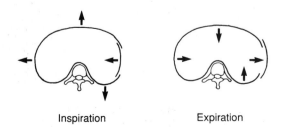

Inspiration   Expiration

Figure 6.3 – Lateral flail segment

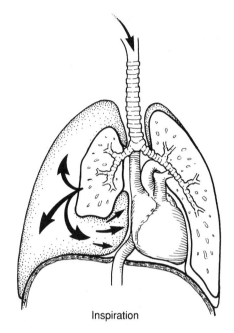

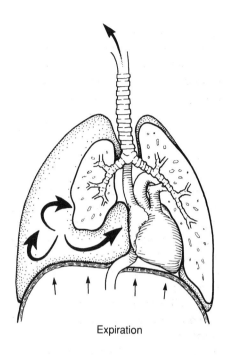

Figure 6.4 – Tension pneumothorax

decompression of the pneumothorax must never be delayed whilst an x-ray is performed to confirm the diagnosis, as the patient may die whilst waiting. The clinical signs of a tension pneumothorax include:

- Respiratory distress
- Deviation of the trachea away from the side of the pneumothorax
- Absent breath sounds on the side of the pneumothorax
- Hyper-resonance to percussion on the side of the pneumothorax
- Distended neck veins
- Cyanosis

Once diagnosed or suspected clinically, the immediate treatment is decompression with a needle to convert the tension pneumothorax to a simple pneumothorax. Connect either a needle or a cannula to a 20 ml syringe. Insert the needle through the anterior chest wall on the side of the pneumothorax at the **second intercostal space in the mid-clavicular line** (Fig. 6.5). Aspiration of air confirms the diagnosis. Disconnect the syringe and leave the needle or

cannula in situ. If no air is aspirated, withdraw both the needle and syringe, **and remember that you may now have created a pneumothorax**.

If air is aspirated, the immediate urgency of the situation has been relieved, and an intercostal chest drain should be sited on the affected side in the **fifth intercostal space anterior to the mid-axillary line**. Place the drain above the rib to avoid injury to the intercostal vessels which run below the rib (Fig. 6.6). Insertion must be

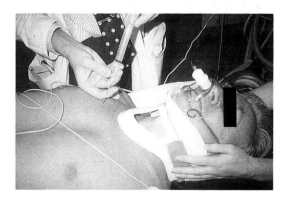

Figure 6.5 – Needle aspiration of a tension pneumothorax at the second intercostal space, mid-clavicular line.

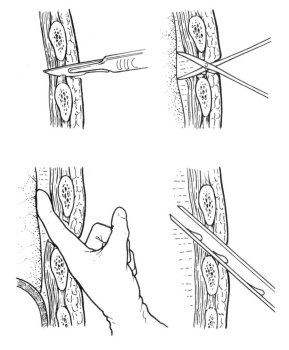

Figure 6.6 – Insertion of an intercostal chest drain ; 1. incise the soft tissues down to pleura, 2. Blunt soft tissue dissection, 3. Finger-sweep, 4. Drain insertion (without trocar).

made using a blunt dissection technique, inserting a finger into the pleural space to sweep in a circular motion ensuring that the lung is not adherent to the pleura. **On no account should the drain be inserted using a trocar.** Once in place the drain should be connected to underwater sealed drainage, and the drain secured with strong sutures.

Open pneumothorax (sucking chest wound)

Large defects in the chest wall do not usually seal themselves as do smaller wounds, but remain open and are aptly described as sucking chest wounds. If the wound is large enough (more than two-thirds the diameter of the trachea) then air will preferentially pass through the wound rather than through the trachea with each inspiration, following the path of least resistance. Air will thus accumulate in the pleural space impairing ventilation. The

wound will be seen and heard to 'suck' with each breath.

Once a sucking chest wound has been detected clinically the management is straightforward. A dressing of any sort, e.g. a gauze square, should be placed over the wound and secured with tape on three sides. This acts as a flutter-valve; as the patient inhales the dressing is sucked over the wound preventing air entering, and during exhalation the untaped side of the dressing allows air to escape.

An intercostal chest drain should then be inserted on the same side, away from the wound, if possible in the fifth intercostal space anterior to the mid-axillary line. The drain should not be placed through the wound as it may follow the track of the wound into underlying structures. If the wound is on the posterior chest wall, the dressing may be held against the wound on all four sides if the patient is turned back into a supine position following its placement. This then has the ability to allow air to accumulate in the thorax and a tension pneumothorax may develop (equivalent to taping the dressing on all four sides). Therefore an intercostal drain pack must be open ready to insert the drain immediately.

Once the drain is in situ and the patient stabilized, the chest wound can be sutured. If the patient presents with an impaling object still in situ, this should be left in place until it can be removed at urgent thoracotomy (Fig. 6.7).

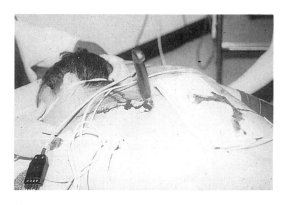

Figure 6.7 – Do not remove this penetrating object in the Accident Department!

Massive haemothorax

Massive haemothorax is defined as more than 1500 ml of blood lost into the thoracic cavity. It is most commonly due to penetrating injuries that damage major blood vessels within the chest. It can also result from blunt trauma, major lacerations to the lung and trauma to the intercostal or internal mammary vessels.

On clinical examination the patient will exhibit signs of severe hypovolaemia and hypoxia with respiratory distress. Breath sounds over the affected side will be decreased or absent, and the percussion note will be dull. The neck veins may be flat secondary to hypovolaemia or distended due to decreased venous return. A chest X-ray is mandatory, but interpretation of this usually supine film may be very difficult; up to 1000 ml of blood may be present in the thoracic cavity with an apparently normal x-ray.

The management of massive haemothorax requires simultaneous replacement of the circulating blood volume with decompression of the haemothorax. Intravenous access should be established with at least two large bore cannulae (14 gauge) and rapid infusion of fluids commenced. Clear fluids should be replaced as soon as possible with type-specific blood. Once intravenous infusion has commenced the chest is decompressed with the insertion of an intercostal chest drain. A large bore drain should be used (38 French gauge), as the large volume of blood to be drained will clot in a narrower drain. The drain should be placed in the fifth intercostal space anterior to the mid-axillary line, using the technique described for tension pneumothorax.

Continual blood loss via the drain of more than 200 ml/hour is an indication for thoracotomy. There is a greater risk of injury to the major vessels, the heart and the hilar structures if a penetrating wound is medial to the nipple on the anterior chest wall, or medial to the scapula on the posterior chest wall.

Cardiac tamponade

The pericardium is a fibrous, non-distensible sac. Injury to a coronary vessel or the myocardium can cause bleeding within the sac, which can only accommodate a small amount of blood before cardiac activity and filling is severely restricted. Therefore removal of only a small volume of blood (15–20 ml) can greatly improve cardiac function.

Traumatic cardiac tamponade usually results from penetrating injuries, although it can be secondary to blunt trauma. Diagnosis requires a high index of suspicion, as many of the 'classic' signs may be absent. It should always be considered in patients with the potential for tamponade who do not respond to the usual resuscitative measures for haemorrhagic shock.

The patient is usually short of breath, restless and cyanosed. The classic signs of cardiac tamponade are known as Beck's triad; increased venous pressure, decreased arterial pressure and muffled heart sounds. However, distended neck veins may be absent if the patient is hypovolaemic, and even normal heart sounds are difficult to hear over the noise of the resuscitation room. Pulsus paradoxus, a fall in the systolic blood pressure of more than 10–15 mmHg during inspiration, is another inconsistent sign of tamponade, and can be caused by other problems (the commonest cause is bronchospasm). A classic sign of cardiac tamponade is Kussmaul's sign – a rise in the venous pressure with inspiration when breathing spontaneously. The ECG may show non-specific changes, including ST segment and T wave changes. The chest x-ray may show a globular shaped heart outline (Fig. 6.8)

On suspicion of cardiac tamponade, the appropriate surgeons and the operating theatre should be immediately notified. Pericardiocentesis may be performed via the subxyphoid route, using a cannula over a needle. The ECG should be constantly monitored. The needle, with a syringe attached, is inserted below the xyphoid and slowly advanced towards the tip of the scapula, continually aspirating the syringe (Fig. 6.9). If blood is aspirated from the pericardial space, attach a three-way tap to continue drainage. **Note that a negative tap does not exclude a cardiac tamponade.**

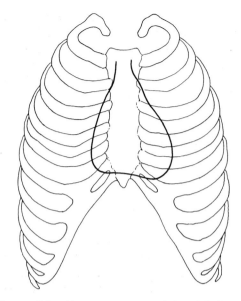

Figure 6.8 – X-ray appearance of the globular shaped heart of cardiac tamponade.

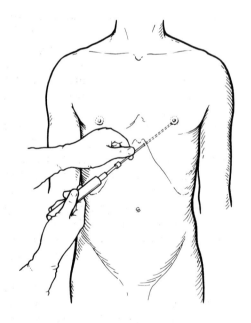

Figure 6.9 – The approach of needle pericardiocentesis (subxiphoid approach)

Pulmonary contusion

Pulmonary contusion, which is almost indistinguishable pathologically from adult respiratory distress syndrome (ARDS), results from a severe blunt injury to the chest. The patient may complain of anterior chest wall pain, and show signs of respiratory distress. Sometimes frothy, blood-stained sputum may be produced. Arterial blood gases may show a decreased partial pressure of oxygen, and increased partial pressure of carbon dioxide. The chest x-ray changes, which tend to follow the arterial blood gas changes by approximately 24 hours, are areas of opacification.

The pathological changes which occur in pulmonary contusion include interstitial oedema with capillary damage, and interstitial and alveolar accumulation of fluid and blood. These changes lead to decreased lung compliance and hypoxia.

This potentially lethal condition requires close and careful monitoring. This occurs largely after the patient has left the Accident Department, in an Intensive Care or high dependency unit, and is aimed at maintaining adequate ventilation and pain control. Not all patients require intubation and ventilation; however early intubation should be considered in certain patients. These include patients with impaired level of consciousness, pre-existing lung disease, skeletal injuries requiring stabilization, and those patients who remain hypoxic despite oxygen therapy and analgesia. Consideration of intubation should also be made in patients who are to be transferred to other hospitals, or where available monitoring is limited.

As with many chest injuries, the signs and symptoms of pulmonary contusion may initially be very subtle, and the importance of the mechanism of injury should not be overlooked.

Myocardial contusion

Myocardial contusion is a difficult diagnosis to make, and a high index of suspicion is required if this potentially lethal injury is not to be missed.

The contusion occurs secondary to blunt chest trauma which should be suggested by the mechanism of injury, e.g. a high speed road traffic accident in which the chest hits the steering wheel with considerable force. The patient will often complain of anterior chest wall pain, and on examination a tachycardia may be present which appears out of proportion to the blood loss. A friction rub may sometimes be elicited. The degree of cardiac depression and consequent decreased cardiac out-put is directly related to the mass of cardiac contusion.

The diagnosis is made by a combination of the history, the examination findings and results of investigations. ECG abnormalities are variable, but the commonest are an unexplained sinus tachycardia, atrial fibrillation, multiple premature ventricular ectopic beats, right bundle branch block, and ST segment changes. The index of suspicion should be raised further if a chest x-ray shows signs of pulmonary contusion, fractures of the first two ribs, the sternum or the clavicles.

These patients are at a high risk of developing sudden, potentially life-threatening dysrhythmias, and therefore should be admitted for cardiac monitoring, high flow oxygen and analgesia. Serial cardiac enzyme measurements and echocardiography may be performed at a later stage, but are not required for the initial diagnosis and admission.

Diaphragmatic ruptures

Up to 60–70% of normal ventilation is dependent upon proper function of the diaphragm, and therefore traumatic rupture can cause serious ventilatory problems. However, the initial signs and symptoms may be minimal or absent, and are often masked by other injuries. As always, early diagnosis requires a high index of suspicion.

Diaphragmatic rupture occurs more commonly on the left, because of the protective effect offered by the liver on the right. Blunt trauma tends to produce large radial tears that lead to herniation, but penetrating trauma produces small tears that may take many months or years to develop into hernias. An accompanying pelvic fracture in blunt trauma increases the incidence of diaphragmatic rupture.

The diagnosis is usually made on the chest x-ray findings, because of the appearance of bowel or the nasogastric tube in the chest.

However, this will be missed if the x-ray is misinterpreted as showing acute gastric dilatation, loculated pneumothorax or an elevated left hemidiaphragm. The diagnosis can also be made by the appearance of peritoneal lavage fluid in an intercostal drain, or the nasogastric tube in the chest on a CT scan.

Diaphragmatic rupture can be confirmed by contrast radiography.

Minor chest wall injuries

These are a frequent presentation to the Accident and Emergency Department. The injury may have been sustained in a road traffic accident, on the sports field or in a fall. The usefulness of radiography in the diagnosis of rib fractures is limited, and therefore a careful clinical assessment is important.

The patient will complain of pain, usually well localized, which may be exacerbated by deep inspiration, coughing or laughing. It is important to elicit a history of pre-existing lung disease, as this group of patients are at a higher risk of developing problems such as respiratory tract infections.

An examination of both the chest wall and respiratory system should be made. Localized tenderness on palpation is usually elicited, and the fracture site or crepitus may be felt. Pain will be increased on springing the rib cage. Examine the respiratory system, particularly for signs of pneumothorax, collapse or haemothorax. If signs of respiratory compromise are present, arterial blood gas measurements should be made.

A chest x-ray is not always necessary, and this should be explained to the patient. Up to 50% of rib fractures will not be apparent on x-ray, and fractures of costal cartilages will not be seen. An x-ray need only be taken to exclude or confirm injury to structures within the chest, based upon the examination findings.

The importance of minor chest wall injuries lies in the fact that the pain they cause may prevent the patient coughing or breathing effectively. This will predispose some patients, particularly those with pre-existing lung disease, to the development of lower respiratory tract infections. Therefore the mainstay of treatment is adequate analgesia. The majority of patients can be treated as out-patients, often with a combination of paracetamol and a non-steroidal anti-inflammatory agent. Occasionally, particularly in the elderly, admission is required for analgesia, local anaesthetic blocks and physiotherapy.

Patients being discharged should be given advice regarding the importance of regular analgesia, deep breathing exercises, coughing and the avoidance of cough suppressants and smoking. They can expect the pain to improve after about 5 days, but may experience discomfort for up to 6 weeks.

Sternal fractures

These fractures are commonly seen as an unfortunate consequence of the protective nature of three-point seat belts. Even apparently minor fractures may be associated with cardiovascular injury, particularly myocardial contusion, and therefore all patients should have careful examination of the cardiovascular system, and a 12-lead ECG performed.

Hospital policies differ as to whether these patients require admission for cardiac monitoring and serial cardiac enzyme measurements, and therefore it is wise to seek a senior opinion regarding the patient's management. They are painful injuries, and the patient will require adequate analgesia to ensure effective chest wall movement can occur.

7
Head injuries

Applied anatomy

The scalp

The scalp consists of five layers (Fig. 7.1):

1. Skin
2. Subcutaneous tissue
3. The galea aponeurosis
4. Loose areolar tissue
5. Pericranium.

The scalp has a very good blood supply and lacerations can be a major source of blood loss, especially in children. The loose areolar tissue can allow sub-galeal haematomas to collect. However, hypotension in a patient with a head injury must **never** be assumed to be due to head injury.

The skull

The skull is in effect a rigid, inflexible bony container for the brain, made up of the vault (calvarium) and the base. The thickness of the skull and therefore the protection offered to the underlying brain varies; it is very thin in the temporal regions. Areas of the skull that have an uneven inner surface can cause injury to the brain as it moves within the skull during trauma.

The meninges (Fig. 7.2)

The outer layer of the meninges is the **dura** which is attached to the inner surface of the skull. Between the dura and the next layer, the **arachnoid**, is a potential space called the **subdural space**. Haemorrhage and resulting haematomas can occur in this space, usually from the bridging veins that lie within it. The dura also forms the venous sinuses that drain blood from the brain which are a further source of potential blood loss.

The potential space between the dura and the skull is the **epidural** or **extradural space**, and contains the meningeal arteries. Injury to these vessels may produce an **extradural haematoma**.

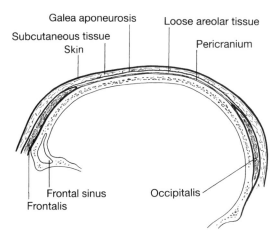

Galea aponeurosis   Loose areolar tissue
Subcutaneous tissue
Skin   Pericranium

Frontal sinus   Occipitalis
Frontalis

Figure 7.1 – The layers of the scalp

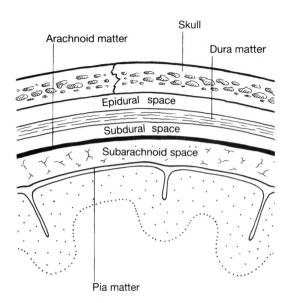

Figure 7.2 – The meninges

The innermost layer of the meninges is the **pia** which is attached to the surface of the brain. The space between the arachnoid and the pia is the **subarachnoid space**. This is where cerebrospinal fluid circulates.

The brain

The brain occupies approximately 80% of the intracranial cavity, and is made up of the cerebrum, the cerebellum and the brain stem. It is partially divided by reflections of the dura. The **falx cerebri** is the dural reflection that divides the cerebrum into right and left hemispheres. The **tentorium cerebelli** partially divides the brain into the cerebrum above (anterior and middle fossae) and the cerebellum and brain stem below (posterior fossa).

The brain stem is made up of the midbrain, the pons and the medulla. The midbrain occupies the tentorial hiatus, an opening in the tentorium. The IIIrd cranial nerve, the oculomotor nerve, also passes through this opening. The midbrain, with the upper pons, contains the reticular activating system which is responsible for 'wakefulness'. Any increase in the supratentorial pressure can force the uncus (the medial aspect of the temporal lobe) through this opening (Fig. 7.3). This **uncal or tentorial herniation**

compresses the oculomotor nerve, leading to an **ipsilateral fixed and dilated pupil**.

The medulla connects the brain to the spinal cord, and contains the cardiorespiratory centres. The cerebellum is in the posterior fossa and surrounds the pons and medulla.

The cerebrospinal fluid

The cerebrospinal fluid (CSF) cushions the brain and spinal cord against trauma. It also provides a fluid pathway for chemical substrates to reach the brain and for metabolites to be removed to the circulation. There is approximately 150 ml of CSF in the cranial cavity, of which 25–30 ml is in the ventricles. CSF is formed by the choroid plexus in the ventricles and having circulated through the ventricular system and the subarachnoid space, it is absorbed by the arachnoid villi into the venous system.

Pathophysiology of head injury

Brain injury due to trauma can be divided into primary and secondary brain damage. Primary injury is that sustained at the time of impact. Secondary brain injury occurs from potentially treatable and avoidable factors. Common management errors fall into two main groups:

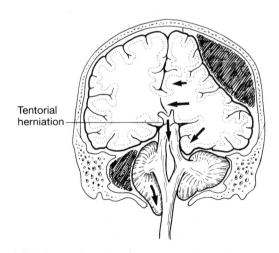

Figure 7.3 – Tentorial herniation as a reflection of supratentorial pressure increase

1. Delayed diagnosis and treatment of intra-cranial haematomas.
2. Failure to diagnose and correct systemic hypotension and hypoxia.

Optimal management minimizes secondary brain injury and decreases the overall morbidity and mortality.

The normal, uninjured brain is able to regulate its own blood supply and maintain constant perfusion despite wide variations in cerebral perfusion pressure. This is known as cerebral autoregulation (Fig. 7.4). **Cerebral perfusion pressure is the difference between mean arterial blood pressure and intracranial pressure.** The seriously-injured brain loses this ability of auto-regulation, and the cerebral perfusion pressure becomes the main determinant of cerebral blood flow.

Permanent ischaemic neuronal damage results if normal perfusion is interrupted for more than a few minutes. Intracranial haematomas increase the intracranial pressure and therefore lower the cerebral perfusion pressure and consequently cerebral blood flow. Similarly, if the brain is subjected to either hypoxia or hypoperfusion, swelling and oedema result, increasing the intracranial pressure and therefore decreasing cerebral blood flow. A vicious cycle is thus established. Systemic hypotension also decreases cerebral blood flow in the injured brain **directly** by decreasing cerebral perfusion pressure as the mean arterial blood pressure falls.

Therefore if secondary brain injury is to be prevented, it is vital priority is given to the **early correction of systemic hypoxia and hypotension**.

Patterns of head injury

Focal lesions

Focal lesions include fractures, haematomas, haemorrhages and contusions. The importance of their diagnosis is that they are often treatable by emergency surgery.

Extradural (epidural) haematomas

An extradural haematoma is a collection of blood between the inner surface of the skull and the dura (Fig. 7.5). The vast majority of extradural haematomas are due to a skull fracture which tears a meningeal artery, usually the middle meningeal artery. A tear through a dural sinus can also produce an extradural haematoma.

It is a relatively uncommon injury, especially in the elderly where the dura is closely applied to the skull. As the underlying brain injury is often minimal, early evacuation is often associated with a good outcome. However, if the

THE INTRACRANIAL PRESSURE–VOLUME CURVE

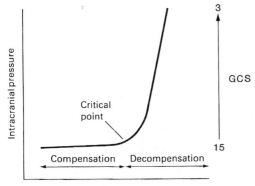

CBF=MAP−ICP

Figure 7.4 – Cerebral autoregulation (CBF, cerebral blood flow; MAP, mean arterial pressure; ICP, intracranial pressure; GCS, glasgow coma scale)

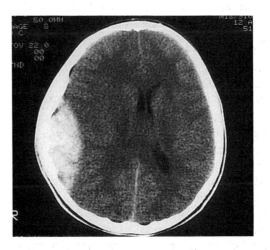

Figure 7.5 – Extradural haematoma

haematoma is not drained secondary brain injury develops which will be rapidly fatal.

The classical history of an extradural haematoma is a period of loss of consciousness, followed by a lucid interval, and then a second decrease in the conscious level. However, **this is the exception rather than the rule**, and the majority of extradural haematomas do not present with this history. They are often associated with linear fractures of the parietal or temporal areas but this is not a prerequisite for their diagnosis.

Acute subdural haematoma

A subdural haematoma is a collection of blood beneath the dura and overlying the arachnoid and the brain (Fig. 7.6). It is four times more common than extradural haematoma following trauma. The haematoma usually results from tears of the bridging veins or lacerations of the brain's surface.

Associated underlying brain injury is common and therefore the prognosis is often poor. However, early evacuation of the haematoma can improve the outcome. Patients with brain atrophy either due to ageing or alcoholism are particularly susceptible to subdural haematomas because the bridging veins are more easily torn.

Subacute subdural haematomas may become clinically apparent at any time between 24 hours and 14 days after the injury, and should be suspected when a patient presents in a state of collapse with no apparent cause.

Intracerebral haemorrhage

The effects of this injury depend upon the site and extent of the haemorrhage and associated injuries of the brain. If combined with contusion an expanding mass lesion can result. This is especially dangerous if it occurs in the temporal lobe as herniation can occur without an overall increase in intracranial pressure.

Penetrating injuries (Fig. 7.7)

The energy transferred to the tissues by any penetrating missile is given by the formula $E = 1/2\ mV^2$ (where E is the energy of the missile, m is its mass and V is the velocity). Therefore bullet wounds inflict injury far beyond their point of impact because of their high velocity and consequent energy. Outcome depends upon the extent of these injuries, but patients presenting in coma have a poor prognosis.

Injuries sustained due to penetrating injuries such as daggers, darts etc. are treated as any other head injury, but the penetrating object **must be left in situ** until operation.

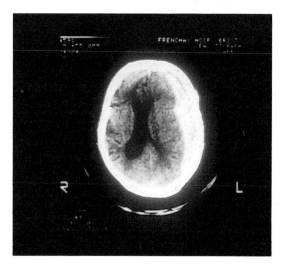

Figure 7.6 – Subdural haematoma

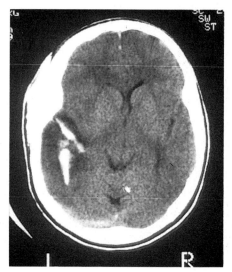

Figure 7.7 – Penetrating injury to the skull

Contusions

Contusions may occur anywhere in the brain, but the frontal and temporal lobes are particularly common sites. As contusions may occur anywhere in the brain, in any size or number, their effects are wide-ranging. They may occur directly under the site of impact or on the contralateral side as the brain moves within the skull (contrecoup injury).

The area of contusion is usually haemorrhagic and surrounded by oedema, often with overlying subarachnoid haemorrhage. If the degree of oedema is sufficient, herniation may result. Contusions commonly cause unconsciousness with or without focal neurological signs depending upon the site.

Skull fractures

At the point of impact in head injury the skull may fracture (Fig. 7.8). Skull fractures are common; linear non-depressed fractures in themselves do not require specific treatment.

However **the identification of a fracture increases the chance of having or developing an intracranial injury** (see Table 7.1), and all such patients should be admitted for neurological observation (see below).

Not all patients with skull fractures have intracranial injury; conversely not all patients with intracranial injury have a skull fracture. As always, treat the patient and not the x-ray. Normal x-rays should not be interpreted as falsely reassuring.

Table 7.1 Risk of development of intracranial haematoma

Level of consciousness	Presence of fracture	Risk of haematoma
GCS 15	No fracture	< 1:1000
GCS < 15	No fracture	1:100
GCS 15	Fracture	1:30
GCS < 15	Fracture	1:4

GCS = Glasgow Coma Scale, see page 68 for details.

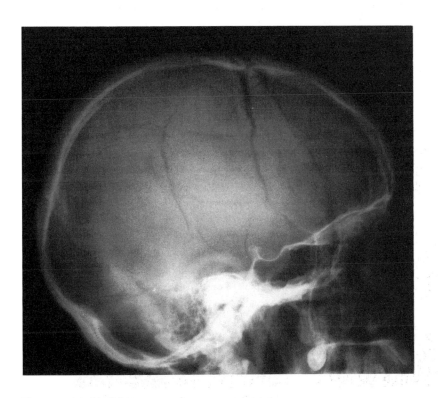

Figure 7.8 – Skull fracture

The management of a patient with an obvious severe head injury should not be delayed by obtaining skull x-rays. If the patient will be undergoing a CT scan then a skull x-ray is unnecessary.

Depressed skull fractures are those in which the skull is depressed by a distance greater than its width at that point (Fig. 7.9). Such fractures may require surgical elevation of the fragment and a neurological referral is therefore required. Depressed fractures have a high risk of epilepsy as a sequela.

Compound skull fractures are those in which the overlying skin is breached. If the **dura** has also been lacerated then the fracture is referred to as an **open fracture**. These injuries are at risk of developing infection and require urgent neurosurgical referral.

Basal skull fractures can occur at any site around the base of the brain but the petrous temporal bone is the commonest site. **The diagnosis is a clinical one as fractures are rarely visible on skull x-rays**. Physical signs suggestive of basal skull fractures are bruising of the mastoid process (Battle's sign), periorbital bruising (racoon eyes, Fig. 7.10) and bleeding behind the tympanic membrane (haemotympanum). Cerebrospinal fluid at the ears or nose is also suggestive of basal skull fracture.

Diffuse lesions

When subjected to acceleration or deceleration, the brain moves within the skull and can be subjected to stretching and shearing forces that may interrupt brain function. The extent of injuries sustained covers a wide spectrum from mild concussion to diffuse axonal injury.

Concussion

Concussion is a transient loss of consciousness following a blunt injury to the head. The duration of unconsciousness is usually brief (from seconds to minutes), although it may last longer. The loss of consciousness is due to impairment of the reticular activating system, and is caused by rotation of the cerebral hemispheres on the brain stem. Although when examined the patient may describe symptoms of headache, dizziness or nausea, a neurological examination will not show localizing signs. Some amnesia for the incident may persist.

Diffuse axonal injury (DAI)

Diffuse axonal injury involves a tearing or shearing of axonal tracts at the time of impact. It results in microscopic changes throughout the brain known as retraction balls, their site and magnitude being determined by the direction and degree of force applied to the head. DAI occurs frequently in severe head injuries and has an overall mortality of 33%. Prolonged coma is associated with a poor neurological outcome.

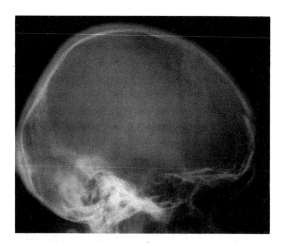

Figure 7.9 – Depressed skull fracture

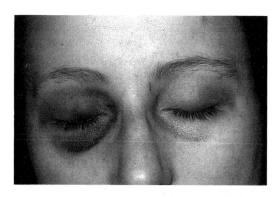

Figure 7.10 – Basal skull fracture – periorbital haematoma

Management of major head injuries

Although management may be divided into that for major and minor head injuries, and aids in its explanation, it is an arbitrary subdivision. **It must be remembered that what initially appears to be a minor head injury can rapidly deteriorate to become a major head injury. ALL** head injuries have this potential, and must therefore be managed with this in mind.

The initial assessment and management of seriously head-injured patients should be carried out by experienced medical staff, following the principles of the Advanced Trauma Life Support System (ATLS). **Airway, breathing and circulatory management must take priority over a detailed neurological assessment of the patient** (Fig. 7.11). The principles of resuscitation are the same for adults and children.

History

A history of the mechanism of injury must be obtained from the pre-hospital personnel before they leave the hospital, preferably in a written report. This is important as, for example, a patient injured in a fall rather than a road traffic accident has a four times greater chance of having an intracranial haematoma. A history from bystanders of the patient's condition immediately following the incident is also important, including loss of consciousness, respiratory effort and speech, as these form baseline observations.

Airway (with cervical spine control)

An obstructed airway rapidly leads to increased carbon dioxide (CO_2) and decreased oxygen (O_2) levels with deleterious consequences for the brain. Therefore assess, secure and maintain a patent airway. Foreign bodies and secretions such as blood or vomit should be removed with wide bore suction or manually. Oxygen should be delivered at 15 litres per minute via a mask with a reservoir bag.

All unconscious patients with a head injury should be assumed to have a cervical spine injury

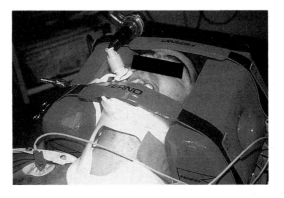

Figure 7.11 – The initial management of the head injury must include airway, breathing and circulation

until this has been excluded. In-line cervical spine immobilization should be maintained at all times with a stiff cervical collar, sand bags and tape. An exception to using sand bags and tape is the 'thrasher' in whom it is preferable to use a collar alone and seek the cause of the thrashing.

Certain patients will require intubation with a cuffed oral endotracheal tube (except in children when an uncuffed tube is used). All patients with a head injury should be assumed to have full stomach and have rapid sequence induction performed, preferably by an experienced anaesthetist. In-line manual cervical spine immobilization should be maintained during this procedure. Indications for intubation in severe head injury are:

1. Coma, i.e. GCS less than or equal to 8 (not obeying, no eye opening, not speaking).
2. Absent gag reflex on suction.
3. When airway protection is needed, e.g. copious bleeding into the airway, multiple facial fractures etc.
4. Ventilatory insufficiency (based on blood gases)

Pao_2 < 9kPa on air
Pao_2 < 13kPa on oxygen
$Paco_2$ > 6kPa

5. To allow hyperventilation with increased intracranial pressure (only after consultation with a neurosurgeon).

Breathing

The adequacy of breathing should be assessed both clinically and by arterial blood gas analysis. Actively seek and treat life-threatening injuries such as a tension pneumothorax. Remember that although pulse oximetry is useful, it is inaccurate when the patient is poorly perfused and gives no indication of the CO_2 level.

It is essential to ensure that not only is the airway patent but that adequate oxygen delivery occurs. Furthermore, if the $Paco_2$ is allowed to rise through ventilatory insufficiency, cerebrovasodilatation occurs leading to increased intracranial blood volume and intracranial pressure. Any patient who is intubated should be ventilated, aiming for a $Pao_2 > 15\,kPa$ and $Paco_2$ of 4.0-4.5 kPa.

Uncorrected hypoxia leads to metabolic failure, oedema and increased intracranial pressure and is associated with a dismal outcome.

Circulation

In order that sufficient oxygen is delivered to the brain an adequate systemic blood pressure is necessary. The injured brain loses its autoregulatory capacity and thus its perfusion becomes directly dependent upon the systolic blood pressure and intracranial pressure. If the cerebral blood flow is insufficient, oedema and further increased intracranial pressure result.

Never assume that brain injury is the cause of hypotension. Intracranial bleeding almost never results in shock (except very rarely in babies). Progressive hypertension with bradycardia is a response to a rapid and potentially lethal rise in the intracranial pressure (the Cushing response).

Neurological assessment

The neurological examination should establish the severity of the head injury and determine which patients may require urgent operation. The most important factor of the examination is that it should be repeated at regular intervals (every 10 minutes) to determine if the patient is stable, improving or deteriorating (Fig. 7.12). The neurological examination should assess:

1. Level of consciousness.
2. Pupillary function.
3. Asymmetry of limb movement.

The level of consciousness is assessed using the **Glasgow Coma Scale.**

The Glasgow Coma Scale
A   Eye opening response
Spontaneously   4
To speech (not necessarily to a request
for eye opening)   3
To pain (stimulus not to face)   2
None   1
B   Best motor response
Obeys commands   6
Localizes to painful stimuli   5
Flexion withdrawl to painful stimuli   4
Abnormal flexion to painful stimuli
(decorticate)   3
Extension to painful stimuli (decerebrate) 2
None   1
C   Verbal response
Orientated   5
Confused conversation   4
Inappropriate words   3
Incomprehensible sounds   2
None   1

Several important points need to be borne in mind when using the Glasgow Coma Score (GCS). The response to painful stimuli should be assessed by pressure on the supraorbital nerve if limb responses are absent, and the **best** motor response recorded. If the pupils cannot be assessed because of periorbital swelling this should be documented. Likewise verbal and motor response cannot be measured in a patient who is intubated and paralysed by drugs, and this should also be recorded. The GCS should be modified for children.

A normal GCS is 15, and the worst possible score is 3. A patient in coma is defined as having a GCS of 8 or less (no eye opening, no ability to follow commands, no word verbalizations).

NEUROLOGICAL OBSERVATION CHART

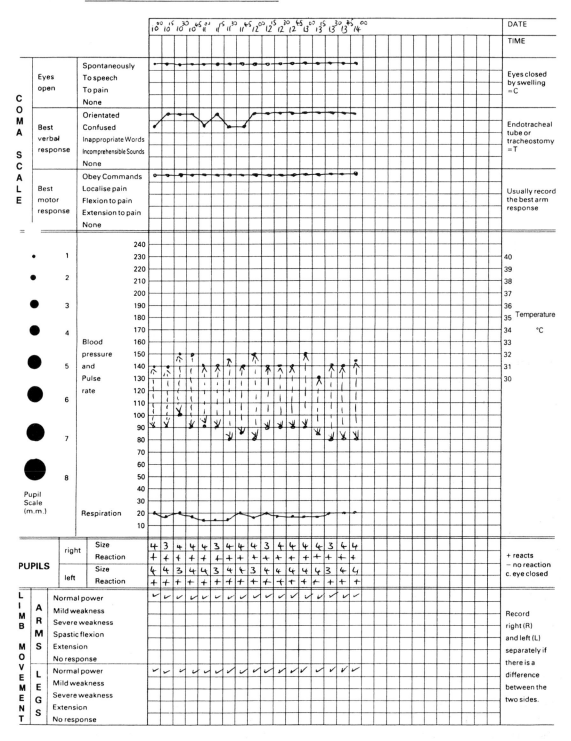

Figure 7.12 – Neurological observation chart

Pupils are assessed for their equality and response to light. It is important that a bright light source is used. An enlarging pupil **together with a decreasing level of consciousness** is strongly suggestive of increasing intracranial pressure with uncal herniation. **The neurological examination must be repeated regularly if signs of neurological deterioration are to be detected.**

Management

The initial aim of management is to prevent intracranial insult secondary to hypoxia and hypovolaemia. Next decide which patients need neurosurgical consultation. The following guidelines have been formulated by a group of British neurosurgeons.

Criteria for consultation with a neurosurgical unit

1. Skull fracture in combination with:

   (a) Confusion or decreased level of consciousness.
   (b) Focal neurological signs.
   (c) Fits.
   (d) Other neurological signs or symptoms.

2. Confusion or other neurological disturbance persisting for more than 6 hours even in the absence of a skull fracture.
3. Coma (GCS <8) continuing after resuscitation.
4. Suspected open injury of the vault or the base of the skull.
5. Depressed fracture of the skull.
6. Deterioration in the level of consciousness, or focal pupil or limb signs.

Indications for CT scanning in head injury

A CT scan should not detract from the priorities of resuscitation. Resuscitation of the patient prior to and during the CT scan is essential. In order to obtain a high quality scan the majority of patients will require sedation.

Interpretation of CT scans is difficult and is best supervised by a neurosurgeon or experienced radiologist. Indications for CT scanning include:

1. Coma (GCS < 8).
2. Skull fracture with a decreased level of consciousness.
3. Unequal pupils.
4. Lateralizing neurological signs.
5. Open head injury.
6. Clinical neurological deterioration.
7. Fractures in the area of the middle meningeal artery.

Skull x-rays are not a priority if CT scanning is clinically indicated.

Drugs used in the management of major head injury

Mannitol

Mannitol is a powerful osmotic diuretic, and can be useful in reducing intracranial pressure. However, it is not without its problems and therefore should **only be used in consultation with a neurosurgeon**. It is usually used as an interim measure whilst awaiting neurosurgical assessment. The dose is 0.5–1.0 g/kg, usually given as 250–400 ml of a 20% solution in adults. The patient must have a urinary catheter in situ.

Steroids

The use of steroids in head injuries is controversial and they should **not** be given except on the advice of a neurosurgeon.

Management of seizures following head injury

Fits are common early in the course of serious head injuries and do not necessarily lead to epilepsy in the long term. Prolonged or frequent fits are associated with cerebral hypoxia and increased intracranial pressure.

1. Intravenous diazepam 5–10 mg can be given but carries a risk of respiratory depression.

2. Phenytoin 5–10 mg/kg can be given intravenously over 10 minutes with ECG monitoring. This should be followed by an infusion of 250–500 mg over four hours.

3. If fitting continues after the loading dose of phenytoin then clonazepam 0.25 mg can be given after each fit.

Antibiotics

Prophylatic antibiotics are only indicated in a few cases:

1. Basal skull fracture.
2. Open vault fracture.
3. Suspected meningitis.

Intravenous penicillin in high doses is suitable.

The restless patient

The restless patient should **never** be treated with drugs until other causes have been excluded including **hypoxia, hypovolaemia, pain, a full bladder and metabolic disturbance.**

Opiates and some other sedatives may mask changes in the conscious level and should be avoided. If the patient is in pain, paracetamol or dihydrocodeine are suitable. Agitation can be helped by chlorpromazine 10–25 mg intravenously, given slowly as it may cause hypotension.

Management of minor head injuries

Only 1% of patients who attend the Accident and Emergency Department with a head injury are admitted. The 99% who are discharged must be judged to have a head injury of insufficient severity to require admission. The decision to discharge is therefore an extremely important one and should never be under-estimated. In order to aid in this management, certain criteria have been published by a group of British neurosurgeons which are discussed below. **The notes made must be clear and comprehensive.**

History

As in major head injuries a detailed history is vitally important. Many patients seen with head injuries are children and a clear history must be obtained from the accompanying adult. Details of falls must include the height from which the fall occurred, and the surface on to which the impact occurred, e.g. concrete, carpet, the sharp edge of a table. In motor accidents the mechanism of injury should include details of the speed, injuries to others involved and head protection worn by cyclists or motor cyclists.

Determine whether the patient has lost consciousness and for how long. Information from witnesses can be useful in determining the duration of unconsciousness. In children it is often useful to ask if the child cried immediately.

A period of amnesia, both before and after the injury, is common and the duration should be recorded. Document any nausea and vomiting. Ask specifically about symptoms of drowsiness, dizziness, visual symptoms, agitation and headache. Symptoms such as dizziness are common but are self-limiting and should be improving by the time the patient is seen in the Accident and Emergency Department.

Determine whether alcohol has been consumed and **beware of the drunk who has sustained a head injury. Do not attribute abnormal examination findings to alcohol.** A brief past medical history should be taken, and details of drug history and allergies. **Remember tetanus status** in any patient with a breach of the skin.

Examination

Examination includes assessment of the level of consciousness measured by the GCS, pupillary function and focal neurological signs as in major head injury. Remember that to have a GCS of 15 a patient must be orientated in time, place and person. Carefully examine the head for lacerations, swelling, haematomas and abrasions. Beware the 'boggy' haematoma, which is suspicious of an underlying fracture.

Wounds should be thoroughly examined for tissue loss and foreign bodies, and a gloved finger used to palpate the base of the wound for a palpable fracture. **Remember that head injuries do not cause hypotension.** However, scalp wounds in the elderly may bleed profusely and the patient may require intravenous resuscitation. The ears and nose should be examined for CSF leaks. Examine the fundi by ophthalmoscopy. Visual acuity should be measured and recorded.

Sharp missiles must not be removed until an x-ray has proved beyond doubt that the missile has not penetrated the skull.

Criteria for skull x-ray following head injury (Fig. 7.13)

1. Loss of consciousness or amnesia at any time.
2. Neurological symptoms or signs.
3. CSF or blood from the nose or ear.
4. Suspected penetrating injury or pronounced scalp bruising or swelling.
5. The patient who has consumed alcohol.
6. Difficulty in assessing the patient, e.g. the very young, post-ictal, drug overdose.
7. Non-mobile infants (the likelihood of abuse is higher)
8. Significant mechanism of injury.

Note that **simple scalp laceration is not a criterion for skull x-ray.**

A patient should not be sent home to return for an x-ray in the morning. Nor should a drunk be left in a cubicle to 'sober up'; he may be dead when you come to try to wake him up.

Interpretation of skull x-ray

The three standard skull views are:

1. **Postero-anterior**

● to show fractures of the frontal bones.

2. **Brow-up lateral**

● to show fractures of the vault;
● to show fluid levels in the sphenoid sinus;
● to show intra-cranial air.

3. **Towne's view**

● to show occipital bone fractures, and shifts of the calcified pineal gland.

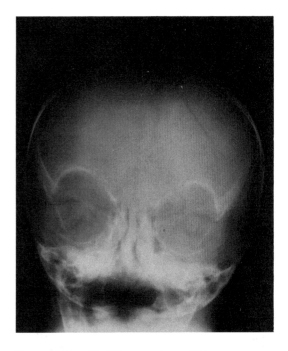

Figure 7.13 – Skull fracture in a child

Various lines on the skull x-ray need to be distinguished.

Sutures

● tend to be symmetrical.

Blood vessels

● may have cortical margins of bone;
● can be bilateral;
● may taper or branch.

Fractures

● usually sharp, straight, well-defined translucent lines;
● do not usually taper or branch;
● do not usually branch;
● can run across blood vessels or sutures.

Turn the lateral view on its side to look for **fluid levels** in the sinuses (Fig. 7.14), which may be the only sign of a basal skull fracture, and a frontal aerocele, which may indicate a sinus fracture. Examine the soft tissue shadow of the skull x-ray with a bright light if foreign bodies are suspected in a wound. If any doubt exists as to whether a fracture is present, the x-rays must be reviewed by a senior colleague or senior radiologist. **All patients with a skull fracture should be admitted for observation.**

Criteria for admission following recent head injury

1. Confusion or any other decrease in the level of consciousness at the time of examination.
2. A skull fracture on x-ray.
3. Neurological signs or headache or vomiting.
4. Difficulty in assessing the patient, e.g. alcohol, very young.
5. Other medical conditions, e.g. haemophilia.

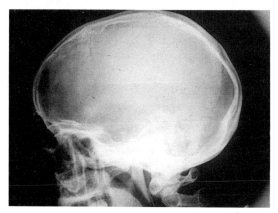

Figure 7.14 – Fluid level associated with a skull fracture

6. The patient's social conditions or the lack of a responsible adult or relative.

Note that post-traumatic amnesia with full recovery is not an indication for admission.

If the patient is discharged, full **verbal and written head injury advice** should be given to both the patient and a responsible adult. The written advice should be in the form of a standard comprehensive 'head injury card', warning of signs and symptoms to look out for, and to return immediately if any of these develop.

Post-concussional syndrome

The post-concussional syndrome is a common sequel to a minor head injury. The term refers to a group of symptoms including headache, dizziness, tiredness, difficulties in concentration, memory problems, depression and anxiety. Up to 50% of patients sustaining a mild head injury will develop some of these symptoms, with most becoming asymptomatic over the following few months.

Many studies have shown that the initially held belief that symptoms were related to compensation claims are false as compensation is not an issue for the vast majority of patients. There is evidence of both structural and functional brain changes following a minor head injury. These physical changes are thought to coexist with psychological and social factors, all contributing to the syndrome.

8

Applied anatomy and physiology of the spine

Applied anatomy of the spine

Vertebral anatomy

The vertebral column is composed of seven cervical, 12 thoracic, five lumbar and four sacral vertebrae with a variable number of coccygeal segments (Fig. 8.1). There are a number of curves to the column that are normally present when viewed from the side; the thoracic segment has a gentle anterior convexity whilst the cervical and lumbar segments have a concavity or lordosis.

An individual vertebra (Fig. 8.2) is composed of:

1. The vertebral body.
2. Two pedicles, from which arise facets to form the facet joints.
3. Two transverse processes.
4. Two laminae.
5. A spinous process.

The vertebral bodies are connected by intervertebral discs, composed of a peripheral annulus fibrosus and a central nucleus pulposus. A nerve root emerges from the spinal canal

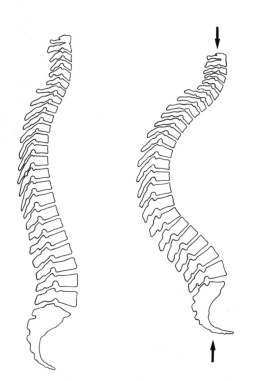

Figure 8.1 – Lateral view of the vertebral column

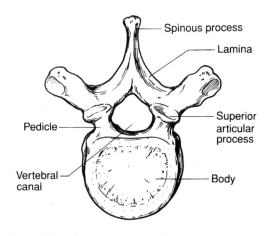

Figure 8.2 – A typical vertebra

through a space, the **intervertebral foramen**, enclosed by vertebral body and disc, pedicles and facet joints; it is important to recognize this anatomical pattern when dealing with compressed nerve roots.

Stability of the vertebral column

The bony vertebral column itself has no intrinsic stability. It greatly depends upon the supporting ligaments and muscles to provide its stability (Fig. 8.3). The important ligaments are:

1. The anterior longitudinal ligament, running along the front of the vertebral bodies.

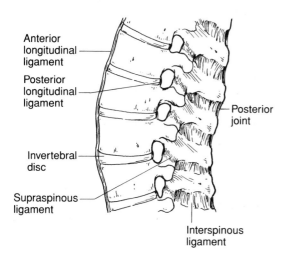

Anterior longitudinal ligament
Posterior longitudinal ligament
Invertebral disc
Supraspinous ligament
Posterior joint
Interspinous ligament

Figure 8.3 – The supporting elements of the vertebral column

2. The posterior longitudinal ligament, which runs along the back of the vertebral bodies and thus forms an anterior relation of the spinal canal.
3. The very important **posterior ligament complex**, composed of the ligaments connecting the laminae and spinous processes of the vertebrae. These are very strong and damage to the complex commonly results in spinal instability.

When dealing with spinal trauma, a useful concept is that of dividing the bony and ligamentous spine into three **columns** – anterior, middle and posterior (Fig. 8.4).

1. The **anterior column** constitutes the anterior portion of the vertebral bodies with the associated anterior longitudinal ligament.
2. The **middle column** is made up of the posterior portion of the vertebral bodies, the posterior longitudinal ligament and most of the pedicles.
3. The **posterior column** forms the rest of the spine, comprising the remainder of the pedicles, the laminae and spinous processes, and importantly, the **posterior ligament complex**.

In general terms, an injury involving only one column is stable, whereas failure of two or more columns results in an unstable injury pattern. Note, however, that **a column may fail due to purely ligamentous disruption**, and thus radiographs must not be interpreted purely in terms of fractures. The spatial

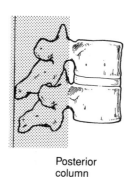

Anterior column   Middle column   Posterior column

Figure 8.4 – The columns of the spine

patterns and any clues of ligamentous disruption must be sought.

Spinal cord and root anatomy

The spinal cord is the continuation of the brain stem and extends caudally as far as the first lumbar vertebral level. Below this level the spinal canal is occupied by the **cauda equina**, the collection of nerve roots as they approach their exiting intervertebral foramina. As a consequence of this difference in the length of vertebral column and spinal cord, vertebral segmental levels do not correspond with cord levels (Fig. 8.5). For example:

Vertebral level	Cord level
C1	C1
C7	C8
T6	T7
T9	L1
T11	S1
L1	S4

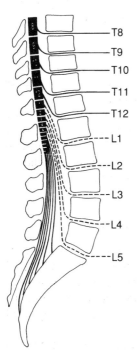

Figure 8.5 – Differing lengths of the vertebral column and the spinal cord

In addition, although each nerve root exits at its respective intervertebral foramen, the nerve roots pursue an oblique course through the spinal canal from cord to foramen, e.g. the S1 nerve root exits from the cord at the level of T11 but exits from the spinal canal at S1. This long oblique course endangers it in trauma at any level from T11 to S1.

Neurological examination in spinal trauma

Neurological injury

Neurological injury may manifest itself in a number of ways. An important discrimination to make in the context of spinal trauma is between:

1. **Damage to the spinal cord** – cord damage implies upper motor neurone injury with, in the **chronic** state, hypertonicity, exaggerated reflexes and clonus.
2. **Damage to the spinal nerves within the spinal canal** – spinal nerves exist at all levels of the cord, passing from the cord to the intervertebral foramen. Below the level of the conus medullaris (the caudal termination of the cord at L1 vertebral level) the nerves collectively form the **cauda equina**. Spinal nerve damage implies lower motor neurone injury with hypotonicity and absent reflexes.

Thus, injury at a high vertebral level will result in predominant cord injury with possible spinal nerve injury for one to two segments. At the thoraco-lumbar junction, injury will result in a mixed cord/spinal nerve deficit. Below the level of L1 injury results in purely spinal nerve damage. In general terms the prognosis for spinal nerve injuries is better than for cord injury.

Spinal shock

Spinal shock, or cord concussion, is a transient condition that occurs following spinal cord injury. Subsequent to injury the spinal cord may become temporarily functionless with flaccidity and an absence of reflex responses. The condition typically lasts 48 hours, although it may be as long as several days or weeks.

When the phase of spinal shock passes the cord demonstrates its true anatomical pattern of injury. If there is a complete cord transection the signs of an upper motor neurone lesion are manifest with hyper-reflexia, hypertonicity and clonus. The return of the **anal sphincter reflex** commonly heralds the end of the phase of spinal shock and should therefore be sought when examining the patient with spinal injury – if the reflex has returned with hypertonicity, hyper-reflexia and no evidence of motor control, it is highly likely that there has been a complete cord injury with little hope for recovery.

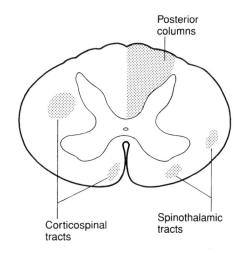

Figure 8.6 – The major tracts within the spinal cord

Neurogenic shock

Neurogenic shock is a cardiovascular phenomenon and should not be confused with spinal shock. The condition occurs in high cord lesions where the sympathetic supply to the heart and the peripheral vessels is lost resulting in a combination of **hypotension with bradycardia**. Most causes of shock result in a tachycardia and so this combination is highly indicative of cord injury in the trauma setting. This condition will require the judicious use of fluids and vasopressor agents.

The major tracts within the spinal cord

In terms of diagnosis in the context of trauma, there are three major tracts within the spinal cord (Fig. 8.6):

1. The **corticospinal tracts** – these are the major motor pathways and supply the ipsilateral musculature.
2. The **posterior columns** – these convey the impulses for vibration, proprioception and fine touch discrimination ipsilaterally.
3. The **spino-thalamic tracts** – these convey the impulses of pain and temperature contralaterally.

Complete and incomplete cord injury

It is essential for any doctor dealing with spinal trauma to be able to differentiate between complete and incomplete cord injuries. The first factor to take into account is that following significant spinal injury the cord, whether completely or incompletely damaged, may pass into a phase of spinal shock. Hence the nervous system below the level of the lesion may be functionless for a short period.

The presence of any voluntary motor or sensory function below the level of injury implies that a lesion is incomplete. Whilst all spinal-injured patients must have excellent care, those with an incomplete injury must be very carefully monitored as any deterioration in their neurological status may imply a correctable factor such as a haematoma within the canal.

The bladder in spinal injuries

In addition to a local reflex arc within the lower spinal cord (S234) the bladder is also influenced by higher centres to allow voluntary control of micturition. The bladder may therefore be influenced by local denervation and by cord transection.

When the sacral nerve roots S234 are damaged the bladder loses its reflex activity. This results in incomplete voiding of urine and ultimately **overflow incontinence.** However, interruption of the spinal cord above the S234 level results in a loss of voluntary micturition – the reflex pathway for voiding is still present and the result is a **reflex bladder** which automatically empties once the bladder volume reaches a critical level.

Examination of the spinal injury patient

When examining a patient with a suspected spinal injury, remember the following points:

1. **Examine the whole patient**. A cord lesion may mask other injuries if there is a loss of sensation, e.g. intra-abdominal injury. Neurogenic shock is only rarely a cause of shock in the trauma setting and hypovolaemia should always be excluded. Respiratory function may be compromised by a high cord lesion.

2. Any neurological deficit must be carefully assessed and the examination should be repeated frequently. All three of the major cord tracts should be evaluated (see above). The autonomic nervous system must also be included – a rectal examination is mandatory as is evaluation of the bladder.

3. The aim of the neurological examination is to establish an anatomical level of damage and to detect any trends towards improvement or deterioration. It is vital to differentiate between a complete and an incomplete cord transection, and remember that this can only be established with any certainty once the phase of spinal shock has passed.

4. Remember that pressure sores can develop very quickly in insensate areas. Great care needs to be taken immediately within the Accident and Emergency Department to prevent such pressure sores.

9
The cervical spine

Cervical spine injuries: evaluation and assessment

Initial assessment

The importance of the diagnosis of cervical spine injuries cannot be over-emphasized. The **unconscious or intoxicated patient** with any remote history of trauma should be assumed to have a cervical spine injury until proved otherwise. Unprotected movement of the head and neck in cervical spine injuries may precipitate catastrophic neurological deterioration. Although care needs to be taken with the **conscious patient** involved in trauma, their reflex muscle spasm in the presence of a spinal injury usually protects them from injudicious handling.

A cervical spine injury should always be suspected in the presence of any injury above the level of the clavicle, high speed trauma **or any unconscious or intoxicated patient.** The patient may have obvious pain in the region, hold his head in his hands or have a torticollis.

If there is any suspicion of a cervical spine injury, the patient's neck **must** be immobilized so as to prevent any further damage. In-line manual immobilization (Fig. 9.1) should be employed prior to the application of a hard collar and further restraint with sandbags and tape (Fig. 9.2). In this way, if further lifesaving measures are required, the cervical spine is protected until further evaluation can take place.

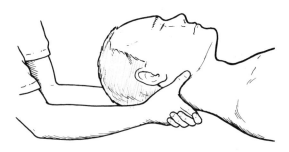

Figure 9.1 – Manual immobilization of the neck

Most authorities now recommend radiological examination of the cervical spine prior to examination. This is essential in the unconscious patient although in the cooperative talking patient an initial examination may be

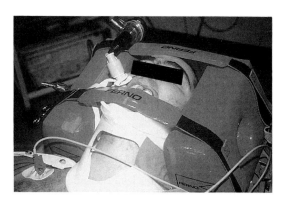

Figure 9.2 – Hard collar, sandbags and tape

worthwhile. An initial **lateral 'scout' x-ray of the cervical spine** is the first film to be taken; this excludes over 90% **but not all** injuries. **All seven cervical vertebrae and the C7/T1 junction must be visualized** (Figs 9.3, 9.4). Failure to check the lower cervical spine, where fracture-dislocations are common, is **negligent and dangerous**. If the initial film does not visualize the C7/T1 junction, two manoeuvres may be employed:

1. Manual traction on both upper limbs so as to depress the shoulders.
2. A **swimmer's view** may be performed (Figs 9.5, 9.6) – this gives a confusing view of the spine but allows the orientation of the lower cervical spine to be assessed.

Once the lateral film has been taken, further mandatory views are the **anteroposterior** and **open mouth views.** The open mouth view allows for assessment of the upper two cervical vertebrae (Figs 9.7, 9.8). If there is any doubt further imaging can be performed, e.g. oblique views

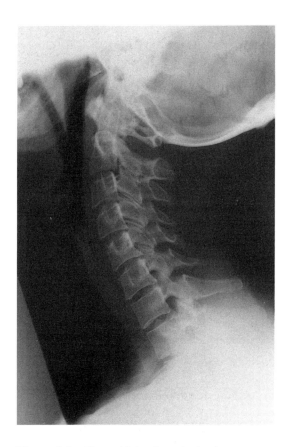

Figure 9.4 – Normal lateral cervical spine x-ray

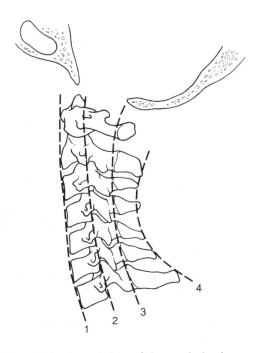

Figure 9.3 – Lateral view of the cervical spine – note the four continuous lines, 1. front of the vertebral bodies, 2. front of the spinal canal, 3. back of the spinal canal, 4. tips of the spinous processes

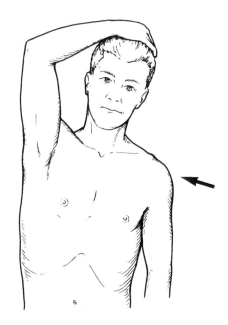

Figure 9.5 – Swimmer's view of the cervical spine – technique

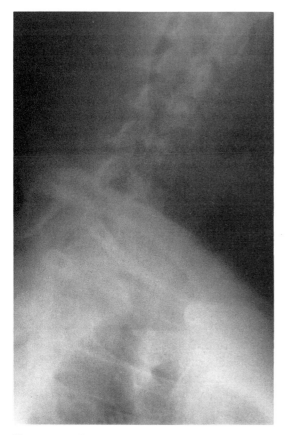

Figure 9.6 – Swimmer's view of the cervical spine

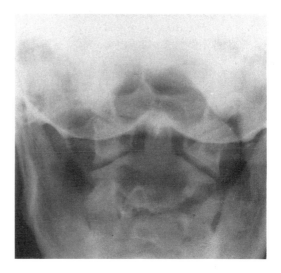

Figure 9.8 – X-ray of an open-mouth view

there is a cervical spine injury, continue to immobilize the patient and seek assistance.

Examination of the patient should include a thorough local examination (for example, many facial fractures are associated with cervical spine injuries) and a detailed neurological examination (see Chapter 8). Remember that it is of vital importance to differentiate an incomplete from a complete cord lesion. Any change in the neurological status must be recognized.

How to interpret a cervical spine x-ray

On the lateral film:

1. Are all seven cervical vertebrae and the top of the first thoracic vertebra adequately visualised? If necessary pull on both shoulders or take a swimmer's view. Remember that it is **mandatory** to see down to the C7/T1 interspace.
2. A straight and rigid spine, rather than the normal lordotic curve, suggests a cervical injury.
3. Trace the following four lines through the x-ray (Fig. 9.3):

- The front of the vertebral bodies.
- The front of the spinal canal.
- The back of the spinal canal.
- The tips of the spinous processes.

(especially for facet joint dislocations), CT and MRI scanning. Flexion/extension films, which may demonstrate instability of the spine, should only be performed by experienced orthopaedic personnel. **If you have any doubt** as to whether

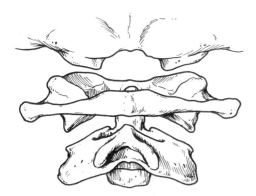

Figure 9.7 – Diagram of an open-mouth view

The four lines should follow a gentle lordotic curve. Any interruption in the line suggests a fracture or dislocation.

4. Look at the bony architecture:

- Check that the contour and height of each of the vertebral bodies is normal.
- Look for fractures of the pedicles, facets, laminae and spinous processes.
- Are there any teardrop fractures on the front of the vertebral bodies (Fig. 9.9, see below)?

5. Check the dimensions of the prevertebral shadow. The normal maximum diameter at C2–4 is 10 mm and from C5–7 is 15 mm. Shadows greater than this suggest injury due to haemorrhage etc. (Fig. 9.10). However, the absence of soft tissue swelling does not exclude skeletal injury.

6. Check the interspinous distances – separations of greater than 3 mm suggest ligamentous disruption.

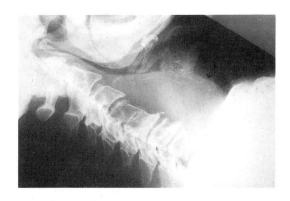

Figure 9.10 – Gross swelling of the prevertebral soft tissues

7. Check the distance between the atlas and the dens; it is normally less than 3 mm in adults, although it can be as large as 5 mm in children. Larger values indicate disruption of the atlas or the transverse ligament.

8. Finally check the clivus-odontoid line to exclude an atlanto-occipital dislocation.

The anteroposterior film (Fig. 9.11) is less useful, but:

1. Look for fractures of the vertebral bodies.
2. Check that the trachea and all the spinous processes are in the midline.

The open mouth view should be routinely requested in suspected cervical spine injury (Figs 9.7, 9.8). It allows visualization of C1 and C2 with the teeth out of view.

1. Look at the odontoid peg and ensure that it is not fractured. Beware misinterpretation of the os terminalum, the ossification centre for the tip of the odontoid peg, as a fracture.
2. The outer edges of the lateral masses of the atlas (C1) should not extend beyond the lateral masses of the axis (C2). Extension beyond this point indicates a fracture of the atlas.

Injuries of the upper cervical spine

Injuries to the atlas and axis (and their ligaments) can be more conveniently considered

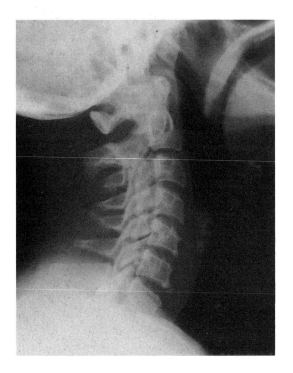

Figure 9.9 – Tear-drop fracture, lower border C6

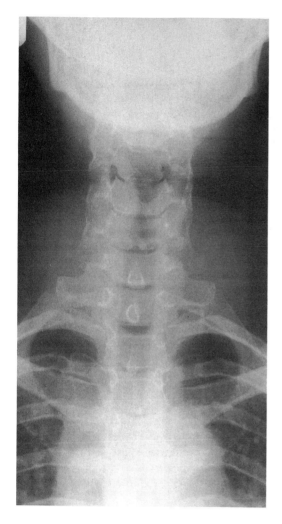

Figure 9.11 – Normal AP view of the cervical spine

separately from injuries of the other cervical vertebrae. The main injury patterns are:

1. Atlanto-occipital injuries.
2. Fractures of the atlas.
3. Odontoid peg fractures.
4. Transverse ligament injuries.
5. Fractures of C2 (other then the odontoid peg).

Clearly all suspected cervical spine injuries must be immediately referred and on no account should reduction be attempted by junior personnel.

Atlanto-occipital injuries (Fig. 9.12)

Separations of the occiput from the C1 vertebra rarely present as most injuries result in death at the scene of injury. The condition more commonly presents as a non-traumatic condition in patients with rheumatoid arthritis. The injury must be carefully reduced with skull traction.

Fractures of the atlas

Fracture of the atlas is commonly termed **Jefferson's fracture**. It is usually as a result of **axial compression** of the head upon the neck. The most common fracture pattern is for the ring to fail in four places (Fig. 9.13). Not uncommonly there is an associated fracture of the odontoid peg.

The patient is often in great pain, and there may be occipital symptoms due to compression

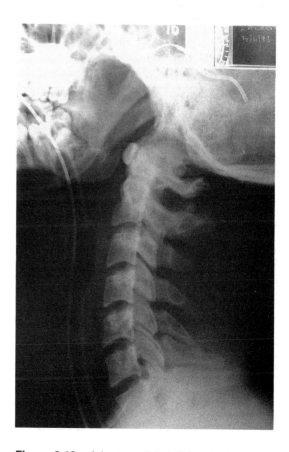

Figure 9.12 – Atlanto-occipital dislocation

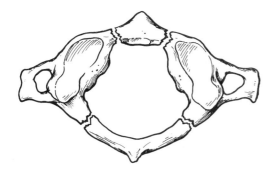

Figure 9.13 – Fracture of the atlas

of local nerves. Surprisingly many cases are neurologically intact. However, damage may occur to the vertebral artery which passes over the atlas, and this may precipitate brain stem and cerebellar infarction.

The most useful x-ray is the open mouth view, which demonstrates outward shift of the lateral masses of the atlas. Look for any associated odontoid fractures. The lateral film may demonstrate fractures of the posterior arch of the atlas. Further imaging may be useful, e.g. oblique views, CT and MRI imaging. Two pitfalls to avoid in interpretation are:

1. The posterior arch of the atlas is often cartilaginous in children up to the age of 3 years – this may be confused for a fracture.
2. Incomplete fusion of the posterior arch is a relatively common variant – this is usually in the midline. Fractures of the arch of the atlas are rarely in the midline, and this can help in differentiating the two.

Fractures of the atlas are potentially unstable. Treatment is generally conservative with treatment in a collar or skull traction, although in some cases a C1–C2 fusion is necessary.

Odontoid peg fractures

The odontoid peg, or dens, is an extension of the body of the axis (C2) that articulates with the anterior arch of the atlas and is held there by the transverse ligament. The peg and its associated ligaments are the primary stabilizers of the atlanto-axial joint.

Odontoid fractures are not uncommon and are being recognized with increasing frequency. They are the result of high energy trauma. The injury occurs in children as well as adults. Eighty per cent are as a result of **sudden flexion** of the cervical spine, although 20% are associated with **sudden extension**. They may be associated with Jefferson (atlas) fractures, and other cervical spine fractures occur in up to 25% of cases. Head and facial injuries are common coexisting injuries. Odontoid peg fractures are usually not associated with a neurological deficit – this is because they constitute a self-selected group of patients who have survived, many patients dying at the site of injury.

Anderson and D'Alonzo have classified odontoid peg fractures into three varieties (Fig. 9.14):

Type 1   Fractures of the upper third of the peg.
Type 2   Fractures at the junction of the peg with the body of C2.
Type 3   Fractures essentially of the body of C2 at the base of the peg.

The most useful radiological view is the **open mouth view**. This usually clearly demonstrates the fracture. Be careful not to be fooled by some radiological variants.

1. Remember that the os terminalum, the ossification centre of the tip of the peg, does not fuse until the age of 12, and may appear deceptively like a fracture. Nonfusion may also occur in the adult.
2. The ossification centre of the body of the peg usually fuses to the body of C2 at 3–6 years.
3. The peg may be congenitally absent or poorly formed.

The injury is potentially unstable. Most of the injuries can be treated conservatively, although many type 2 fractures go on to non-union and so fusion is advocated by many for the latter group.

Transverse ligament injuries

The transverse ligament restrains the odontoid peg against the anterior arch of the atlas. The

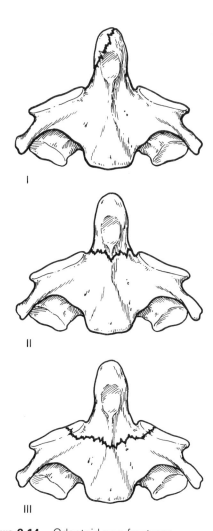

Figure 9.14 – Odontoid peg fractures

normal atlas to dens interval is 3 mm (5 mm in children). Traumatic rupture of the transverse ligament (as a result of a severe sudden flexion force) is rarely seen as the result is almost always cord compression and inevitable death. Cases more commonly seen are as a result of minor trauma in a patient with erosive rheumatoid arthritis. The management of these cases is outside the scope of this book, but many require an atlanto-axial fusion.

Other fractures of the axis

The main fracture pattern of the axis (other than the odontoid peg) is fracture through the pedicle. There are two main mechanisms involved:

1. **Extension and distraction of the neck** This is commonly termed a **hangman's fracture**, in that this was the mechanism of death in judicial hanging. In accidental trauma there is high rate of cord compression and inevitably death.

2. **Extension and compression of the neck** This fracture is usually not associated with significant cord compression but is potentially unstable as there is often a spondylolisthesis of C2 upon C3 (Fig. 9.15).

The injury needs to be handled very carefully as there is a great risk of cord compression with poor neck control. The injury most commonly seen, due to compression, often coexists with other cervical spine injuries, and the rest of the neck needs to be thoroughly reviewed.

Injuries of the lower cervical spine

Injuries of the lower cervical spine can be conveniently reviewed in terms of the mechanism of

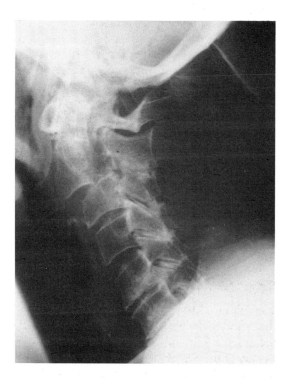

Figure 9.15 – Spondylolisthesis of C2 on C3

injury. The main forces involved are flexion, extension, compression and rotation. Most injuries are a combination of two of these with one force predominating.

Injuries due to a predominantly flexion force

These are described in ascending order of neurological severity.

Crush fracture of a vertebral body

A crush fracture of a vertebral body is due to a combination of **flexion and compression**. The fracture pattern is a **stable** one with wedging of the anterior body with the posterior portion undisturbed (Fig. 9.16). Note that to come into this category there must be no involvement of the posterior complex (i.e., increased separation or fracture of the spinous processes). Cord involvement is rare although roots at that level may be involved leading to lower motor neurone lesion in the arms.

Stability of the fracture can be checked with dynamic flexion/extension lateral x-rays but these should only be undertaken by experienced personnel. Nearly all of these fractures can be treated symptomatically in a collar or cast.

Posterior complex ligament tears

These can be very difficult to diagnose. The x-rays may show very little in the way of bony damage but look carefully for evidence of separation of the spinous processes by more than the normal distance of 3 mm. Some avulsion fractures of spinous processes form part of such posterior complex damage. Such injuries are **potentially unstable** in that should further flexion force be applied to the neck, neurological compromise may occur. If there is any doubt about such an injury, immobilize the neck and seek advice. Most of the injuries can be treated by immobilization in a collar.

Unifacetal dislocations

A unifacetal dislocation implies that one of the facet joints has 'jumped' resulting in some forward shift and rotation of one vertebra upon another (Fig. 9.17). **For this to occur there must also be some damage to the posterior complex soft tissues** and thus the injury is **potentially unstable**. The injury does not usually cause any neurological deficit.

The history is usually one of **flexion with rotation**. The patient is often in pain with a 'cock-robin' attitude with the chin rotated to the side contralateral to the dislocated facet. Root symptoms at the level of the dislocation may

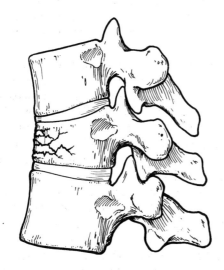

Figure 9.16 – Crush fracture

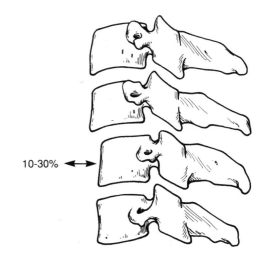

10-30%

Figure 9.17 – Unifacetal dislocation

be present. Cord involvement is not common. On the lateral x-ray the most obvious feature is overlap of one vertebra upon another by 10–30% (Fig. 9.17). The anteroposterior film may show a loss of continuity of the lines of the spinous processes, implying rotation of the vertebra.

The management of these injuries must be performed by experienced personnel. They usually require reduction by traction and some, with severe posterior complex damage, require surgical stabilization.

Bifacetal dislocations

These are severe injuries that are commonly associated with paraplegia. Both facet joints 'jump' and again, there is **damage to the posterior ligament complex**. The injury is very unstable and if not associated with any neurological deficit must be handled with the utmost care. The lateral x-ray demonstrates forward shift of one vertebral body upon another of **more than 50%** (Fig. 9.18). There is a high incidence of intervertebral disc expulsion into the spinal canal with this injury, and for this reason immediate reduction is not always advised. **Immediate assistance** from senior personnel is required to allow management to proceed.

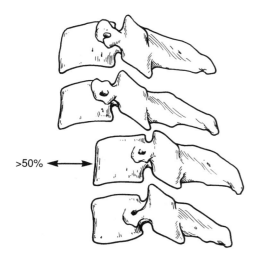

>50%

Figure 9.18 – Bifacetal dislocation

Fracture – dislocations of the cervical spine

These are the most serious of all flexion injuries and have a very high rate of cord compression. As well as facet joint disruption there is a fracture of the body of the vertebra with gross shift and instability. Clearly any patient with an incomplete neurological deficit needs to be handled very carefully. Most injuries require reduction and surgical stabilization.

Injuries due to a predominantly extension force

(Note that fractures of odontoid peg and 'hangman-type' fractures of the axis are predominantly extension injuries – see p. 85 above.)

Extension injuries resulting in ischaemic cord damage

Many elderly patients have a degenerate cervical spine with many osteophytes. Relatively trivial hyperextension forces can cause a number of pathological processes within the region, including tears of the anterior longitudinal ligament, cord stretching and thrombosis of the local vessels. The latter can result in a number of cord syndromes, the commonest of which is the **central cord syndrome** (see below). As the patient may only show subtle radiological signs, it is important to be aware of this mechanism of injury.

The **central cord syndrome** is due to ischaemic cord damage more centrally than peripherally (Fig. 9.19). As the lower limb corticospinal tracts run laterally in the cord, the upper limb is affected more than the lower limb. The patient generally complains of pain in the neck and weakness in the arms. Bladder function is usually spared.

Clinically, take great care in the elderly patient with neck injuries. Forehead bruises and lacerations imply an extension force to the neck. X-rays may appear remarkably normal. Look for any evidence of avulsion fractures on the front of the vertebral bodies (due to avulsion of the anterior longitudinal liga-

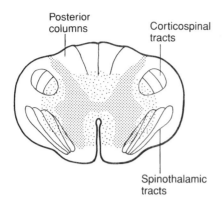

Figure 9.19 – Central cord syndrome

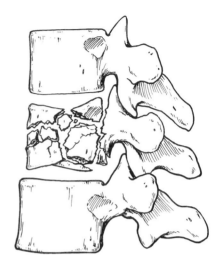

Figure 9.20 – Burst fracture

ment) and for enlargement of the prevertebral shadow on the lateral film.

These injuries are largely stable. The injury itself is treated symptomatically with analgesia and a collar. Attention is directed towards management of the neurological lesion.

Vertebral body fractures due to extension

Vertebral body fractures due to extension have more wedging posteriorly than anteriorly. However, in addition, there is the risk of intervertebral disc prolapse into the spinal canal. Many of these patients require urgent decompression and stabilization. Therefore be aware of the patient with neurological deficit who has a wedge-type body fracture with more of the wedging posteriorly.

Injuries due to a predominantly compressive force

(Fractures of the atlas also fall into this group, see above.) True compressive fractures of the cervical spine are rare, as most injuries usually involve a flexion or extension force. However, true axial loading can occur, and results in **burst fractures** of the vertebral body (Fig. 9.20). Take care to distinguish these from wedge or crush fractures that occur as part of a flexion or extension force. The danger with burst fractures lies in the possibility of bone and/or disc extrusion into the spinal canal. The posterior complex is usually unaffected and therefore the injury is a stable one.

Be aware of this mechanism of injury in patients who have a history of compression of the vertex or vertex lacerations etc. As the anterior cord is more at risk of damage, the motor supply of the upper limbs is most affected, followed by that to the lower limbs. The dorsal columns, supplying the modalities of vibration and proprioception, are affected last.

Treatment is usually a period in traction, although surgical decompression and stabilization is required if there is any neurological deficit.

Miscellaneous injuries

Avulsion fractures of the spinous processes

Sudden severe muscular contraction may avulse the supraspinous and interspinous ligament from the spinous process. This has been termed **clay shoveller's fracture of the spine**. It must be distinguished from anterior and middle column injuries with spinous process fractures as part of the posterior complex injury. The injury is stable and can be treated symptomatically in a cervical collar.

Soft tissue injuries of the neck

Soft tissue injuries of the neck are frequently seen in the Accident and Emergency Department, mostly as a result of road traffic accidents. Optimal initial management may decrease the morbidity of these injuries. In your assessment, ensure that you exclude any **fracture of the cervical spine** or a **cervical disc prolapse**.

Mechanism of injury

There is a divergence of opinion as to the mechanism of soft tissue injuries of the neck in road traffic accidents. Typically, the driver of a stationary or slowly moving vehicle is shunted from the rear by another vehicle. In some cases there is a second impact with a vehicle ahead of the driver. This is classically said to result in a **hyperextension–hyperflexion force** to the cervical spine. However, many authorities now feel this is incorrect and that rotational forces are also responsible; the use of seat belts accentuates any rotational force.

Diagnosis

Immediately following a road traffic accident as depicted above, frequently there is no complaint of neck pain. Discomfort in the cervical region gradually begins after 6–8 hours and is typically more severe the following day. Thus the patient may present to the Accident and Emergency Department after a short delay.

The cervical symptoms are usually concentrated at the base of the neck and in the midline posteriorly. Common associated symptoms are frontal and occipital headache, interscapular and shoulder pain and low back ache. **If there are any segmental upper limb ('root') symptoms, leg weakness or bladder problems, suspect either a fracture of the spine or a cervical disc prolapse.**

Examination usually reveals a very stiff cervical spine with a decreased range of movement. Point tenderness of the midline is absent although palpation of the free border of one of the trapezius muscles may be painful. **It is mandatory to perform a neurological examination of the upper and lower limbs and to determine that bladder and anal function is normal.**

It is wise to radiograph all soft tissue injuries of the neck following road traffic accidents, although your unit may have its own policy. The normal lordotic curve of the spine is frequently replaced by a rigid linear pattern. Exclude any skeletal injury and remember to visualize the entire cervical spine including as far caudally as the C7/T1 interspace. Any pre-existing degenerative disease of the spine should be noted as this worsens the prognosis of the injury.

Management

The long-term prognosis of soft tissue injuries of the neck is depressing, many never obtaining a full recovery. Poor prognostic signs are early onset of pain, interscapular and low back pain and root symptoms in the upper limb.

Any fractures must be promptly referred. A cervical disc prolapse can be difficult to diagnose but any patient with upper limb symptoms (e.g. paresthesiae, numbness or weakness) and lower limb long tract signs (upper motor neurone signs such as weakness, hypertonicity and hyper-reflexia) should be suspected as having a central disc prolapse and should also be referred immediately.

The majority of patients that you will see have no objective neurological signs. The clinical syndrome may be due to a number of factors such as muscle and ligament tears or lateral disc prolapse. Your hospital may have its own policy as to management of these cases. It has been appreciated that prolonged immobilization worsens the prognosis. Optimal management involves explanation of the diagnosis, prescription of analgesia and anti-inflammatories and the application of a soft cervical collar **for a short period.** Physiotherapy follow-up is useful and, in any event, the patient should be instructed to mobilise the neck after 2–3 days. Routine fracture clinic referral is not indicated.

10

The thoraco-lumbar spine

Thoraco-lumbar spine fractures and dislocations

Thoraco-lumbar injuries are very easy to miss in the patient with multiple trauma. All patients who have sustained significant trauma must be assumed to have sustained an injury to the back. The patient should be placed on a spine board in the emergency setting and moved only by log-rolling with no rotational or bending forces applied to the spine (Fig. 10.1). It is usually not possible to obtain good-quality radiographs with portable x-ray equipment in the Accident and Emergency Department – the best policy is to maintain immobilization

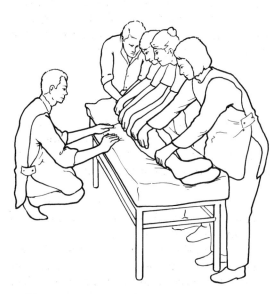

Figure 10.1 – Log-roll of a trauma patient

of the back until the patient can be safely taken to the main x-ray department. Note that this may be some days following admission if the patient has undergone early major surgery.

Most of the thoracic spine, from T1 to T10, is highly stable due to the orientation of the facet joints and the presence of the bony rib cage. Where significant fractures and dislocations occur in this region, very high energy is involved and the neurological deficit rate is high. The T10–L1 segment has a large 'stress riser' placed upon it by virtue of the fact that an immobile segment of the spine meets a mobile area – this explains the high incidence of injuries in this region.

It is important to remember that the conus medullaris, the end of the spinal cord, is at the level of the L1 vertebra. Lesions at this level are a mixture of cord (upper motor neurone) and cauda equina (lower motor neurone) deficits. (See Chapter 8 for full details.)

Thoracic spine fractures

Clinical examination of the thoracic spine can play a helpful role in injuries in this region; the posterior ligament complex, often involved in unstable fractures, can be easily palpated and pain, tenderness, swelling etc. is usually evident. To do this, the patient needs to be carefully log-rolled. Remember that log-rolling requires a minimum of **four** personnel.

The main categories of thoracic spine fractures are:

1. Crush fractures of the vertebral body.
2. Burst fractures of the vertebral body.
3. Fracture-dislocations of the thoracic spine.

Crush fractures of the thoracic spine

Crush fractures are due to **compression in flexion**. The vertebral body is wedged anteriorly with the posterior margin left undisturbed (cf. burst fractures). The injury is common in the elderly with osteoporotic and pathological bone, where relatively trivial trauma may result in a crush fracture. Younger patients require a great deal of energy to produce the fracture, e.g. falls from a height. Note that there is an association between fractures of the calcaneum and wedge fractures of the spine. Most occur in the thoraco-lumbar region.

The most helpful x-ray is the lateral film (Fig. 10.2). Where the loss of anterior vertebral body height is less than 50%, the injury is stable and can be treated symptomatically with a few days' bed rest. Loss of more than 50% implies a degree of instability that may require operative stabilization, especially if there is evidence of posterior ligament complex involvement.

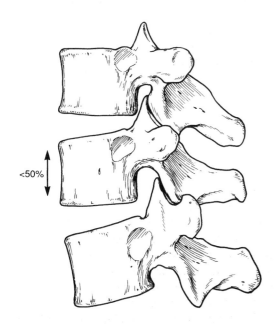

<50%

Figure 10.2 – Crush fracture of a vertebral body

Burst fractures of the thoracic spine

Burst fractures are due to an **axial load** (whereas crush fractures have a component of flexion). High energy trauma is responsible for these fractures, and there is the risk of vertebral body and intervertebral disc expulsion posteriorly into the spinal canal. Many are associated with posterior ligament complex damage and are thus **unstable**. Note that any degree of posterior body wedging implies a burst fracture rather than a crush fracture, and this difference is important in terms of management.

Burst fractures with any neurological deficit may require urgent decompression. Otherwise they may be treated conservatively, although surgical stabilization may be indicated.

Fracture-dislocations of the thoracic spine

These fractures are very serious and are nearly always associated with paraplegia. Any degree of vertebral body shift implies posterior complex damage. Most injuries of this type have body, pedicle and/or laminar fractures. Look for signs of potential instability such as fractures or wide separations of the spinous processes. The management of these injuries is outside the scope of this book. However it cannot be over-emphasized that a detailed neurological examination must be performed to determine if the neurological lesion is complete or incomplete (see Chapter 8). Urgent specialized management is required to maximize the chances of neurological recovery.

Lumbar spine fractures

The lumbar spine, as well as the T11–T12 vertebral segments, has more mobility than the thoracic spine and injuries are therefore more common. The main injury patterns are:

1. **Crush or wedge fractures** (Fig. 10.3) – the management of these injuries is similar to those in the thoracic spine.
2. **Fracture-dislocations of the lumbar spine** – these injuries are similar mechanically to those in the thoracic spine. Note however that the prognosis is often better

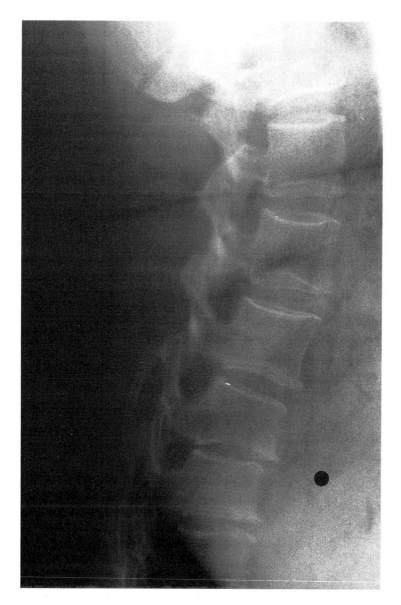

Figure 10.3 – Crush fracture of a lumbar vertebral body

as the cauda equina rather than the spinal cord is involved.

3. **Fractures of the transverse processes of the lumbar vertebrae** – the psoas and the quadratus lumborum muscles are attached in part to the transverse processes of the vertebrae in this region. Violent muscular contractions may result in avulsion fractures of the transverse processes (Fig. 10.4). The injuries are stable and may be treated symptomatically. However, retroperitoneal haematoma is a common sequel and may result in a paralytic ileus.

Back pain – diagnosis and management

One of the commonest emergency presentations is the patient with back pain. Although such a patient is often a 'heart-sink' for the doctor, the patient is often in a great deal of pain and dis-

history and examination will pick these up. Examples include:

1. Cardiovascular, e.g. abdominal aortic aneurysm.
2. Respiratory, e.g. lower lobe pneumonia, pulmonary embolus.
3. Gastrointestinal, e.g. pancreatitis, perforated peptic ulcer.
4. Urinary, renal or ureteric colic.

Intraspinal causes

Acute back strain

This is a common symptom that is generally short-lived and self-limiting. The onset may be preceded by a minor traumatic event. The patient complains of low back pain without any nerve root symptoms. Rest for a short period is advocated followed by an exercise programme. The old adage that the patient should take to bed for 2 weeks is now discredited as there is evidence that mobilization after 2–3 days is beneficial. The patient can be given simple analgesics and should not require referral.

Long-term mechanical back pain

This, unfortunately, is a very common problem that is a frequent source of disability and cost in terms of employment days lost. It is often managed poorly. The term mechanical back pain encompasses a wide variety of conditions that manifest as long-term low back pain but with no evidence of nerve root irritation or entrapment and without evidence of a progressive underlying pathology. Symptoms are often present for many years.

This book cannot deal in detail with the management of mechanical back pain. No one treatment has proved success. Physiotherapy, facet joint injections, manipulations, acupuncture and a number of other treatment modalities may be helpful. Surgery, except in a few selected cases with degenerative disc disease for which spinal fusion may be advocated, **is not indicated** and may worsen the prognosis of the condition.

The patient requires a full explanation of the condition, and should be told that the

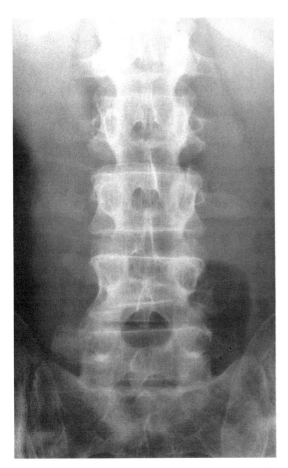

Figure 10.4 – Fracture of the transverse process of L3

tress. Any doctor dealing with the condition should be able to manage the patient appropriately and be able to select out those that require further expert help. This chapter aims to give a systematic method for dealing with the acute management of back pain – the patient with significant pathology must be recognized and given appropriate referral. On the other hand, 'blanket referral' of all patients with back pain will overload the specialist services.

Classification of back pain

Extraspinal causes

Never forget that back pain may be a symptom of extraspinal disease. In most cases a thorough

symptoms may be present for a considerable period but should be reassured that the condition will not worsen. Most patients do not require specialist referral and can be managed by the General Practitioner. Many would say that if a referral is necessary it should be to a rheumatologist or orthopaedic physician rather than an orthopaedic surgeon. It is certainly not appropriate to refer mechanical back pain patients as 'urgent' referrals to the fracture clinic.

Root pain

This is a symptom which must be specifically sought when dealing with back pain. The commonest cause of root pain is intervertebral disc prolapse although other pathologies (e.g. tumour, spinal stenosis, spondylolisthesis) may be responsible.

Be careful to differentiate root pain from referred pain. Root symptoms are experienced in a segmental distribution, and for the common levels of L5/S1 and L4/5, **radiate below the knee**. Referred pain from local back pathology, e.g. facet joint dysfunction as in mechanical back pain, may radiate into the buttocks and thigh but does not extend below the knee. Remember, however, that high lumbar lesions (e.g. intervertebral disc prolapse at L2/3) may cause symptoms in the anterior thigh alone.

Be aware of the **cauda equina syndrome**. This constitutes a **surgical emergency**. Whilst most disc prolapses are peripheral, thereby compressing the nerve root near the root canal (Fig. 10.5), a central disc prolapse may compress the whole of the cauda equina (or the cord if above the level of L1 – rare). The syndrome is represented by bilateral sciatica, saddle anaesthesia (in the S2–4 distribution), overflow incontinence and loss of anal tone (Fig. 10.6). A catch for the unwary is that the patient may not have significant root pain at presentation and may even say his pain has improved. Urgent decompression is necessary or permanent bladder dysfunction will ensue. **It is therefore mandatory to look for saddle anaesthesia and perform a rectal examination in all patients with back pain.**

In the younger age group root pain in association with back pain is often primarily assumed to be associated with disc prolapse. This is the one group of patients where 2 weeks of bed rest may be beneficial. Up to 90% will settle with conservative treatment. If symptoms are still present after 6 weeks orthopaedic referral is appropriate as decompression of the nerve root may then be needed. Early referral is desirable if there is progressive neurology or significant motor or reflex loss. **Any evidence of bladder dysfunction, saddle anaesthe-**

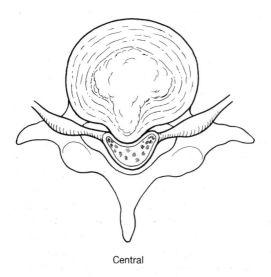

Central

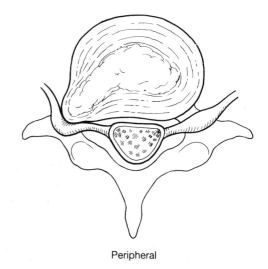

Peripheral

Figure 10.5 – Disc prolapse – central and peripheral

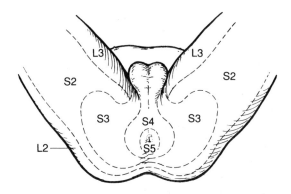

Figure 10.6 – Note that the lower sacral nerve roots innervate the perineum

sia or loss of anal tone may be indicative of a central disc prolapse as part of acute cauda equina syndrome and demands emergency referral.

Older patients with root pain usually do not primarily have disc pathology although this may be contributory. Although many have lateral recess stenosis with osteophytes etc., a number may have an underlying pathology such as tumour. Early referral is therefore necessary in this group.

Neurogenic claudication

Neurogenic claudication is a condition that is easy to miss unless you think of it. The patient complains of ill-defined but largely segmental root symptoms in one or both legs on walking which is relieved after a short period (but not immediately) of rest. The condition is largely due to lateral recess stenosis most often caused by degenerative change with osteophytes etc. The symptoms are similar to vascular intermittent claudication but in neurogenic claudication the distance to pain is more variable and the rest period to pain relief longer. Patients have a classical stooped posture in which position the nerve roots are less compressed. **On examination there are usually no abnormal signs** – straight leg raise is usually unrestricted as there is nerve root entrapment rather than irritation. Hence the importance of an accurate history.

Referral on an elective basis is needed as the patient may benefit from nerve root decompression.

Intraspinal pathology

Local pathology is a not uncommon cause of back pain and should always be considered in any patient with back pain of recent onset. Examples include tumour (usually metastases), infection, inflammatory causes such as ankylosing spondylitis and primary neurological disease. Crush fractures without trauma (i.e. pathological fractures) are most commonly due to osteoporosis or osteomalacia but may be due to underlying tumour or other bone pathology (e.g. myeloma). Structural pathology of the spine (e.g. spondylolisthesis, spondylolysis) can also be included in this group although the pain may not necessarily be due to the structural abnormality.

A patient complaining of constant unremitting pain, and especially **night pain**, should be suspected of having an underlying pathology. An initial series of baseline investigations, including x-ray, full blood count (FBC), ESR and CRP is usually abnormal. It can be difficult to differentiate this group of patients from those with mechanical back pain.

Diagnosis in back pain

As with all diagnostic manoeuvres, a diagnosis is made from a history, examination and special investigations. Nowhere are history and examination more important than in back pain as most patients will have normal investigations (including x-rays).

The history of the problem is usually the most helpful in establishing a diagnosis. The age and occupation of the patient are important to note. Beware young and old patients presenting with back pain as they have more chance of an underlying pathology. The site of the pain and any radiation into the legs **must** be noted; **differentiate between referred and root pain** (see above). Charts that the patient fills in demonstrating the pain and its radiation, together with functional activity scores, are very helpful. The onset and duration of symptoms may give a clue in aetiology; gradual onset of progressive symptoms is suspicious of an underlying pathology. **Beware the patient with unremitting night pain** as this is very indicative of a serious problem. Pain on walking may indicate neurogenic claudication. Remember also to carry out a full systematic review to exclude extraspinal aetiologies.

Examination should proceed in a systematic fashion, and should include:

1. A full general examination of the patient to exclude extraspinal causes of the back problem.

2. The back should be examined. Is there any paraspinal muscle spasm or wasting? Is there a deformity, e.g. a compensatory scoliosis? Are there any scars of previous operations? The range of movement of the back should be assessed.

3. Examination of the legs is essential in establishing whether there is any root involvement.

(a) Any **limitation of straight leg raise** should be noted. This test detects any nerve root **irritation**. The test is only positive if the manoeuvre elicits **true segmental symptoms**. Back pain, referred leg pain or hamstring tightness do **not** denote nerve root irritation. The nerve root does not move until the leg is raised 30°, hence symptoms between 0–30° should be viewed with suspicion. If the straight leg raise is positive, it implies nerve root irritation of one of the nerve roots forming the sciatic nerve, i.e. L4–S3. The pain distribution can then give a clue as to which nerve root is being compressed (see below).

(b) The **femoral stretch test** is similar to the straight leg raise (Fig. 10.7) in that it implies nerve root irritation except that it applies to the nerve roots forming the femoral nerve (i.e. L2–4).

(c) Each modality of nerve function should then be evaluated:

  (i) muscle wasting and motor power (according to the MRC grading);

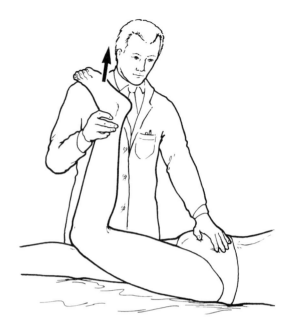

Figure 10.7 – The femoral stretch test

  (ii) sensory deficit (pain and proprioception);

  (iii) somatic reflexes, i.e., the knee jerk (L2/3) and the ankle jerk (S1).

4. **The bladder function, anal tone and saddle area sensation must always be examined so as to exclude a cauda equina syndrome** (see above).

5. Note that there are a number of collective signs that, if elicited together, may indicate 'non-organic pathology' or functional overlay. The manoeuvres should not elicit symptoms in the presence of back and/or root pain. Examples include:

(a) Pain immediately on straight leg raise – remember that the nerve root does not move until 30° of leg raise.

(b) An inability to fully straight leg raise but the ability to sit forward to 90°. This is a very useful manoeuvre when, for example, telling the patient that you would like to examine the back.

(c) Pain in the back on axial head pressure.

(d) Inconstant pattern of pain distribution or movement required to produce symptoms.

X-rays are not always required in low back pain. Your hospital may have its own guidelines as to when back x-rays are required. Quite large doses of radiation are required to visualize the spine. Remember that young females may be pregnant! If there is any history of significant trauma, if there is a long history of pain, or if there are 'hard' or progressive neurological signs, x-rays are useful and should be obtained. AP, lateral and coned lumbo-sacral views are the standard projections. Look in particular for the loss of the normal spinal curvature, fracture, bone pathology (e.g. osteoporosis, osteolysis), spondylolisthesis and non-osseous change.

Investigations are usually inappropriate in the acute setting and should ideally be performed if specialist referral is required. 'Blanket' mass testing is certainly not appropriate. The FBC, ESR and CRP, if normal, are good indicators that serious underlying pathology is not present. False-positives, however, are common.

The common segmental patterns of the lumbo-sacral nerves

As an aid to the diagnosis of root symptoms and signs, given below are the most useful patterns in establishing neurological abnormality for the commonly affected nerve roots.

1. **S1 nerve root**

Motor • plantarflexion of the foot and toes
• eversion of the foot (also L5)

Sensory • lateral aspect of the foot
Reflex • ankle jerk

2. **L5 nerve root**

Motor • dorsiflexion of the great toe (exclusively L5)
• dorsiflexion of the ankle (also L4)
Sensory • lateral aspect of the calf and medial aspect of the foot
Reflex • none

3. **L4 nerve root**

Motor • extension of the knee (also L3)
• inversion of the foot (exclusively L4)
• dorsiflexion of the ankle (also L5)
Sensory • medial aspect of the calf
Reflex • knee jerk (also L3)

4. **L3 nerve root**

Motor • extension of the knee (also L4)
Sensory • anterior thigh
Reflex • knee jerk (also L4)

5. **L2 nerve root**

Motor • flexion of the hip (also L3)
Sensory • proximal anterior aspect of the thigh
Reflex • none

Part III
The Upper Limb

11

Applied anatomy of the upper limb

The bones of the upper limb

The bones of the upper limb are shown in Figs 11.1–11.3

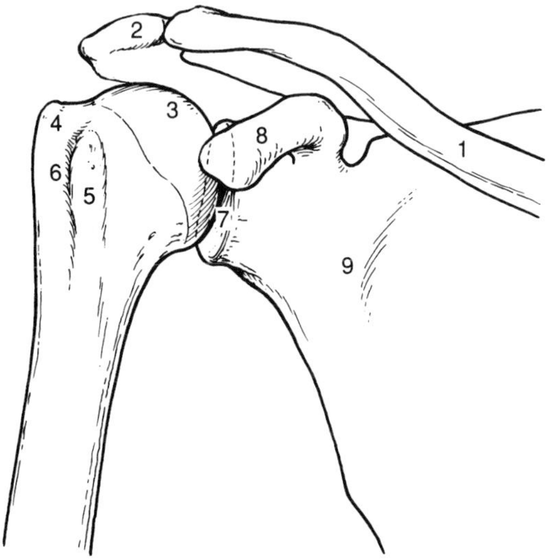

Figure 11.1 – AP view of the shoulder region
1. Clavicle
2. Acromion
3. **Humeral head**
4. Greater tuberosity
5. Lesser tuberosity
6. Bicipital groove
7. Glenoid fossa
8. Coracoid
9. Scapula

The nerves of the upper limb

Space permits only an outline of the nerve supply of the upper limb.

The brachial plexus (Fig. 11.4)

The upper limb derives its nerve supply from C5–T1 segments of the spinal cord. The anterior primary rami from these levels combine to form the brachial plexus, situated in the root of the neck through to the axilla.

Damage to the entire brachial plexus is a devastating injury. (See Chapter 12.)

The axillary nerve (C5,6)

The axillary nerve arises from the posterior cord of the brachial plexus and passes through the axilla towards the neck of the humerus. Through its course it winds around the neck of the humerus and supplies the **deltoid muscle** and **the skin overlying the deltoid** ('regimental badge area').

The axillary nerve is most frequently damaged by dislocations and fractures of the proximal humerus. Following trauma, because of pain, it may be difficult to assess the integrity of deltoid; the area of anaesthesia over the regimental badge area gives the best clue of nerve injury. If possible, deltoid can be assessed by abducting the upper arm against resistance with the arm at right angles to the trunk.

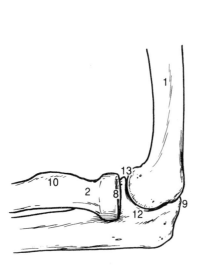
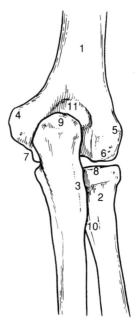

Figure 11.2 – AP and lateral views of the elbow
1. Shaft of humerus
2. Radial neck
3. Ulna
4. Medial epicondyle
5. Lateral epicondyle
6. Capitellum
7. Trochlea
8. Radial head
9. Olecranon
10. Radial tuberosity
11. Olecranon fossa
12. Trochlea notch within ulna
13. Coronoid process of ulna

The radial nerve (C5,6,7,8 T1)

The radial nerve arises from the posterior cord of the brachial plexus and supplies the extensor compartments of both the upper arm and the forearm. The nerve divides just below the elbow into:

(a)　the posterior interosseous nerve – supplies most of the extensor musculature of the forearm;
(b)　the superficial radial nerve – supplies sensation to the radial aspect of the dorsum of the hand (see below).

The nerve is most commonly damaged in the upper arm by fractures of the humerus or prolonged pressure on the arm (e.g. 'Saturday night palsy' whilst under the influence of alcohol). The clinical picture is one of a 'wrist drop' with paralysis of the wrist extensors. Lesions high in the arm also have weakness of extension at the elbow (triceps). Sensory loss is minimal as the median and ulnar nerves in the hand have a wide overlap of innervation with the radial nerve. The most consistent sensory loss is on the dorsum of the hand over the first dorsal interosseous muscle.

The ulnar nerve (C7,8 T1)

The ulnar nerve arises from the medial cord of the brachial plexus. It supplies:

(a)　some of the muscles of the flexor compartment of the forearm;
(b)　**nearly all the intrinsic muscles of the hand, entirely by T1;**
(c)　sensation on the ulnar aspect of the forearm and hand.

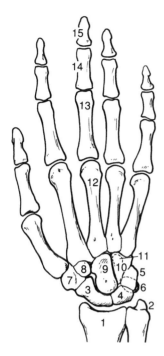

Figure 11.3 – AP view of the wrist
1. Distal radius
2. Ulnar styloid process
3. Scaphoid
4. Lunate
5. Triquetral
6. Pisiform
7. Trapezium
8. Trapezoid
9. Capitate
10. Hamate
11. Hook of hamate
12. Metacarpal shaft
13. Proximal phalanx
14. Middle phalanx
15. Distal phalanx

The ulnar nerve is injured as a result of trauma most commonly at the level of the wrist or around the elbow.

At the level of the wrist the nerve may be damaged by lacerations or more rarely by car- pal injuries. The consequence of a 'low' lesion is clawing of the hand. The intrinsic muscles of the hand (lumbricals and interossei) are lost so that the interphalangeal joints cannot be extended nor the metacarpo-phalangeal joints

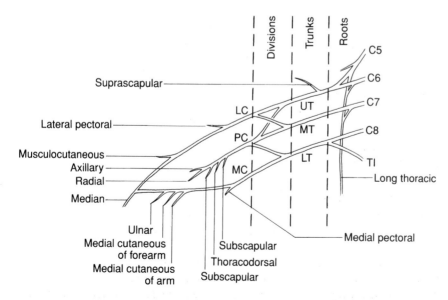

Figure 11.4 – diagramatic representation of the brachial plexus
UT, MT, LT – upper, middle and lower trunks
LC, PC, MC – lateral, posterior and middle cords

flexed. The unopposed flexor digitorum profundus (its part destined for the little and ring fingers is supplied by the ulnar nerve but proximal to the wrist) results in unopposed flexion of the fingers.

At the level of the elbow the nerve runs superficially posterior to the medial epicondyle. It may be damaged by elbow fractures and dislocations as well as by soft tissue injuries. The consequences of a 'high' lesion are, paradoxically, less severe than low lesions. The ulnar half of flexor digitorum profundus is lost so that the ring and little fingers are straighter.

As confirmation, for low lesions test abduction of the fingers. To distinguish a high from low lesion, test flexion at the distal interphalangeal joint of the little finger – if present the profundus complex is working. In addition to motor loss, there is a variable sensory loss on the ulnar aspect of the hand (see below).

The median nerve (C6,7,8 T1)

The median nerve arises from both the medial and lateral cords of the brachial plexus. It supplies most of the forearm flexor musculature

and innervates a few intrinsic muscles of the hand in addition (the thenar muscles and the lateral lumbrical muscles). It has an important sensory supply to the lateral aspect of the hand (see below).

The median nerve is most commonly damaged at the level of the wrist by lacerations etc. Injury may also occur around the level of the elbow, typically following dislocation of the elbow and supracondylar fracture of the humerus. The typical clinical consequence is of 'the pointing index finger sign' due to loss of the long flexors of the digit. The other fingers are usually flexed. Test for lesions by evaluating the long flexors of the index finger and also the abductor pollicis brevis, supplied exclusively by the median nerve. The most consistent sensory loss is over the fingertips of the thumb and index finger.

Segmental and peripheral sensory supply to the upper limb

The segmental sensory supply is summarized in Fig. 11.5 and that by peripheral nerves in Fig. 11.6.

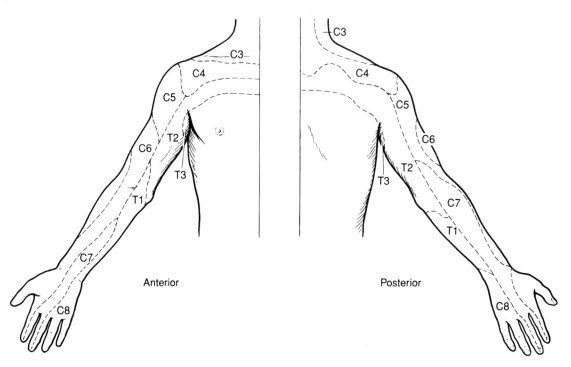

Figure 11.5 – Segmental sensory distribution of the upper limb

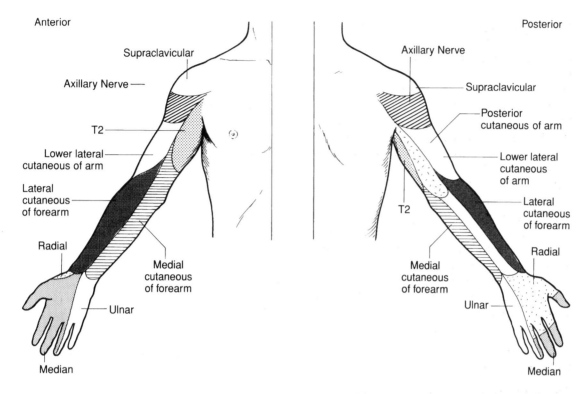

Figure 11.6 – Peripheral nerve sensory supply to the upper limb

12

The shoulder region

Injuries of the brachial plexus

The brachial plexus is described in Chapter 11. Traumatic injuries to it are of three major types: closed complete lesions, closed incomplete lesions and open lesions.

Closed complete lesions

Complete brachial plexus lesions are devastating injuries and result in a flail, useless and often painful upper limb. The most frequent cause is motor-cycle accidents where the neck is forcibly flexed away from the arm or where the arm is restrained in a collision. In most cases there are other injuries, reflecting the energy involved in the accident. **The lesions are often associated with major vascular and other injuries which are life-threatening.** Early referral is mandatory.

Closed incomplete lesions

Many injuries of the shoulder girdle may be associated with partial lesions of the brachial plexus, often of isolated cords or trunks. If noted, immediate referral is necessary.

Open lesions of the brachial plexus

These are now far less common, but were frequent in times of war. Most are now caused by assault or industrial accident. Clearly urgent exploration is required by senior personnel.

Injuries of the sterno-clavicular joint

The medial end of the clavicle can dislocate in either an anterior or posterior direction.

Anterior dislocation of the sterno-clavicular joint

The mechanism of injury underlying anterior dislocation of the sterno-clavicular joint (SCJ) is usually a fall on to the shoulder or the outstretched hand.

The diagnosis is a clinical one, palpating the prominent medial end of the clavicle on examination. The differential diagnosis is of a fracture of the medial end of the clavicle. The radiograph request should specify views of the sterno-clavicular joint; however, the films are difficult to interpret.

The management of the majority of these injuries is conservative, with acceptance of the subluxed position. Rest the arm in a sling for a short period prior to mobilization. If gross displacement is present manipulation under anaesthesia may be necessary.

Posterior dislocation of the sterno-clavicular joint

This is an extremely rare injury, the medial end of the clavicle passing posterior to the sternum to lie retrosternally. It is usually secondary to direct trauma. The dislocation may be accompanied by fractures of the upper ribs.

Posterior SCJ dislocation is potentially a dangerous injury. Underlying great vessels may be injured or the clavicle may exert direct pressure on the trachea or innominate vein. Therefore ensure that the patient is haemodynamically stable and seek senior advice.

Fractures of the clavicle

Fracture of the clavicle occurs mainly in children and young adults; it is the commonest fracture of childhood. Rapid union and re-modelling of the fracture are the rule, and long-term complications are rare.

The commonest mechanisms of injury are either a **fall on the outstretched hand**, where the force of impact is directed upwards along the shaft of the arm, or a **direct blow to the clavicle**. Sports injuries are common.

The patient presents with pain around the shoulder, and supports the injured side with the other arm. Pain and tenderness on palpation are usually well localized to the clavicle itself, and a painful lump or deformity is often palpable. There is a decreased range of movement of the shoulder because of pain.

The clinical diagnosis is supported by radiographs. Request an anteroposterior view of the clavicle (Fig. 12.1); a lateral film is usually not helpful. The commonest fracture site is the middle third or junction of the middle and lateral thirds. The lateral fragment will often be displaced inferiorly by the pull of the arm, whilst the medial fragment is pulled superiorly by sternomastoid. Greenstick fractures are common in children and are easy to miss.

In the vast majority of patients, the only treatment required is support of the arm in a broad arm sling and analgesia. Reduction of the fracture is rarely required. **A collar and cuff sling should not be used** as this will increase the downward pull on the lateral part of the clavicle. Follow-up should be arranged at the next fracture clinic. Even grossly displaced fractures heal extremely well, although the patient should be warned that they will have a palpable bump at the fracture site.

Immediate referral is warranted:

(a) where the fracture is open;
(b) in those injuries that are displaced so much that the viability of the overlying skin is at risk;
(c) in fractures of the distal clavicle beyond the coraco-clavicular ligament which may require internal fixation (Fig. 12.2).

Dislocations of the shoulder joint

There are three major forms of shoulder dislocation:

1. Anterior dislocations (over 90% of cases).
2. Posterior dislocations.
3. Luxatio erecta.

Anterior dislocation of the shoulder

Anterior dislocation of the shoulder (glenohumeral joint) is a common injury seen most often in young adults or the elderly. Anterior dislocation of the shoulder usually follows a **fall on the outstretched hand**, as the force of the impact is directed upwards along the extended arm. Occasionally it results from **forced internal rotation of the shoulder**, for example when the arm is held in an arm-lock.

The humeral head comes to lie anterior to the glenoid. During this process, the shoulder capsule and rotator cuff may be torn or the glenoid labrum avulsed. The dislocation may be accompanied by fractures of the humeral head or neck.

Do not attempt to reduce an old shoulder dislocation in the Accident and Emergency Department – there is a high risk of fracture. Refer the patient to the next fracture clinic. In addition, patients with recurrent dislocation of the shoulder are most appropriately referred to the unit in which their elective care is based.

Diagnosis

The patient usually presents in severe pain. If the problem is one of recurrent dislocation they may be only too aware of what has happened to

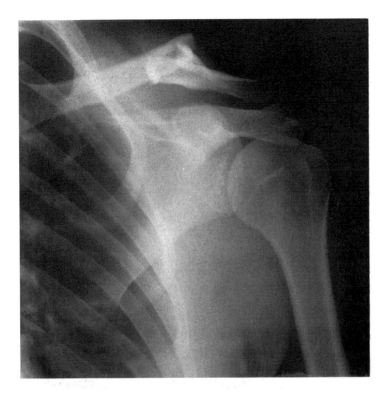

Figure 12.1 – Fracture of the clavicle

their shoulder. The injured shoulder is supported by the other arm, and the patient is often reluctant to allow anything but the minimum of examination because of the degree of

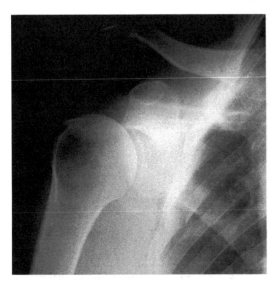

Figure 12.2 – Fracture of the distal clavicle – these fractures require surgical stabilization.

pain. On inspection the shoulder has a more squared contour than the normal side due to the prominent acromion (Fig. 12.3). On palpation, a gap is felt beneath the acromion, and the humeral head may be palpable in the axilla.

As always, sensation and circulation should be assessed and documented. In particular the radial pulse and **the integrity of the axillary, or circumflex nerve should be established**. Normal sensation over the 'regimental badge' area of the upper arm and deltoid abduction indicate a functioning circumflex nerve (Fig. 12.4). **These tests must be repeated and documented after reduction.** Rarely partial brachial plexus palsies may occur, therefore ensure the integrity of all the nerves of the upper limb.

The clinical diagnosis is supported by radiography. Even if the diagnosis seems obvious on examination, **radiographs are necessary to exclude accompanying fractures** (Fig. 12.5). This is an exception to the rule where a dislocation should be reduced prior to radiography. A fracture (e.g. of the greater tuberosity) does not normally prevent reduction of the dislocation

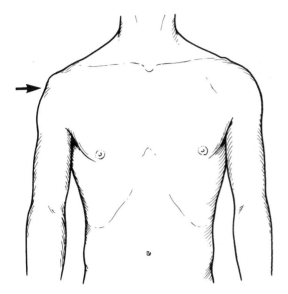

Figure 12.3 – Dislocation of the right shoulder – note the loss of the rounded contour with prominence of the acromion.

and usually aligns satisfactorily when reduction is attained. Ideally anteroposterior and axillary views should be taken, but pain often precludes the latter view. A translateral view will suffice.

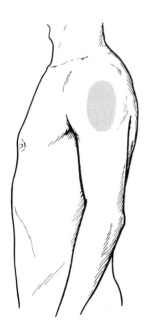

Figure 12.4 – the sensory distribution of the axillary nerve

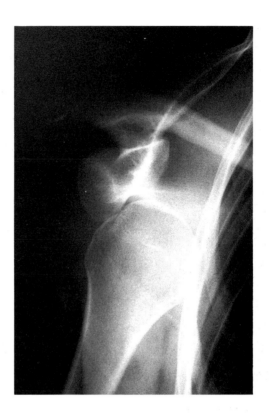

Figure 12.5 – Anterior dislocation of the shoulder

An anteroposterior view does not on its own exclude a gleno-humeral dislocation.

Facilities for reduction

Reduction of the dislocation is usually performed in the Accident and Emergency Department. The emphasis at all times should be on safety and this must never be compromised because of time or staffing pressures.

Alternatives available for facilitating reduction are:

1. Relaxation techniques.
2. Inhalation analgesia, i.e. 50% nitrous oxide/50% oxygen.
3. Intravenous sedation.
4. General anaesthesia.

The method selected will depend upon the experience and preferences of the doctor, staff availability, patient suitability and any anticipated problems. A patient who has suffered multiple dislocations should not always be assumed to be an easy reduction; the shoulder joint may be lax, but the patient's fear and anticipation following repeated previous manipulations may lead to great difficulty in obtaining sufficient relaxation.

The most common method employed is intravenous sedation. This is a safe procedure if several rules are **always** obeyed.

1. Full resuscitation facilities must be available **in the same room**, not down the corridor.
2. The doctor must be fully familiar with all the resuscitation equipment; this equipment must be checked prior to **every** reduction.
3. Reduction under intravenous sedation is a **two**-doctor technique as one doctor must always be available to look after the airway if necessary.
4. The outdated cocktail of long-acting drugs such as pethidine and diazepam should **not** be administered. This is not a safe technique in the Accident and Emergency Department.
5. Short-acting drugs, e.g. midazolam and/ or fentanyl (a short-acting opiate) should be used and the doctor must be familiar with their dosage on a milligramme per kilogramme basis.
6. Intravenous drugs should be administered slowly, titrating to effect. Remember that the elderly have a slower circulation time.

Reduction techniques

The most commonly employed techniques for reduction of anterior dislocations of the shoulder are Kocher's method, the Hippocratic method and gravitational traction. **All methods require an adequate degree of muscle relaxation at the shoulder.**

The Kocher's technique (Fig. 12.6)

The Kocher's technique used today is really a modification on that originally described by Kocher, as his description included no mention of traction. This is a two-person technique, the first person performing the manipulation whilst the assistant provides counter-traction.

The injured arm is supported with the elbow flexed at 90°. Steady firm traction is applied in the line of the humeral shaft. Counter-traction is applied in the axilla by the assistant; this can be with either a sling, such as a rolled up towel, or with the assistant's hands in the axilla. Take care with the technique of counter-traction so as not to damage the structures of the axilla, e.g. the brachial plexus.

Whilst continuing to apply steady traction, the manipulator then slowly and steadily abducts and externally rotates the humerus as far as possible. If the 'clunk' of reduction is not felt, the arm is then adducted and internally rotated to finish lying across the body. If this is unsuccessful, ensure that the patient is completely relaxed and repeat the above steps,

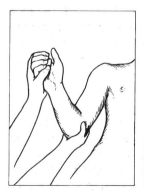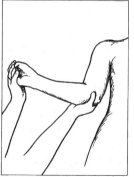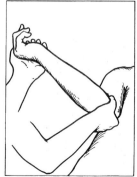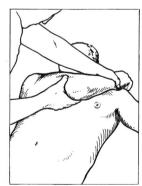

Figure 12.6 – Kocher's technique for reduction of anterior shoulder dislocations. Note the initial traction, subsequent abduction with external rotation and the final adduction with internal rotation.

ensuring that maximal abduction and external rotation are obtained. The whole procedure should be a steady, smooth and continuous process. If unsuccessful, the patient may be inadequately relaxed or there may be a mechanical block to reduction. Consider an alternative method of reduction or manipulation under general anaesthesia.

The Hippocratic technique (Fig. 12.7)

This is a one-operator technique, although remember that the overall management is two-person if intravenous sedation is being used.

Direct traction is applied on the extended arm in the line of the humerus by the operator. Meanwhile the operator applies counter-traction by placing the heel of his stockinged foot in the axilla which thus acts as a fulcrum. This is often easier if the operator sits on a stool to bring himself up to the same height as the patient. Care must be taken with the degree of pressure exerted by the foot because of the risk of neurovascular injury. Again, the process is smooth and continuous.

Gravitational traction

The patient lies prone on the trolley with the injured arm hanging unsupported down towards the floor. A sandbag placed beneath the ipsilateral clavicle can aid reduction. The pull of gravity in a relaxed patient can result in reduction, but time must be allowed for this to occur. **This method is not suitable when intravenous sedation is being employed** as careful monitoring of the patient and the airway is not possible in the prone position.

Post-reduction management

Once reduction has been attained, the arm is placed in a broad arm sling held close to the side of the body either by a bandage or the patient's clothes. The patient should be told to rest the arm in the sling.

All patients must have **a post-reduction radiograph** taken and **the integrity of the axillary nerve** reassessed.

Occasionally anatomical reduction is not obtained by one of these methods, and the patient should be referred for reduction under general anaesthesia. Rarely, a dislocation with an accompanying grossly displaced fracture may require open reduction and internal fixation if closed reduction has failed.

Those patients in whom reduction has been attained should be followed up at the next fracture clinic, and discharged home with suitable analgesia. All patients who have received intravenous analgesia should be carefully observed in the Accident and Emergency Department until they have made a **complete recovery**.

Posterior dislocation of the shoulder

This is a much less common injury than the anterior dislocation, and is more difficult to diagnose. It must always be considered in a patient who on clinical examination appears to have a considerable injury to the shoulder but who has an apparently 'normal' AP radiograph.

Diagnosis

Posterior dislocation is most commonly seen in patients who have sustained a direct blow to the front of the shoulder, or in those who have suffered an epileptic fit or electric shock, where the shoulder is flung in abnormal directions with considerable force. **Active exclusion of a posterior dislocation of the shoulder should always be**

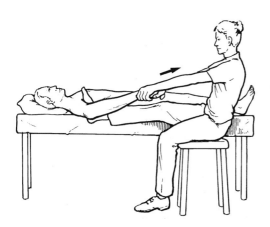

Figure 12.7 – Hippocratic technique for reduction of anterior shoulder dislocations.

made when assessing a patient following a fit or electric shock.

The patient complains of pain and limited range of movement of the shoulder. The humerus is internally rotated and held fixed in this position. On looking at the shoulder from above, the normal rounded contour anteriorly is lost, and the shoulder appears flat at the front. The coracoid process is more prominent than normal. However the shoulder may appear normal on examination.

Two radiographic views of the shoulder are essential, as the AP view in a posterior dislocation can appear deceptively normal (Figs 12.8, 12.9). The humeral head normally has an asymmetrical appearance because of the greater and lesser tuberosities. In a posterior dislocation, this asymmetry is lost because of the internal rotation, producing the appropriately named **'light-bulb sign'**. This is a subtle sign that must be specifically sought. **An axillary view must be taken** (Figs 12.10, 12.11), and the humeral head can be clearly seen lying behind the glenoid. For this view to be taken, adequate analgesia may be necessary.

Reduction

The same criteria for safe reduction apply as described for anterior dislocation. A two-person technique is employed.

The operator applies steady traction on the arm in 90° of abduction (Fig. 12.12). Maintaining traction, the arm is externally rotated. At the same time, an assistant may apply pressure to the back of the humeral head in an anterior direction.

Failure to achieve reduction, or an unstable reduction, necessitates referral.

Following successful stable reduction the arm is placed in a broad arm sling held to the side of the body either with a bandage or the patient's clothes. Post-reduction radiographs are essential as is a **check of the integrity of the axillary nerve**. Follow-up should be arranged for the next fracture clinic.

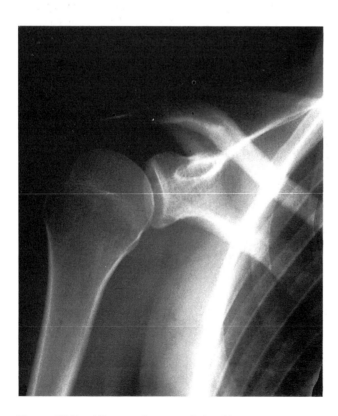

Figure 12.8 – AP x-ray of a normal shoulder

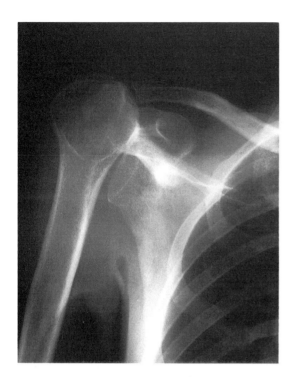

Figure 12.9 – Posterior dislocation of the shoulder Note the 'light bulb sign'.

Other dislocations of the shoulder

Luxatio erecta

In this rare injury, the humeral head comes to lie beneath the glenoid. On examination there is an obvious deformity with the arm held in abduction. Reduction is achieved by applying traction in abduction and then swinging the arm into adduction.

Habitual dislocators

These patients may present to the Accident and Emergency Department with a dislocated shoulder either as a result of deliberate self-dislocation or because of problems with proprioception secondary to repeated trauma. Minimal trauma is required for the shoulder to dislocate. Such patients are usually able easily to reduce the dislocation themselves and rarely require any form of sedation. Most cases are difficult to manage. They should **not** be referred to an emergency fracture clinic as their problem is an elective one.

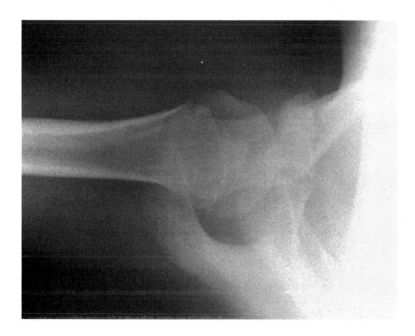

Figure 12.10 – X-ray of axillary view of the shoulder

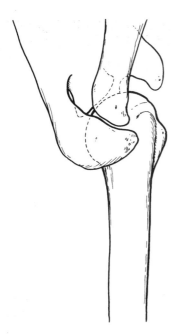

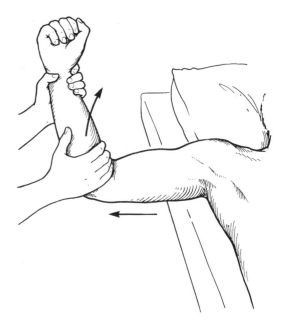

Figure 12.11 – Diagram of axillary view of the shoulder.

Figure 12.12 – Posterior dislocation of the shoulder – method of reduction.

Injuries to the acromio-clavicular joint

The acromio-clavicular joint (ACJ) may either subluxate or dislocate. In subluxation of the joint, the acromio-clavicular ligaments are torn, allowing the clavicle to displace upwards. In the more severe dislocation, the conoid and trapezoid ligaments, which anchor the clavicle to the conoid process, are torn (Fig. 12.13).

Diagnosis

These injuries most often occur in young adults. They are usually caused by a fall directly on to the point of the shoulder, and commonly occur

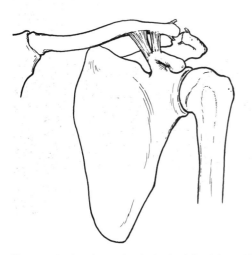

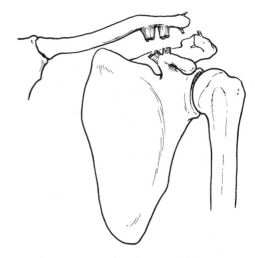

Figure 12.13 – Acromio-clavicular joint injury. Note that in subluxation the conoid and trapezoid ligaments are intact whilst in dislocation they are torn.

during sport. The patient presents with pain in the shoulder, supporting the injured side with the other arm. The lateral end of the clavicle may be more prominent than normal. The pain is usually well localized to the ACJ and a step at the ACJ may be palpable. The patient has a decreased range of movement of the shoulder because of pain.

ACJ injury is a clinical diagnosis supported by radiography (Fig. 12.14). The x-ray should be requested as 'ACJ-weight-bearing views'. The radiographer will then take films of both ACJs whilst the patient holds heavy weights in both hands, and display both these views on the same film for comparison (Fig. 12.15). The weights open up the injured joint making diagnosis by comparison with the normal side easier.

Treatment

The vast majority of these patients require no more than rest in a broad arm sling and anal-

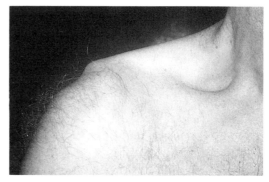

Figure 12.14 – Clinical appearance of an acromio-clavicular dislocation.

gesia, followed by mobilization as the pain allows, with follow-up in the fracture clinic. Very occasionally, a patient with severe disruption of the joint with pressure on the surrounding skin may require internal fixation of the joint.

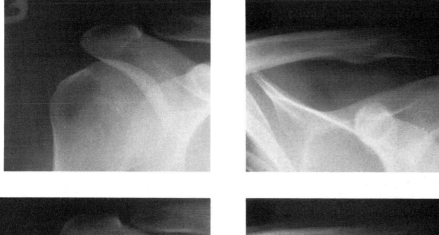

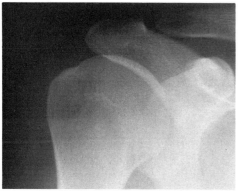

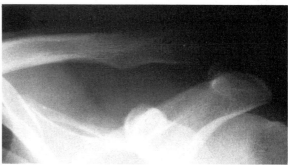

Figure 12.15 – Acromio-clavicular dislocation. Note that in the lower photographs the patient carries a weight so as to accentuate any displacement.

Fractures of the scapula

Fractures of the scapula are caused by falls on to the scapula or a direct blow. Fractures of the scapular blade are particularly associated with high energy trauma. The patient presents with localized tenderness and a decreased range of movement of the shoulder. **Scapular fractures may be associated with other significant injuries.** It is important to exclude accompanying rib fractures and to assess carefully the respiratory system for underlying lung injury.

The clinical diagnosis is confirmed by radiography, requesting specific scapular views (Fig. 12.16).

The majority of cases are managed by initial rest in a broad arm sling with analgesia, followed by mobilization as the pain allows and follow-up in the fracture clinic.

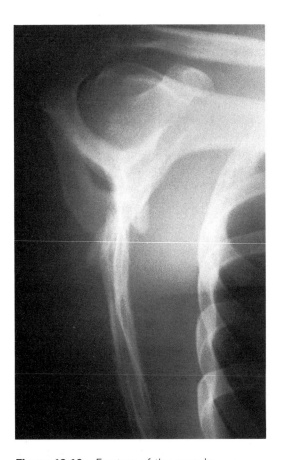

Figure 12.16 – Fracture of the scapula

Fracture of the glenoid, being intra-articular, should be referred, as internal fixation may be necessary.

The acutely painful shoulder

The shoulder is particularly prone to developing stiffness following trauma. Soft tissue injuries of the shoulder are common and frequently misdiagnosed. Accurate early diagnosis will result in correct management and optimal conditions for promoting maximal recovery.

Rotator cuff tears

The rotator cuff is made up of four muscles:

1. Supraspinatus – initiates abduction.
2. Infraspinatus – externally rotates the shoulder.
3. Teres minor – externally rotates the shoulder.
4. Subscapularis – internally rotates the shoulder.

Tears to the rotator cuff can follow falls, sports injuries, road traffic accidents etc. The exact site of the tear depends upon the direction of the force and the position of the shoulder at the point of impact. The cuff tears more easily if degenerative disease is present, and this is almost a prerequisite for tears.

Rotator cuff tears can be either complete or partial.

Complete tears are less common, and occur more in the older age group. **The patient is unable to initiate abduction** and is tender over the point of the shoulder. Such patients demonstrate the '**drop arm sign**' – the deltoid is able to hold the arm in full abduction; however, as the arm is lowered it suddenly drops to the patient's side at the point when the action of supraspinatus should normally come into play.

Partial tears occur more commonly, and often in a younger age group. If in the early stages it is difficult to differentiate this from a complete lesion because of pain, an injection of local anaesthetic at the most tender spot will allow the patient to abduct, albeit weakly.

Management is usually a combination of rest in a sling initially, with analgesia, followed by physiotherapy. Young patients with complete tears should be referred electively for consideration of assessment and surgical repair.

Persistent pain may be relieved by injection of local anaesthetic and steroids at the most tender spot. It is important to warn the patient that this will aggravate their symptoms before any benefit is felt.

Supraspinatus tendonitis

This is a degenerative condition where the fibres at the distal end of the supraspinatus tendon become relatively avascular. The ischaemic tendon is therefore weakened and small tears may result following relatively minor trauma.

The condition occurs most commonly in middle-aged men, who present with tenderness at the point of the shoulder and restricted movement due to pain. Radiographs may show calcification beneath the acromion.

Treatment is initial rest followed by exercises. Relief may be gained from injection of local anaesthetic and steroids beneath the acromion.

Acute calcific supraspinatus tendonitis

This syndrome has a characteristic rapid onset and recovery. It may be an overuse injury, and any accompanying trauma is usually insignificant.

Degeneration in a small localized area of the supraspinatus tendon results in the deposition of calcium. This may be seen on radiography (Fig. 12.17). Friction due to overuse leads to rapid swelling and increased tension within the tendon, causing **severe constant pain present at rest**. There is virtually no movement possible.

If the condition is recognized early, the patient may benefit from a surgical decompression of the tendon; a 'toothpaste-like' material may be expressed and this will provide a dramatic relief of pain. If left untreated the condition will ultimately resolve but with considerable morbidity. Some would advocate injection of local anaesthetic into the tender area and/or aspiration of the 'toothpaste'.

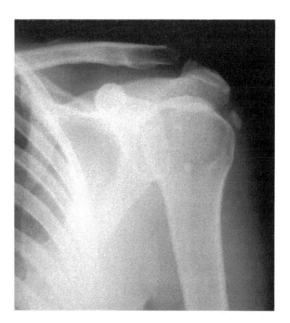

Figure 12.17– Acute calcific supraspinatus tendonitis

Painful arc syndrome

The painful arc refers to pain on abduction between an arc of 60 and 120°. The pain may be worse on lowering the arm, which may drop suddenly as it passes through the horizontal position.

The condition results from swelling of the supraspinatus tendon near its insertion, secondary to degenerative changes or chronic tears. As the arm is abducted the tendon and the subacromial bursa are squeezed between the humeral head and the acromion process, causing the painful arc. This is termed **impingement**. The onset of pain is gradual and may follow a few weeks after injury. Symptoms are difficult to eradicate but may be helped by injection of local anaesthetic and steroids beneath the acromion process.

Frozen shoulder (pericapsulitis, adhesive capsulitis, periarthritis)

Frozen shoulder occurs mainly in the middle-aged and elderly. It may follow either minor trauma or periods of prolonged use or disuse. The pain experienced is constant and generalized rather than localized as in many other soft tissue problems around the shoulder. Pain is felt over the deltoid and may radiate along the dorsum of the arm to the hand.

The onset of pain is gradual and probably starts in supraspinatus. There is great variation in the degree of incapacitation experienced due to the pain. Radiography is normal. Symptoms take several months to subside, and stiffness persists long after the pain has resolved.

Management is a combination of analgesia, heat and cold, injections and gentle exercise. Severe resistant cases may be referred for manipulation under anaesthesia. It is important to warn the patient that progress will be slow over many months.

Rupture of the long head of biceps

This injury is most commonly seen in older men doing manual work. The rupture classically results from attempting to flex the elbow against resistance. Tearing occurs at the junction of a usually degenerate tendon with the muscle belly.

The patient presents with acute pain in the upper arm, with decreased power of elbow flexion. On examination the classic low bulge of the muscle belly is prominent (Fig. 12.18).

Treatment is initial rest and analgesia followed by mobilization. The tendon itself does not heal but good function gradually results. The patient presenting with an acute tear should be referred to the fracture clinic. Surgical repair is not usually advocated except in athletes or those patients who also have a tear of the rotator cuff.

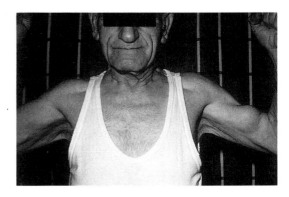

Figure 12.18 – Rupture of the long head of biceps

13
Fractures of the humerus

Fractures of the proximal humerus

Fractures of the proximal humerus may occur in any age group but most commonly in the older female population. The usual mechanism of injury is a fall on the upper limb, either a fall on to the side of the arm or on to the outstretched hand. The force involved is often sufficient to impact the fracture, allowing the patient to move the arm to some extent, and the injury may then be overlooked if not specifically sought. As the shoulder is prone to stiffness, particularly in the elderly, the best management is that which allows early mobilization.

Diagnosis

The patient presents with a painful shoulder, and often supports the injured side with the other arm. If the presentation is delayed, there may be marked bruising of the arm. In an impacted fracture there may be a surprising degree of movement at the shoulder. As always, neurovascular lesions should be excluded. Damage to the axillary nerve is occasionally seen, where the patient is unable to contract the deltoid muscle in attempted abduction and has numbness over the 'regimental badge' area. Treatment of the palsy is expectant and a gradual recovery usually results.

The clinical diagnosis is confirmed by antero-posterior and lateral radiographs. The fracture can involve the anatomical neck (rare), the surgical neck, the greater tuberosity or the lesser tuberosity (Figs 13.1, 13.2). These may occur in combination and be associated with dislocation of the gleno-humeral joint (Fig. 13.3).

The commonest proximal humeral fractures in children or adolescents are greenstick fractures of the surgical neck (Fig. 13.4). In this age group, beware the epiphyseal line which may be mistaken for a fracture line (Fig. 13.5). Another injury seen in childhood is fracture separation of the proximal humeral epiphysis; the shaft shifts proximally and anteriorly whilst the head, with a piece of the metaphysis attached, remains in place.

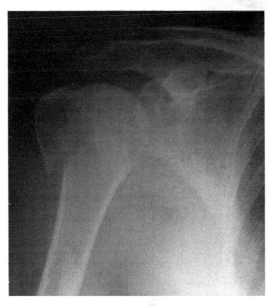

Figure 13.1 – Fracture of the neck and greater tuberosity of the humerus

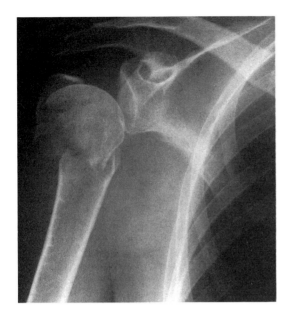

Figure 13.2 – Four-part fracture of the proximal humerus

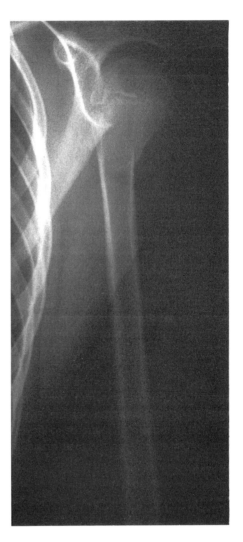

Figure 13.4 – Greenstick fracture of the surgical neck of the humerus

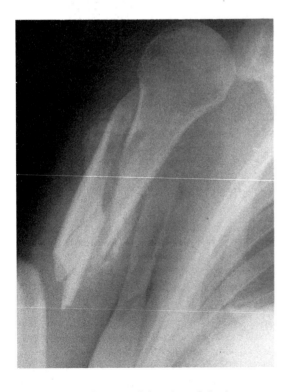

Figure 13.3 – Fracture-dislocation of the humerus

Management

Most fractures of the proximal humerus are managed conservatively, even where displacement is severe. The arm should be immobilized in a sling and the patient referred to the next fracture clinic. Some of the fractures may require internal fixation or the humeral head may have to be replaced with a hemiarthroplasty – these decisions may be left to the time of the clinic attendance. **However, ensure that there is no gleno-humeral dislocation**; such fracture-dislocations will need immediate relocation.

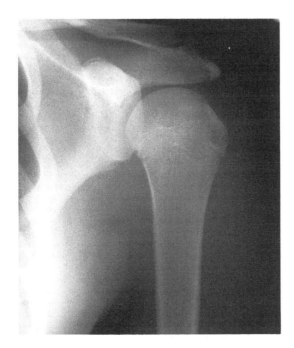

Figure 13.5 – Do not misinterpret epiphyseal lines for a fracture!

Most children's fractures in this region re-model surprisingly well. Even fractures with significant angulation may be left without reduction. If in doubt however, seek senior advice. Most injuries can be referred to the fracture clinic.

Fractures of the shaft of the humerus

These injuries are uncommon in children, but occur in adults of all ages. Whenever a patient with a humeral fracture is seen, it must be remembered that the proximal half of the shaft is a common site for metastatic deposits, and should always be considered as a possible underlying pathology (Fig. 13.6).

There are two main mechanisms of injury. A fall on to the outstretched hand usually produces a spiral fracture, most commonly in the middle third of the shaft. A direct blow to the upper arm produces a transverse fracture which can be at any level.

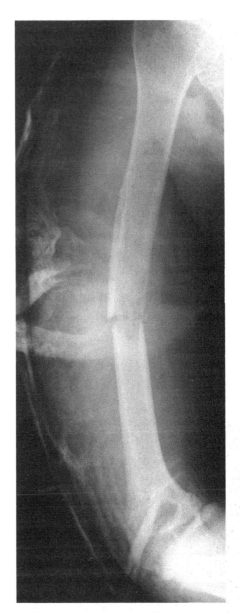

Figure 13.6 – Pathological fracture of the mid-shaft of the humerus. Note the lytic lesion at the fracture site. Transverse fractures of long bones should raise the suspicion of a pathological lesion.

Diagnosis

The patient presents with pain and swelling of the upper arm. The range of movement of the shoulder and elbow is markedly reduced. It is **mandatory** to establish integrity of the **radial** nerve and the brachial artery, which are easily injured in fractures of the shaft. Both modalities of the radial nerve should be assessed; test for power of extension at the wrist (wrist drop) and sensation over the dorsum of the hand in the first dorsal web space.

Radiographs of the whole shaft including the shoulder and elbow joints must be obtained. Both AP and lateral views are needed to assess the degree of displacement and angulation (Fig. 13.7).

Management

The majority of these injuries can be managed conservatively. Perfect opposition of the bone ends is not required and between 25 and 50% bone contact is sufficient. Support of the arm in a collar and cuff sling is often all that is required. An alternative to this is a 'hanging U slab' type of plaster, which may provide more support. The slab extends from the axilla around the elbow to the top of the shoulder, and must be well padded (Fig. 13.8).

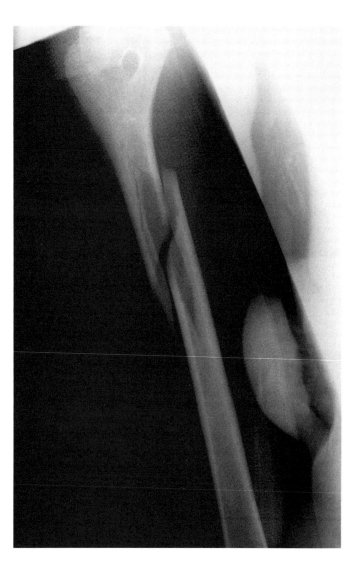

Figure 13.7 – Spiral fracture of the humerus

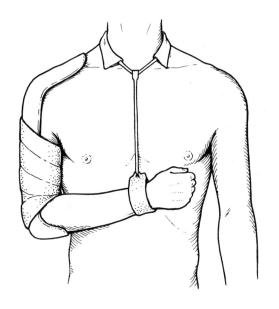

Figure 13.8 – A 'U' slab of the humerus

Indications for referral are:

1. In the elderly living alone who would have difficulty in managing with one arm immobilized.
2. Where there are injuries to both arms.
3. Two or more fractures in the same limb.
4. Pathological fractures (usually require fixation if they are to unite).
5. Gross angulation of the humeral shaft.

Follow-up should otherwise be arranged for the fracture clinic.

14
Injuries around the elbow joint

Fractures of the distal humerus in adults

Supracondylar and intercondylar fractures of the humerus in adults

These fractures of the distal humerus result from a fall on the elbow or on to the outstretched hand. There are two main patterns of injury:

1. Pure supracondylar fractures (Fig. 14.1).
2. Supracondylar fractures with an intra-articular extension (i.e. an intercondylar fracture in which the condyles are split by the upward force of the olecranon, Fig. 14.2).

Pure supracondylar fractures, even if minimally displaced, nearly all require internal fixation. Intercondylar fractures always require fixation.

Fractures of the capitellum and trochlea

These injuries are generally sustained by a fall on the outstretched hand with the elbow extended. Capitellar fractures are often associated with fractures of the radial head.

The patient presents with a swollen, painful elbow. A fullness can often be palpated anteriorly. Movement, particularly flexion, is painful and limited.

Diagnosis is confirmed on radiography. The fracture may be undisplaced or small flake fractures may be seen. With increased force the anterior half of the capitellum and trochlea

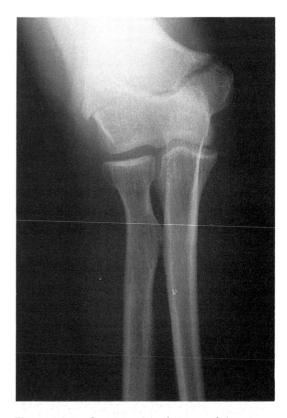

Figure 14.1 – Supracondylar fracture of the humerus

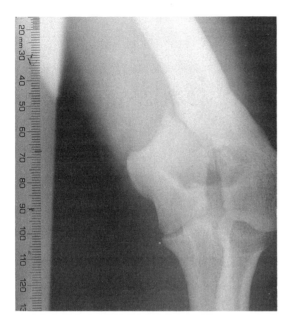

Figure 14.2 – Intercondylar fracture of the humerus

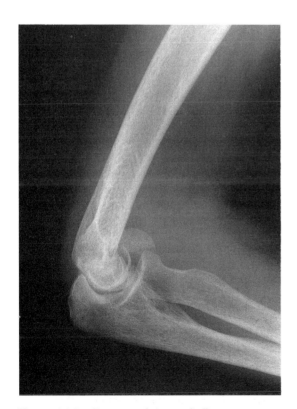

Figure 14.3 – Fracture of the capitellum

are broken off and displaced proximally. The capitellum will be seen lying in front of the humerus with the radial head no longer pointing towards it as normal (Fig. 14.3).

All fractures of the capitellum and trochlea should be referred as interpretation of the radiographs can be difficult. Undisplaced fractures may be treated conservatively. However, most fractures require open reduction and internal fixation.

Fractures of the medial and lateral epicondyles

These uncommon fractures are not usually severely displaced, and management is largely conservative. The arm should be placed in a broad arm sling and referred to the fracture clinic. Those fractures that are displaced should be referred for fixation.

Fractures of the distal humerus in children

Supracondylar fractures of the humerus in children

This is an important, common fracture of childhood. The fracture commonly results from a fall on the outstretched hand, although some are due to falls on to the point of the elbow.

The child is usually in considerable pain, holding the injured arm by their side. On palpation the whole elbow is tender and the exact site of pain may be difficult to localize. **The normal triangular relationship between the olecranon and the epicondyles is preserved** (as opposed to elbow dislocations where this relationship is lost). **A careful assessment of the circulatory and neurological status of the limb is mandatory.**

Radiographic detection of a supracondylar fracture may be difficult. If necessary, compare with the x-ray of the normal arm. Be particularly aware of a greenstick fracture which may appear as no more than a slight buckle in the cortex (Fig. 14.4).

In 90% of cases, on the lateral view, the distal fragment is displaced posteriorly, with anterior angulation, i.e. the distal fragment is tilted

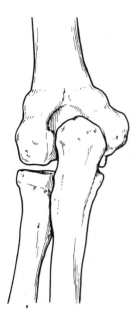

Figure 14.4 – Supracondylar greenstick fracture of the humerus

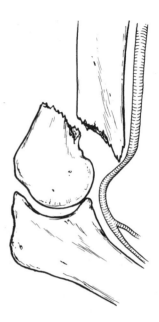

Figure 14.6 – The brachial artery is at risk in supracondylar fractures.

backwards (Fig. 14.5). **The sharp, anterior border of the proximal fragment may cause the adjacent brachial artery to become kinked, contused or severed** (Fig. 14.6). This is the most important consideration in the assessment of a supracondylar fracture.

A true anteroposterior view in extension may be difficult to obtain because of pain. If this is possible the distal fragment may be angulated in either a medial or lateral direction. A flexed AP view may have to be accepted, and will show the normal alignment of the three bones, with the humerus superimposed on the radius and ulna.

In 10% of cases the distal fragment is displaced anteriorly, and this deformity worsens

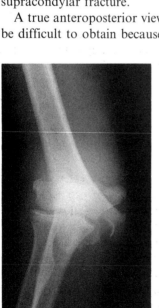

Figure 14.5 – Supracondylar fracture of the humerus

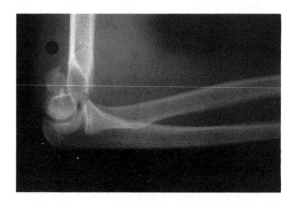

when the elbow is flexed (Fig. 14.7). This injury is usually due to a fall on the point of the flexed elbow.

The most important factor in management is the assessment of the vascular status of the limb. Interruption of the circulation is a **surgical emergency**. If not detected early, ischaemia of the forearm muscles may result in **compartment syndrome** of the forearm and permanent deformity (**Volkmann's ischaemic contracture**). Nerve injuries in supracondylar fractures, especially of the median and ulna nerves, may occur.

If there is no neurovascular deficit, a decision must be made as to whether the fracture requires manipulation. Undisplaced fractures require only immobilization in a broad arm sling or long arm back slab, flexing the elbow as the radial pulse allows. Displaced fractures should be manipulated if:

1. Any fracture is associated with suspected circulatory impairment.
2. There is more than 50% loss of bony contact of the bone ends at the fracture site.
3. The fracture has a rotational component.

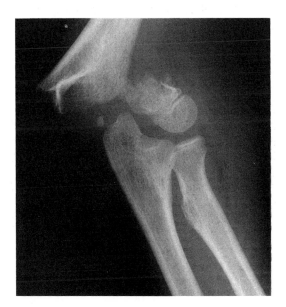

Figure 14.7 – Supracondylar fracture of the humerus with anterior displacement of the distal fragment.

4. There is backward tilting (anterior angulation) of more than 15° on the lateral radiograph. Note that as the normal distal humerus is tilted forwards, a 15° backward tilt results in a humerus that appears 'straight'.
5. There is tilting in a lateral or medial direction of greater than 10° as seen on the AP view. The normal distal humerus has a valgus tilt of 10°.

The above criteria emphasize that it is the degree of angulation rather than the degree of displacement that determines the need for manipulation.

All patients in whom manipulation is required should be referred to senior personnel as these fractures are difficult to manage. The method of reduction is not given for this reason.

Those patients only requiring immobilization should be followed up **the next day** in the fracture clinic. They should be given full instructions to return immediately should any signs of circulatory embarrassment develop.

Fractures of the medial epicondyle

The medial epicondyle appears radiographically at the age of 6 and fuses at around 16 years. Injuries of the medial epicondyle are far more common in children than those of the lateral epicondyle.

The commonest mechanism of injury is a fall on to the outstretched arm. The medial epicondyle is avulsed by either the attached flexor muscles of the forearm or the medial ligament of the elbow (Fig. 14.8). With sufficient force, the medial epicondyle can become trapped within the joint as part of a momentary dislocation of the elbow which then spontaneously reduces. **Always check that the medial epicondyle is in place in childhood elbow dislocations.**

The child presents with a painful elbow with markedly reduced range of movement. Bruising over the medial aspect of the elbow may be seen. The integrity of the **ulnar nerve** must be assessed and documented, because it passes directly behind the medial epicondyle.

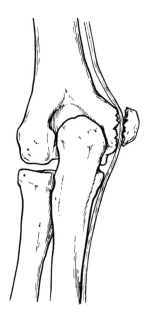

Figure 14.8 – Fracture of the medial epicondyle. Note that the ulnar nerve runs immediately posterior to the fracture.

Both AP and lateral radiographs are necessary. If the medial epicondyle cannot be seen in the radiograph of a child over the age of 6 years, suspect that it is lying within the joint. The fragment may sometimes be confused with a loose body. If any doubt exists, views of the other elbow should be obtained for comparison.

Those fractures in which the fragment is lodged within the joint should be referred for reduction. Undisplaced fractures should be placed in a long arm backslab and reviewed at the following day's fracture clinic.

Fractures of the lateral epicondyle

Fractures of the lateral epicondyle are uncommon in children. The lateral epicondyle appears radiographically at around the age of 11 and fuses at about 14 years.

The injury results from a forced adduction or varus stress being applied to the elbow. Severe displacement is uncommon.

Management follows those guidelines for fractures of the medial epicondyle.

Fractures and dislocations around the elbow

Dislocation of the elbow

Dislocation of the elbow is a relatively common injury in both children and adults and is commonly caused by a fall on the hand with the elbow partially flexed. The commonest injury is posterior dislocation of the ulna on the humerus.

The patient presents with a swollen elbow which is very painful. The important finding on examination is that **the normal triangular relationship between the olecranon and the epicondyles is disrupted**, with the olecranon lying posteriorly to the distal humerus. The patient will resist any movement of the elbow. The integrity of the median and ulnar nerves and the brachial artery should be established. Damage to the artery is rare, but median nerve palsies occasionally occur, usually with a good long-term prognosis.

X-rays will usually reveal the radius and ulna to be dislocated posteriorly on the distal humerus (Fig. 14.9). Accompanying fractures may also be present, most commonly fractures of the radial head or the coronoid process. In children **dislocation may be accompanied by fracture of the epicondyles.** Avoid the pitfall of the medial epicondyle trapped in the joint.

Far less commonly, the radius and ulna may dislocate anterior to the humerus, following a fall on to a flexed elbow. This dislocation is nearly always accompanied by a fracture of the olecranon and is therefore very unstable.

Manipulation of a posterior dislocation can be performed under either inhalational analgesia, intravenous sedation or general anaesthesia. With the elbow flexed, an assistant applies steady gentle traction in the line of the forearm whilst the operator puts his fingers around the epicondyles from behind and pushes the olecranon forwards with his thumbs.

Once reduction is achieved, usually with a satisfying 'clunk', **check that the elbow is stable**. Place the elbow into either a long arm backslab or a broad arm sling. Reassess the neurovascular status of the limb and confirm the reduction

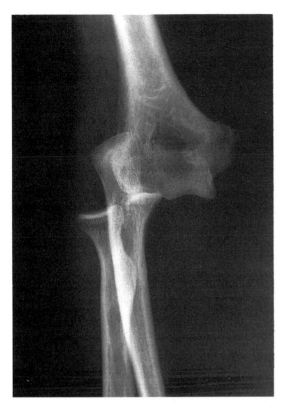

Figure 14.9 – Dislocation of the elbow

on x-ray. The patient should be referred to the next fracture clinic. **Refer any unstable dislocations immediately**.

Fracture of the radial head

This is a common injury seen in all age groups. The usual mechanism of injury is a fall on the outstretched hand. The force of impact is transmitted along the forearm driving the radial head against the capitellum; the capitellum itself may also be injured.

The patient presents with a swollen, painful elbow, supporting it with the other arm. Movement in all directions is painful, especially **pronation and supination**. Extension is restricted. Palpation reveals localized tenderness over the radial head.

A complete assessment should always include examination of the wrist, considering the possibility of the rare **Essex-Lopresti lesion**. In this injury, the interosseous membrane is torn as the radius is driven proximally, resulting in subluxation of the distal ulna at the wrist.

Three patterns of injury are seen:

1. A vertical split in the radial head (Fig. 14.10).
2. A single fragment of bone, which is usually displaced distally.
3. A comminuted fracture.

More than 50% of radial head fractures will be no more than simple cracks, and the majority of the rest are single fragments. These can be managed conservatively in a broad arm sling and referred to the fracture clinic.

Comminuted or severely displaced fractures should be immediately referred for further assessment.

Fracture of the radial neck (Fig. 14.11)

Radial neck fractures occur most commonly in children, with a similar mechanism of injury to those of radial head fractures. Management of radial neck fractures in children depends on the degree of tilting. The angle of tilt beyond which manipulation is needed depends upon the age of the child. All children with radial neck fractures should be referred.

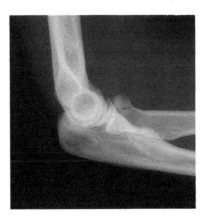

Figure 14.10 – Fracture of the radial head

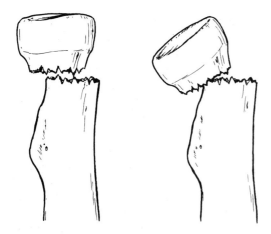

Figure 14.11 – Fractures of the radial neck

Fracture of the coronoid process of the ulna (Fig. 14.12)

Most fractures of the coronoid process are associated with elbow dislocations. If undisplaced they can be treated conservatively. Displaced fractures are associated with instability at the elbow and may require internal fixation.

Fracture of the olecranon

These fractures usually occur in adults, although they are occasionally seen in children. The commonest mechanism of injury is a fall directly on to the point of the elbow. The fracture can also result directly from contraction of the triceps muscle.

The important factor to ascertain is **if the extensor mechanism of the elbow is intact**. The patient presents with a bruised and swollen elbow, and there is localized tenderness over the olecranon. Test whether the patient is able to extend the elbow against resistance; if this is possible then the triceps mechanism is intact.

The diagnosis is confirmed by radiography (Fig. 14.13). Beware of the normal epiphyseal line which may be confused with a fracture. The radiographic findings will depend upon the degree to which the triceps pulls on the proximal fragment. Three appearances are commonly seen:

1. A fracture line with no displacement.
2. A fracture line with separation of the fragments.
3. A comminuted fracture.

An undisplaced fracture in which the extensor mechanism is intact may be treated conservatively. The bone fragments will be held in opposition by the triceps aponeurosis. The arm should be immobilized in a long-arm backslab plaster with review in the fracture clinic.

The majority of other cases should be referred for open reduction and internal fixation.

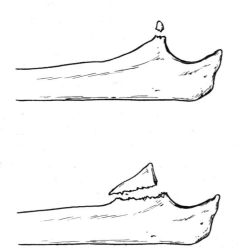

Figure 14.12 – Fractures of the coronoid process of the ulna

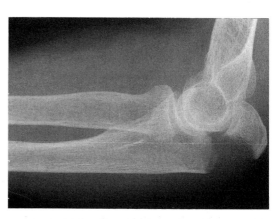

Figure 14.13 – Fracture of the olecranon

The acutely painful elbow

The pulled elbow

This is a frequently seen injury of childhood in which the radial head is pulled from the annular ligament at the elbow (Fig. 14.14). It occurs most commonly in the 2–6 years age group.

The injury can result from any sudden pull on the elbow. Classical causes include a child that falls whilst holding on to its parent's hand, being given 'aeroplane rides', and being pulled out of the path of danger.

The miserable child presents holding the affected arm by the side. A careful history will usually reveal a precipitating incident. Characteristically, gentle palpation of the entire arm (without moving it) reveals no tenderness, unlike the examination findings with a fracture. However any movement of the elbow, especially flexion, immediately produces pain.

It is important to remember that the child is unable to accurately localize pain, and usually complains of a painful wrist. Gentle movement of the wrist in a distracted child will be painless in a pulled elbow.

The diagnosis of a pulled elbow is a clinical one. However, even if a good history for a pulled elbow is obtained, **radiographs should still be taken to exclude a fracture**. A radiograph of a pulled elbow is normal.

Before manipulation warn the parents that the procedure will hurt the child, but only for a few seconds. No analgesia is required. Place the thumb of one hand over the radial head. With the other hand, flex the elbow to 90° and firmly supinate and then pronate the forearm. The 'click' of the head relocating should be felt with the thumb, and occasionally may be heard. If unsuccessful, quickly repeat the above procedure.

Once the head is located the child will not usually start using the arm immediately, but reassure the parents that this should begin over the next couple of hours. A sling is not required. If manipulation fails, the child can still be discharged with advice that spontaneous relocation should occur over the next few days. The parents should be told to return for follow-up.

Olecranon bursitis

This commonly results from pressure or friction on the bursa, usually from leaning on the elbow. Very occasionally the bursitis may be caused by gout, syphilis or tuberculosis. The bursa forms a well-localized swelling over the olecranon. Distinguish this localized swelling from an effusion of the elbow. In addition to the bursal swelling there may be an associated cellulitis.

The bursitis often responds to no more than rest and a firm bandage. Occasionally aspiration under aseptic conditions may be required if the bursitis becomes a nuisance. Chronically enlarged, troublesome bursae may require excision as an elective procedure.

Tennis elbow (lateral epicondylitis)

Despite its name, tennis elbow is only occasionally due to playing tennis, and occurs

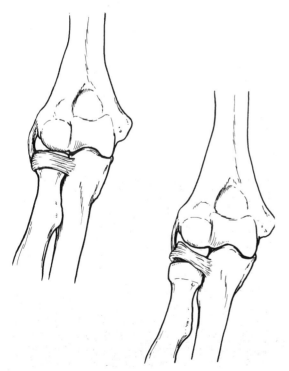

Figure 14.14 – Pulled elbow – the radial head is thrust from the annular ligament

much more commonly in patients whose work involves gripping and twisting. Degeneration of the **common extensor origin** is thought to predispose to this injury. Inflammation occurs at the origin of the extensor muscles of the wrist and fingers secondary to repetitive movements.

The patient presents with chronic pain over the lateral aspect of the elbow radiating down the lateral aspect of the forearm. This is exacerbated by gripping. On examination tenderness is elicited over the anterior aspect of the lateral epicondyle, which is the most proximal point of the common wrist and finger extensors.

If the elbow is extended and the forearm simultaneously pronated whilst flexing the wrist, the pain is exacerbated. This is known as Mill's test. Pain on resisted dorsiflexion of the wrist is a further indicator of lateral epicondylitis.

The symptoms often spontaneously settle over a period of months without any specific treatment. Initial rest and injection of local anaesthetic and steroid can help. Physiotherapy and ultrasound may be of help in particularly chronic or debilitating cases. Surgery is indicated if symptoms are refractory.

Golfer's elbow (medial epicondylitis)

This occurs less frequently than tennis elbow. The pathology lies within the common flexor origin. The treatment principles are the same.

15
The forearm

Fractures of the forearm

Principles of forearm fractures

Fractures of the forearm fall into two basic groups, depending upon the mechanism of injury:

1. Twisting or rotational forces produce spiral fractures of the radius and ulna, often occurring at different levels.·
2. A direct blow produces transverse fractures occurring at the same level.

Note that, unless there is a direct injury, if one of the forearm bones is fractured with displacement, it is likely that the other bone has also fractured **or** there has been a dislocation at the wrist or elbow. **Hence the importance of examination and x-ray of the whole forearm including the wrist and elbow joints.**

The Monteggia fracture-dislocation
(Fig. 15.1)

The Italian surgeon Monteggia first described this **fracture of the ulna with a dislocation of the proximal radius** in 1814.

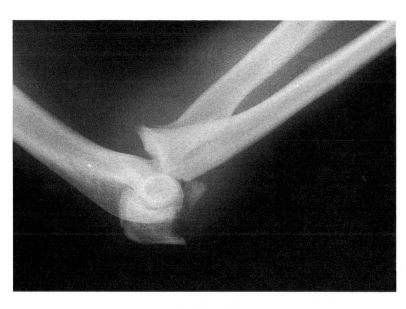

Figure 15.1 – Monteggia fracture-dislocation

The commonest mechanism of injury is a fall on to a forcibly pronated forearm. The proximal radius is levered away from the capitellum as the ulna fractures resulting in its dislocation. Other less common causes include a direct blow to the proximal ulna and a forced hyperextension injury.

The patient presents with a painful forearm with a limited range of movement. The fracture site may be obvious visually or on palpation. Despite dislocation of the proximal radius, **this may not always be apparent clinically** and the patient may not complain of pain around the elbow. **It is important to specifically test for tenderness over the proximal radius**.

When requesting radiographs it is important to ask for anteroposterior and lateral views of the whole forearm, **including the elbow and the wrist joints.** The usual pattern of injury seen is anterior angulation of the ulna with anterior dislocation of the radius. Remember in its normal position the head of the radius points towards the capitellum. Rarely the ulnar fracture angulates posteriorly with posterior dislocation of the radius.

The Monteggia fracture is often missed in children as the ulnar fracture may be only a greenstick injury. It is important to check the position of the radial head on two views and look for kinking or buckling of the ulnar shaft.

Although this fracture-dislocation may be manipulated under anaesthetic, this is both difficult to perform and hold in a satisfactory position. Nearly all adults require open reduction and internal fixation. Children with this fracture pattern in some cases may be treated conservatively, but the manipulation must be performed by experienced personnel.

The Galeazzi fracture-dislocation
(Fig. 15.2)

The Galeazzi fracture was first described in 1935 by an Italian surgeon of that same name. The name describes a **fracture of the radius with dislocation of the distal ulna**.

This injury usually results from a fall onto the outstretched hand. The inferior radio-ulnar

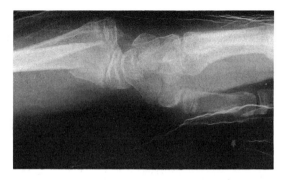

Figure 15.2 – Galeazzi fracture-dislocation. Note the distal ulnar dislocation.

ligament is ruptured, allowing the distal ulna to subluxate or dislocate. Clinical examination of the distal ulna is important as x-rays of this region may be difficult to interpret.

The patient presents with a painful forearm with limited range of movement. Deformity at the fracture site may be visible or palpable. The patient may not complain of pain at the wrist and this should be specifically sought.

As with all forearm fractures, **the elbow and wrist must be seen on two x-ray views.** The radius usually fractures at the junction of the middle and distal thirds. The ulna may be dislocated in either a medial, anterior or posterior direction.

All patients should be referred for consideration of open reduction and internal fixation, as most of the fracture-dislocations are unstable.

Fractures of both the radius and the ulna

This injury most commonly follows a fall on the outstretched hand. However, transverse fractures of both bones can be sustained by a direct blow to the forearm.

The patient presents with a painful forearm, often with an obvious deformity. It is important to detect and document the presence of a radial pulse.

The diagnosis is confirmed on radiography. The displacement seen is usually greater in adults than in children, in whom greenstick fractures are common (Figs 15.3, 15.4).

Accurate alignment is essential to allow full pronation and supination to occur. The degree

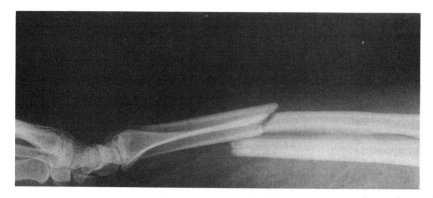

Figure 15.3 – Fractures of the midshafts of both radius and ulna

of angulation is more important than displacement in determining whether the fracture requires manipulation. The following fractures may be treated conservatively:

1. Undisplaced fractures.
2. Fractures that are minimally displaced with **no angulation.**
3. Fractures in children where the degree of angulation is less than 10°, as this will remodel (but remember that it is the clinical deformity of the forearm which is more important).

Such fractures can be placed in an **above-elbow backslab** and reviewed in the fracture clinic.

All other fractures should be referred. Fractures in children can often be manipulated whilst adult fractures usually require open reduction and internal fixation.

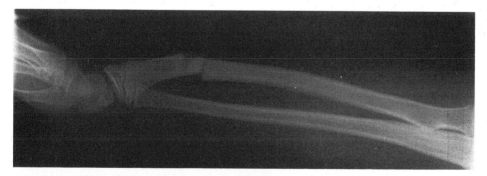

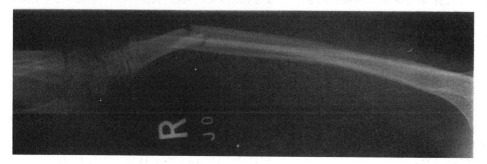

Figure 15.4 – Angulated greenstick fracture of the radius associated with a minimally angulated greenstick fracture of the distal ulna

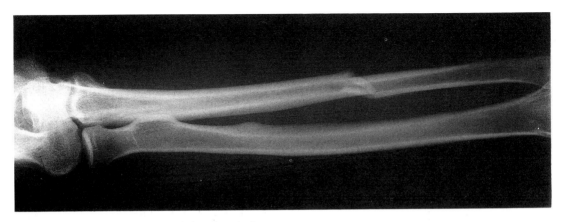

Figure 15.5 – Isolated fracture of the ulna shaft

Isolated fracture of the ulnar shaft (Fig. 15.5)

The most important factor to consider when managing a fracture of this type is to ensure you are not missing a Monteggia injury.

This injury most commonly results from a direct blow to the ulnar aspect of the forearm, as when the arm is raised to protect the face from attack. It can also be sustained when falling and striking the forearm against an object.

The patient presents with a painful forearm, and often a good history suggestive of an isolated fracture of the shaft. Tenderness is elicited over the fracture site. The diagnosis is confirmed by radiography. **It is essential to see the whole length of both bones and the wrist and elbow joints to exclude a fracture or an accompanying dislocation.**

Undisplaced fractures can be placed in an **above-elbow backslab** in mid-pronation with review in the fracture clinic. Displaced or comminuted fractures need referral as there may be an indication for open reduction and internal fixation.

Isolated fracture of the radial shaft (Fig. 15.6)

This is an uncommon fracture, usually resulting from a direct blow to the forearm. **It is essential to exclude an accompanying dislocation of the distal ulna (Galeazzi fracture-dislocation).** Although the fracture may be treated conservatively in children, most adults require open reduction and internal fixation.

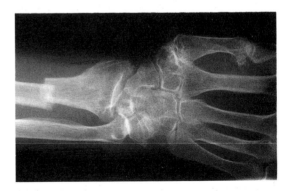

Figure 15.6 – Isolated fracture of the radial shaft

16
The wrist joint

Injuries of the distal radius and associated structures

Introduction and classification

Distal radial fractures are a very common group of injuries, and their initial diagnosis and management is important. Many of the fractures have eponyms, e.g. Colles fractures, Smith's fractures, Barton's fractures etc. However, many authorities feel that the use of such eponyms may allow mal-recognition of fracture patterns. This chapter is organized in terms of the anatomical pattern of injuries, and eponyms are used. However, an introduction to the overall classification of these fractures is given at the outset.

The Frykman classification of distal radial fractures

No classification of distal radial fractures has been devised that is ideal. The Frykman classi-fication (Table 16.1) is probably the most widely used system in operation at present.

Colles fractures

Abraham Colles described this fracture in 1814, and it is essentially a **fracture of the distal radius within 2.5 cm of the wrist joint where the distal fragment is dorsally and radially displaced** (see below for full description). Its name is often overused to describe many other fractures of the distal radius, leading to inappropriate treat-ment. Many feel it should best be used to describe distal radial fractures (of the appropri-ate pattern) in the middle-aged and elderly. Distal radial fractures in younger patients are often very different in their behaviour and should be managed as a separate injury. Because of its common frequency, its descrip-tion will be given in detail. The fracture occurs most often in middle-aged and elderly women with osteoporotic bone, often caused by a fall on the outstretched hand.

Table 16.1 Frykman classification of distal radial fractures

Radial fracture type	Distal ulna fracture	
	Absent	Present
Extra-articular	Type 1	Type 2
Intra-articular involving the radio-carpal joint	Type 3	Type 4
Intra-articular involving the distal radio-ulnar joint	Type 5	Type 6
Intra-articular involving both radio-carpal and distal radio-ulnar joints	Type 7	Type 8

Fracture anatomy

A Colles fracture can be described as a fracture of the distal metaphysis of the radius within 2.5 cm of the wrist joint, with some or all of the following features (Fig. 16.1).

1. The distal radial fragment is dorsally displaced.
2. The distal radial fragment is radially displaced.
3. The distal radial fragment is impacted.
4. Avulsion of the ulnar styloid (caused by avulsion of the insertion of the triangular fibrocartilage of the distal radio-ulnar joint, implying a greater degree of violence).

5. Anterior angulation of the distal radial fragment.
6. Ulnar angulation of the distal radial fragment.
7. Torsional deformity of the distal radial fragment.
8. As a consequence of the above, the radius is 'short'; the radius normally extends further distally than the ulna as seen on an antero-posterior radiograph of the wrist (Fig. 16.2). (This is one of the more reliable methods of assessing need for reduction of a fracture).

A Colles fracture can include any of the above features, but not all are necessary for its diagnosis. The essential features are **dorsal and radial displacement** of the distal radial

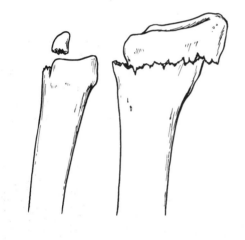

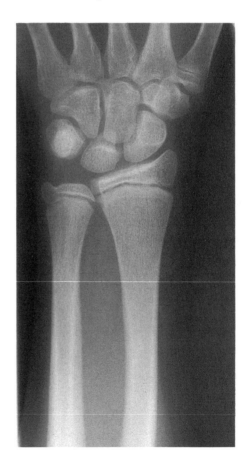

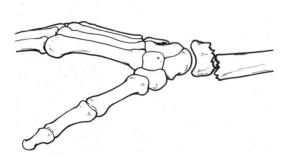

Figure 16.1 – Colles fracture. Note the dorsal and radial deviation of the distal fragment, and the ulna styloid avulsion.

Figure 16.2 – Normal AP x-ray of the wrist. Note that the radius extends further distally than the ulna.

fragment. The fracture may be undisplaced or displaced; the classical description of 'dinner-fork deformity' applies to the displaced fracture (Fig. 16.3). When assessing fractures of the distal radius, it is essential to have knowledge of the normal anatomy of the wrist joint, remembering that, in lateral view, the joint surface of the distal radius has a 10° forward tilt (Fig. 16.4).

Diagnosis

All patients who, following a fall on the outstretched hand, have a painful wrist should be suspected as having a skeletal injury, and thus should be radiographed. While the displaced fracture may have a characteristic 'dinner-fork deformity', the undisplaced or minimally displaced fracture may merely demonstrate pain and tenderness in the region. As with all frac-tures, the associated neurovasculature should be checked; in Colles fractures, any evidence of damage to the median nerve should be specifically sought. In rare cases, the extensor tendons may be acutely damaged. Other bones and joints (e.g. hand, elbow, shoulder) should also be examined.

In most cases, true anteroposterior and lateral radiographs of the wrist joint suffice in establishing a diagnosis (Fig. 16.5). Particular care should be paid to identifying undisplaced fractures or those impacted fractures (Fig. 16.6) with an alteration in the distal radial forward tilt.

Management of undisplaced and minimally displaced fractures

Those fractures not requiring reduction should be initially placed into a plaster backslab (see below for details of application). These fractures are capable of causing significant soft tissue swelling, and careful instructions need to be given, as many of the patients are elderly with

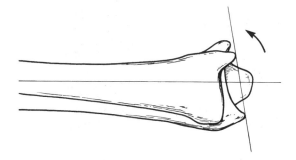

Figure 16.3 – Dinner-fork deformity of the wrist seen in Colles fractures

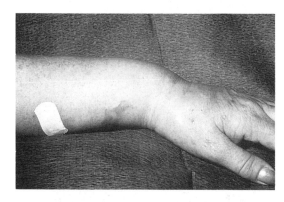

Figure 16.4 – The distal radius normally has a 5–10 degree forward tilt in lateral profile

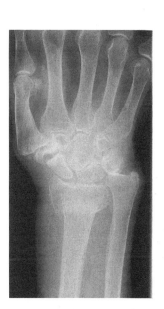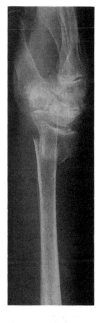

Figure 16.5 – Colles fracture – AP and lateral views

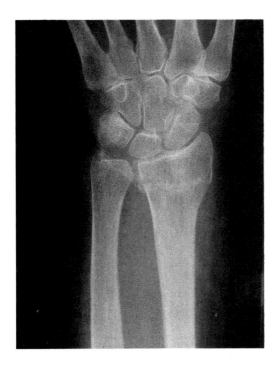

Figure 16.6 – Impacted fracture of the distal radius

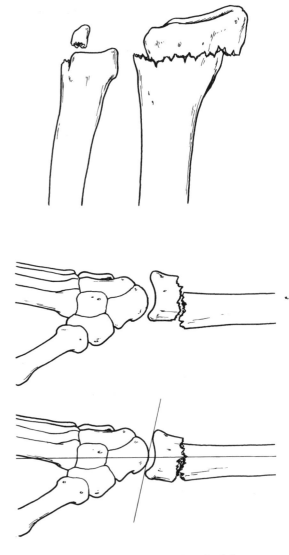

Figure 16.7 – Criteria for reduction. Radial deviation, dorsal deviation or a loss of the normal 10 degree forward tilt of the distal radial joint surface.

comprehension difficulties. These patients should be followed up in the fracture clinic.

Management of displaced fractures – criteria for reduction

A common problem is the decision as to whether reduction is necessary in Colles fractures. Such a decision needs to be made with respect to the physiological age and expectations of the patient. A semi-retired man with an injury to his dominant wrist who regularly does DIY etc. needs a more exacting result than a 95-year-old elderly patient with dementia; **that is to say, do not treat the x-ray but the patient!**

In general terms, the following features indicate the need for reduction (Fig. 16.7).

1. Gross dorsal or radial displacement of the distal radial fragment.

2. 'Shortening' of the radius (see above) – this is a good indicator of the need for reduction.

3. A loss of the normal 10° forward tilt of the distal radial joint surface on the lateral x-ray of the wrist. Many would advise reduction if there is any backward angulation, but this is patient-dependent.

Method of reduction and immobilization

There are many methods of reduction and immobilization of Colles fractures; you should master one that works for you!

Anaesthesia

The following, not necessarily an exhaustive list, are acceptable as methods of establishing anaesthesia for fracture reduction.

General anaesthesia   In the elderly this is rarely required for a primary manipulation of a Colles fracture. However, in younger patients it is very helpful in establishing an accurate reduction with the use of an image intensifier.

Intravenous regional anaesthesia ('Biers Block')   This is probably the most widely practised method in the UK. Many centres now demand an anaesthetist to perform the block, and this has decreased the complication rate of the method. The patient should be fasted as for a general anaesthetic prior to its use. Good analgesia may be obtained with this method, allowing accurate reduction.

Installation of local anaesthetic into the fracture haematoma   This method has its advocates, although its use is criticized by some as it converts a closed fracture into a potentially open one. Analgesia is not as effective as in other methods. However, it can be useful in the elderly patient with a simple fracture pattern.

Intravenous sedation   This can be useful in the very elderly patient with gross displacement, where reduction can quickly be achieved.

Reduction

Again, many methods of reduction abound in every hospital. It is good practice to perform a trial reduction prior to the application of a plaster cast; the definitive reduction within the plaster can then be performed accurately and quickly. Care should be taken with the skin of

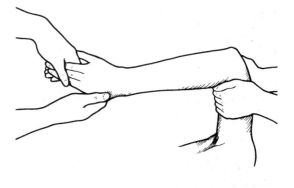

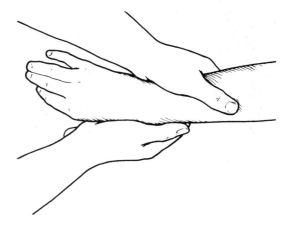

Figure 16.8 – Colles fracture reduction. Initial traction followed by correction of dorsal and radial displacement.

elderly patients; many a disaster has occurred with an enthusiastic reduction degloving the skin of the forearm.

There are two essentials of reduction of a classical Colles fracture (Fig. 16.8).

1. *Disimpaction*   A gentle pull for one minute makes the reduction much easier. In some cases, the deformity may need to be increased as part of this stage to disengage the impacted cortices.
2. *Reduction of deformity*   This implies that the wrist should be **pronated** with correction of, first, dorsal displacement and then radial displacement. Firm pressure should be established on the distal radius towards the ulna. **The fracture is most stable in palmarflexion, ulnar deviation and pronation.**

Immobilization

This is a stage often performed incorrectly, leading to unnecessary remanipulation.

In treating these injuries, the rule of immobilizing joints proximal and distal to the fracture is broken. Theoretically, by immobilizing the elbow joint, rotation at the distal radio-ulnar joint would be prevented. However, a compromise is made, as such immobilization would cause considerable stiffness at the elbow. The plaster should extend **from just distal to the elbow to just proximal to the metacarpophalangeal joints.** This allows full finger flexion and prevents stiffness in the hand.

The forearm should be placed into a backslab rather than a complete plaster to allow the swelling to subside. However, the slab should not be a 'back' slab extending solely around the back of the wrist. It should be more correctly described (as by Charnley) as a **radial slab** (Fig. 16.9). The plaster is attempting to immobilize the radius, and it is futile to leave the radius uncovered ventrally. Another important feature is that the slab should be **moulded** as this decreases the tendency to post-reduction slippage.

Imaging

Ideally, reduction of fractures should be undertaken under image intensifier control. However, in many cases this is not practicable. A minimum should be plain radiographs (anteroposterior and lateral) taken following immobilization. These should be taken and studied before termination of analgesia in case a further reduction is necessary. Criteria for adequate reduction are essentially those features considered prior to manipulation (see above). In younger patients, reduction with the aid of image intensification is helpful to obtain the best possible position.

Instructions to the patient

It is very important, in what is usually an elderly patient, to give clear instructions about the precautions concerning swelling within a plaster slab etc. This is best written down or given to a person looking after the patient. Until swelling of the area is reduced, the limb should be placed within a sling with the wrist above the level of the elbow.

It is very easy for all the joints of the upper limb to become stiff following a Colles fracture.

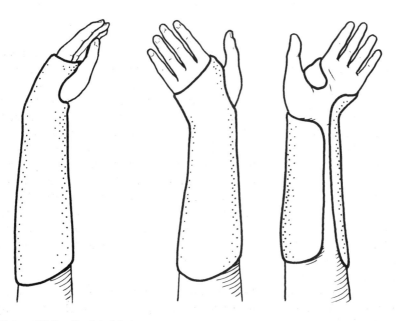

Figure 16.9 – Radial slab

Patients should be encouraged to move all joints not immobilized, from the metacarpophalangeal joints to the elbow and shoulder. This is a very important factor in decreasing the morbidity from these fractures, and should occur as soon as possible. The arm should not remain in the sling for long periods.

Follow-up of Colles fractures

Colles fractures are usually followed up in fracture clinics, although in some hospitals, the Accident and Emergency Service perform this task. The patient should be seen within 2–3 days at the next available clinic. The purposes of this attendance are:

1. A clinical evaluation of swelling of the hand etc. and for any other problems.
2. A check radiograph to ensure continuing adequacy of reduction (**with the plaster slab still applied**).
3. Completion of the radial slab to a full plaster if swelling has subsided.

A common problem is to what degree the fracture should be allowed to slip before re-reduction is contemplated. Re-manipulation is often a difficult procedure, and several studies have shown that it may not help in long-term outcome. If a re-manipulation is considered, it should ideally be performed under general anaesthesia with the aid of an image intensifier. Such a manipulation is unlikely to be of help after 10 days, so that it is important to arrange follow-up appointments before this time.

Displaced fractures should be seen, in addition to the first outpatient attendance, on a further occasion with an x-ray. The number and timing of visits should be allocated according to the stability of the fracture and according to the physiological age and needs of the patient.

The fracture should be immobilized for a period of 5–6 weeks in total within a plaster slab. There should be no routine necessity for an x-ray when the plaster is removed. The fracture should be assessed for clinical union, which in the vast majority of cases occurs by this time. Wrist stiffness should be clearly distinguished

from pain at the fracture site. The range of movement and wrist swelling should be determined, along with the need for any physiotherapy. Many centres hold 'wrist classes', and if available, these are very useful in post-immobilization therapy. Cases should be followed up until recovery is as near complete as can be expected, and any complications (see below) should be positively sought.

Complications of Colles fractures

Early complications

Swelling This is a great hazard in the elderly, and may produce severe skin complications if not recognized. The slab should be released if necessary, even if a re-reduction is later needed.

Acute median nerve compression This is uncommon at this stage. If not caused by tightness of the plaster, operative decompression may be necessary.

Later complications

Loss of fracture reduction This is common, and as stated above, re-reduction is often unfruitful. However, it may be necessary, and should be considered in even small slips in the young patient.

Malunion This is very common. It may result from an inadequate initial reduction or a post-reduction slippage. Common deformities are persisting radial and dorsal displacement of the distal radius, and prominence of the ulnar styloid. The deformities are often unsightly. In many cases this has to be accepted, and only where loss of **function** is seen after a long course of physiotherapy should surgery be contemplated. Surgery should not be considered on anatomical grounds alone, for fear of converting a painless wrist into a painful one! This problem emphasizes the importance of getting it right first time.

Median nerve compression This is not an uncommon finding in the weeks following removal of the plaster. Its presence may imply a level of disorganization at the wrist. Clinical findings are usually sensory with paraesthesiae in the distribution of the median nerve. Ideally, an electromyelogram (EMG) should be performed prior to any surgery to distinguish a difficult case from reflex sympathetic dystrophy (see below), where surgery may worsen the situation. Decompression of the median nerve at the level of the flexor retinaculum may be needed; this is a relatively simple operation and may be performed under local anaesthesia.

Reflex sympathetic dystrophy (Sudek's atrophy)   This complication, although relatively uncommon, can be devastating. The clinical findings may be varied, and there is no definite aetiology, although it is commonly said to be due to dysfunction of the autonomic nervous system. Following removal of the plaster, the distal limb is swollen, painful and tender with a grossly reduced range of motion. Radiographs often show a 'washout' of the bones. Treatment is difficult, and may include physiotherapy and autonomic ablative procedures (e.g. sympathectomy). Pain clinics are often useful. An important point is that surgery should be avoided at all costs, as this commonly aggravates the clinical situation.

Delayed rupture of the tendon of extensor pollicis longus   The aetiology of this is uncertain, but probably involves devascularization of the tendon at the level of the dorsal radial (Lister's) tubercle. Interestingly, it often occurs in cases where displacement is slight. It results in loss of active extension at the interphalangeal joint of the thumb. In the elderly this is often treated conservatively; in the young an extensor indicis proprius tendon transfer may be utilized if the disability demands it.

Prolonged stiffness   This is a very common problem, and in many cases may represent a spectrum of reflex sympathetic dystrophy. Physiotherapy is useful, but may not affect the long-term outcome.

Other fractures around the wrist joint

Fractures occurring in the immature skeleton

Greenstick fractures of the distal radius and ulna

These are very common fractures in childhood, usually caused by a fall on to the outstretched hand. Greenstick fractures are fractures where only one cortex is broken (Fig. 16.10). The important feature to note with these fractures is the presence of **clinical deformity**. Surprisingly, angulated fractures may cause little deformity whilst minimally angulated fractures may appear considerably deformed. **The need for reduction should be based upon the correction of clinical deformity** rather than the radiograph itself.

If not requiring manipulation, the fracture should be immobilized in a plaster backslab, with completion within the next day or so at the time of the fracture clinic appointment.

If the fracture requires manipulation, this should be performed under general anaesthesia with image intensification at hand. The use of intravenous relaxants in Accident and Emergency Departments for children in this setting is not ideal. The method of reduction of these fractures is important. These fractures often require over-correction so as to realign the periosteum satisfactorily although this does **not** imply that the fracture needs to be completely broken, which can cause considerable difficulty. The fracture should then be immobilized in a moulded plaster, either a backslab or a complete plaster split down to skin. Moulding is very important here in preventing re-angulation.

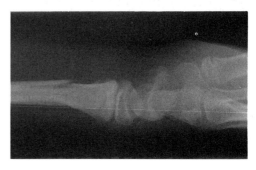

Figure 16.10 – Greenstick fracture of the distal radius

Of vital importance in the follow-up of greenstick fractures that have undergone manipulation, is the realization that children's fractures heal extremely quickly. It is always best if fractures do not re-angulate, but this inevitably does occur in some cases. For this to be recognized, the child needs to be seen at frequent intervals in the fracture clinic for repeat x-rays, and not left for more than one week before the next attendance in the clinic, by which time the fracture may have united!

Some greenstick fractures are difficult to manage, especially where both the radius and ulna have broken, or where the fragments are overlapping. In some cases, closed reduction is not possible and an open reduction is necessary, which may need stabilization with percutaneous K wires. Always beware the Galeazzi fracture-dislocation (see below), where the distal ulna is dislocated in conjunction with the distal radial fracture (Fig. 16.11).

Finally, the saving grace of children's fractures is that their powers of remodelling are very good. Malrotation, however, is least sensitive to remodelling, so close attention should be paid to this.

Fractures involving the distal radial epiphysis

These are another common group of fractures in the immature skeleton. The most common form is a Salter–Harris type 2 injury (see Chapter 3) where the fracture extends through both the distal radial epiphysis and the distal metaphysis (Fig. 16.12). Most are easily reduced under general anaesthesia and immobilized in plaster. Accurate reduction is necessary. Open reduction is rarely required. The prognosis of type 2 injuries is good. Other forms occur more rarely, and may be difficult to manage.

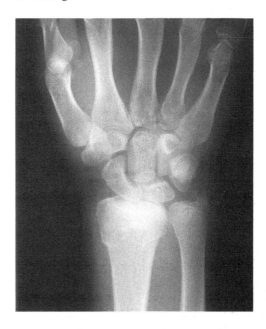

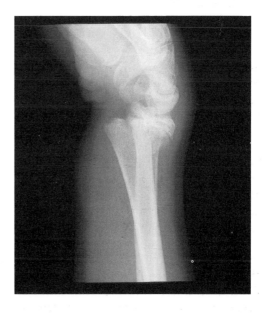

Figure 16.12 – Salter-Harris type 2 fracture of the distal radial epiphysis

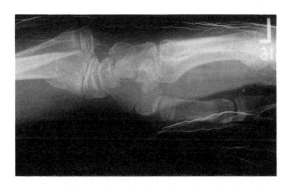

Figure 16.11– Galeazzi fracture-dislocation

Fractures occurring in the mature skeleton

Smith's fractures (including Barton's fracture)

A Smith's fracture is essentially the reverse of a Colles fracture, i.e. a fracture of the distal radius **where the distal fragment is displaced ventrally** – see Fig. 1613 (cf. dorsally in a Colles fractures).

There are three grades of Smith's fractures:

A   Extra-articular fracture.
B   Fracture extending into the dorsal articular surface.
C   Fracture extending into the radio-carpal joint (a Barton's fracture, see Fig. 16.14).

The fractures occur in a wide age group, but tend to be in the elderly. They are usually caused by a fall on the dorsal aspect of the palmar-flexed wrist. A clear distinction should

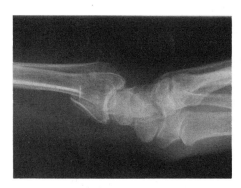

Figure 16.13 – Smith's fracture

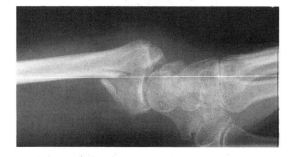

Figure 16.14 – Barton's fracture

be made between Smith's fractures and Colles fractures, as their management is different.

An attempt may be made to treat a Smith's fracture conservatively. Reduction should ideally be under general anaesthetic, although other methods are acceptable. Reduction is obtained by **traction (disimpaction), supination and ventral pressure on the distal radial fragment**. An important difference between a Colles fracture and a Smith's fracture is that the latter demands an **above-elbow plaster** when immobilized. The position of the limb should be in **supination with the wrist dorsiflexed** and the elbow at a right-angle. Initially, either an anterior/radial slab or a split complete plaster may be used.

The problem with conservatively treated Smith's fractures is the significant tendency for re-displacement. A conservatively treated fracture must be regularly checked with serial x-rays for 2–3 weeks to ensure continuing adequacy of reduction. In addition, a careful check should be made for the development of median nerve compression at the wrist – the development of carpal tunnel syndrome is not uncommon with Smith's fractures.

Because of the problem of re-displacement in Smith's fractures, in combination with the need to immobilize the elbow as well as the wrist, and the tendency for median nerve compression, many centres now advocate primary open reduction and internal fixation for displaced Smith's fractures. This of course should be modified according to physiological age etc. If a delay is anticipated prior to surgery, a temporary reduction is helpful. The most common internal fixation device used in this context is a buttress plate placed on the volar surface of the radius. This may be combined with decompression of the carpal tunnel, which may be performed prophylactically.

Fractures of the radial styloid

This is a common fracture, occurring in a wide age group. The usual cause is a fall on the outstretched hand. Most fractures are undisplaced (Fig. 16.15). Special care needs to be taken in clinically distinguishing it from a scaphoid fracture, as both cause pain in the anatomical snuff

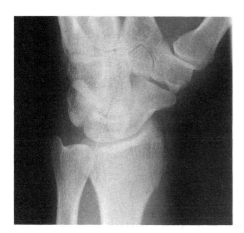

Figure 16.15 – Radial styloid fracture

box. Undisplaced fractures should be immobilized for 4–5 weeks in a below-elbow plaster. Surprisingly, stiffness is common with these fractures following immobilization.

Galeazzi fracture-dislocation

This injury pattern should never be forgotten. A dislocation of the distal ulna occurs in combination with a fracture of the radius (see above). This injury emphasizes the importance of views of joints above and below a fracture.

Injuries of the carpus

Scaphoid fractures

Scaphoid fracture is an important injury, especially medico-legally, and is the most common carpal fracture. It is said to occur most often in young adults. The aphorism that scaphoid fractures do not occur in the immature skeleton is **not** true, a fact that a number of doctors have realized in courts of law! Because of its vascular anatomy (see below), the bone, once fractured, is susceptible to both avascular necrosis and non-union; neglected fractures may result in catastrophic degenerative arthritis at the wrist necessitating fusion of that joint. If a scaphoid fracture is suspected, **always** treat it as such by initial immobilization – specialist clinics can determine if a fracture is present at a later stage.

Applied anatomy (Fig. 16.16)

The scaphoid is part of the proximal row of carpal bones and plays a very important part in wrist dynamics. It articulates with several bones (radius, lunate, capitate, trapezium and trapezoid). Hence, when its anatomy is disorganized, the wrist is often severely compromised.

An understanding of the blood supply of the scaphoid is essential when discussing the pathological changes of the bone. In many, but not all, patients the blood supply to the bone enters distally, with intra-osseous transport of blood to the proximal pole. Hence the proximal pole is susceptible to **avascular necrosis** in some fractures (Fig. 16.17).

Diagnosis

A scaphoid fracture is most often caused by a fall on the outstretched hand, resulting in a hyperextension force on the wrist. In the past,

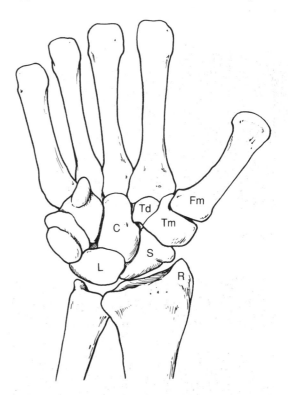

Figure 16.16 - Scaphoid relationships. R = radius, S = scaphoid, L = lunate, Td = trapezoid, Tm = Trapezium, C = capitate, FM = thumb metacarpal.

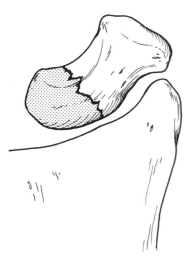

Figure 16.17 – Avascular necrosis of the scaphoid. In some patients the blood supply to the proximal pole enters distally. Thus fractures at the waist may render the proximal pole avascular.

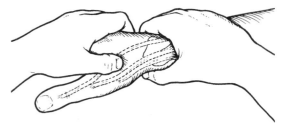

Figure 16.18 – Tender anatomical snuff box – in addition to the scaphoid, the radial styloid and the base of thumb metacarpal are in this region. Fractures of any of the bones results in tenderness.

the classical cause was from a 'kickback' from motor car starting handles etc. Other mechanisms, e.g. blows on to the wrist, are **unlikely** to cause a scaphoid fracture, although it is safest to treat the injury as a scaphoid fracture if suggestive clinical features are present. When a scaphoid fracture is present, a complaint is made of pain on the radial aspect of the wrist. It is also important to note that a scaphoid fracture may coexist with other fractures of the upper limb; its presence should therefore always be sought.

On examination, the wrist may be swollen, especially on its radial aspect. A classic finding is that of '**tenderness in the anatomical snuff box**', i.e. over the scaphoid bone. A number of points should be considered in relation to this.

First, firm palpation of this area is normally uncomfortable (probably due to the course of the superficial cutaneous branch of the radial nerve), and the two sides should be compared.

Secondly, you must understand what bones are present in the area; although the scaphoid is situated centrally in the snuff box, the radial styloid is proximal, and the trapezium and base of thumb metacarpal are distal. Fractures of these other bones also cause pain in the snuff box (Fig. 16.18).

Thirdly, scaphoid fractures often cause tenderness both dorsally and ventrally in the lateral carpus as well as in the snuff box itself. Other fractures in this area rarely share this property.

Radiographic findings

This is a very important aspect, which often causes confusion. The following points should be considered:

1. Whenever a scaphoid fracture is clinically suspected, **special scaphoid views of the wrist should be requested**. Because scaphoid fractures are often difficult to demonstrate, the normal request of two views (anteroposterior and lateral) is **not** sufficient. Scaphoid films consist of two additional, oblique views of the joint to give extra information about the bone. Hence, there should be at least four radiographs taken of the bone.

2. It is important not to overlook a scaphoid fracture that may not be obvious on the initial radiograph. Fractures may not be immediately obvious, but may become so when decalcification occurs at the fracture site. Hence, **the importance of the classic repeat x-ray at 10 days or so after a period of immobilization (see below)**.

3. On a medico-legal viewpoint, once scaphoid views of the wrist have been requested in the Accident and Emergency Department, and even if the initial films do not reveal a fracture, you are essentially obliged to treat the injury as a scaphoid fracture. This should be remembered lest all patients are given these views of the joint!

Management of the suspected scaphoid fracture

This is a common clinical situation. **All patients seen soon after injury with clinical features of a scaphoid fracture should be treated as if they have one** by immobilization of the wrist in a 'scaphoid plaster'. Many authorities would regard it as negligent to not follow this plan. The patient should then be seen at 10–14 days in the fracture clinic, at which time the plaster should be removed, the patient re-examined, and further radiographs taken. A number of possibilities may follow.

1. A fracture may be confirmed radiologically (see below).
2. Radiographs are negative and the clinical features have settled (i.e. tenderness has subsided). The injury may be diagnosed as a sprain, with the plaster discarded.
3. Radiographs are negative but clinical features continue. In this case, the optimal management is to continue immobilization and to arrange a **bone scan** of the region. A scaphoid fracture will reveal itself after 36–48 hours on bone scan, and this is a useful way of firmly establishing the presence or absence of a fracture.

With a scaphoid plaster, the wrist should be in the 'beer glass' position (Fig. 16.19), with the wrist dorsiflexed, pronated and in moderate radial deviation, with the thumb in abduction. The plaster should extend from just below the elbow to (a) proximal to the metacarpophalangeal joints of the fingers and (b) to just short of the interphalangeal joint of the thumb (so that the joint is functional). Most centres now utilize a complete cast, although an anterior slab is acceptable. If complete, the plaster should be split, or at least warning instructions given to the patient to return for plaster splitting if necessary. The bony areas of the wrist should be adequately padded.

Management of the established scaphoid fracture

The common sites of scaphoid fracture are shown in Fig. 16.20. Fractures at the level of

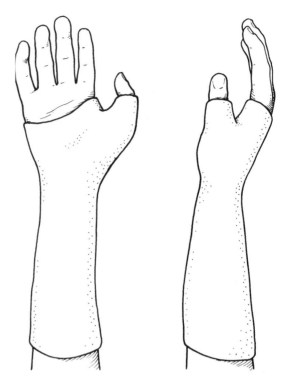

Figure 16.19 – Scaphoid plaster

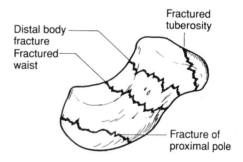

Figure 16.20 – Scaphoid fractures – common sites

the waist are most common, with fractures also noted at the distal and proximal poles. Displacement and fracture site bears some relation to the risk of subsequent avascular necrosis.

Non-displaced and minimally displaced fractures (Fig. 16.21)

Non-displaced and minimally displaced fractures should be immobilized initially for a period of 6 weeks. If a fracture is confidently diagnosed at the time of the injury, the plaster

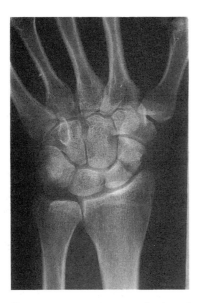

Figure 16.21 – Minimally displaced scaphoid fracture

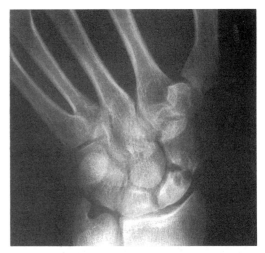

Figure 16.22 – Pathological fracture of the scaphoid through a cyst – the displacement is such that internal fixation with bone grafting is advised.

need not be removed at the subsequent clinic review until 6 weeks following injury. At this time, the wrist should be examined and further radiographs taken. Two outcomes are common:

1. The fracture is radiologically united with clinical features subsided – the wrist should be mobilized, but it is prudent to x-ray the wrist again after a further period of 6 weeks to ensure continuing union.
2. The fracture has not united – most authorities would advise a further period of immobilization for 6 weeks.

If non-union is present at 12 weeks post injury, most would advise internal fixation and bone grafting of the fracture. This is often performed using a **Herbert screw**.

Significantly displaced fractures of the scaphoid (Fig. 16.22)

If a scaphoid fracture is significantly displaced, the risks of non-union and avascular necrosis are high if the injury is treated conservatively. Ideally, such fractures should be treated by internal fixation primarily, again using a Herbert screw.

Old scaphoid fractures presenting as acute wrist pain

It is not uncommon for an old untreated or inadequately treated scaphoid fracture to present with acute wrist pain many years later, or as an incidental finding on a radiograph. The presentation may be that of non-union, or of avascular necrosis/secondary degenerative arthritis of the wrist joint (Fig. 16.23). Such cases should always be referred on to the fracture clinic, where appropriate advice and follow-up can be offered. Immobilization is not always necessary if the fracture is an old one.

Complications of scaphoid fractures

As well as the complications of any fracture, the following are worthy of mention in scaphoid fractures.

Non-union of the scaphoid

Non-union of the scaphoid is not always symptomatic, and in general terms non-symptomatic cases should be treated conservatively in the absence of avascular necrosis (see below).

Symptomatic non-union, or a non-union complicated by avascular necrosis of the prox-

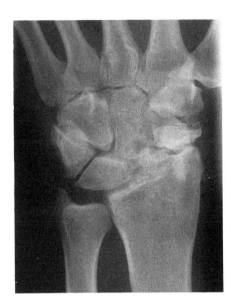

Figure 16.23 – Avascular necrosis of the proximal scaphoid with subsequent collapse and degenerative change

imal segment, should be treated by internal fixation (Herbert screw) and bone grafting.

Avascular necrosis

Because of the blood supply to the bone (see above), the scaphoid is prone to this complication in the proximal segment. The onset of avascular necrosis is usually short (within 3 months). The appearance is characteristic. Surgery should be considered in all cases to prevent secondary degenerative arthritis at the wrist joint. Treatment options include excision of the scaphoid and replacement with a silastic spacer. Primary fusion is an alternative, although less common, option.

Secondary degenerative arthritis

This can be a very disabling condition, and may occur in young working people. It is usually a result of non-union or avascular necrosis. It may occur without a formal history of a scaphoid fracture, with a vague history of a wrist injury in the past. Such an eventuality, if symptomatic, is usually treated by wrist (radiocarpal) fusion, although excision of the proximal carpal row is an alternative option.

Other carpal injuries and carpal instability

Fractures of the carpal bones other than the scaphoid

Isolated fractures of carpal bones other than the scaphoid are rare. The usual initial treatment is immobilization within plaster followed by physiotherapy. If a fracture is seen, always exclude a dislocation within the carpus or significant carpal instability.

Dislocations and fracture-dislocations of the carpus

These form an important group of injuries, and if undiagnosed can cause significant long-term problems. They are not common but their recognition is essential. The group are largely caused by falls on to the outstretched hand.

True lunate dislocation

This is probably the most important of the carpal dislocations, and is the commonest. It is easily missed. There is often an antecedent peri-lunate dislocation (see below). Pain is maximal over the volar surface of the wrist, and there may be symptoms suggestive of median nerve compression. The radiographic findings are important to recognize. Compare the normal anatomy of the wrist to that of a lunate dislocation (Figs 16.24, 16.25). On the lateral view, note that the lunate is displaced with respect to the rest of the carpus in an anterior direction, and that it changes shape to a 'moon-shape'. On the anteroposterior view, note the characteristic change in shape of the bone from its normal quadrilateral shape to a triangular-shaped mass. (Scaphoid fractures commonly coexist with this injury.)

In the management of the condition, the most important factor is recognition of the injury pattern. **These injuries should be immediately referred.** Most lunate dislocations can be managed conservatively by reduction under anaesthesia (preferably general) with image intensification available. One method of reduction is to apply volar pressure over the lunate whilst applying traction to the supinated wrist, flexing the wrist once reduction is obtained. The

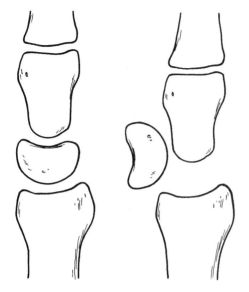

Figure 16.24 – Lunate dislocation – compare normal (left) with lunate dislocation in which the rest of the carpus maintains its relationship with the radius.

reduction should be confirmed radiologically. The wrist is immobilized in flexion, and this may be changed to a neutral position after 2–3 weeks. Because of the considerable swelling associated with this injury, a slab is preferable initially, with completion shortly thereafter. Regular check radiographs in follow-up are mandatory.

If reduction is not possible by closed means, the dislocation should be openly reduced by an experienced surgeon.

There are complications associated with lunate dislocation. The **median nerve** is susceptible to injury, and may require decompression. Should the injury not be recognized, the lunate may undergo **avascular necrosis**, with subsequent degenerative arthritis of the wrist. Avascular necrosis may also occur in cases of successful reduction, so that regular follow-up of lunate dislocations is essential. Should this complication ensue, the lunate may be excised and/or replaced with a silastic implant. Should significant arthritis develop, wrist fusion may be necessary. (Note that the radiological appearance of Kienbock's disease, a form of osteochondritis of the lunate, is similar to avascular necrosis, and may have a shared aetiology).

Peri-lunate dislocation (Figs 16.26, 16.27)

This may represent one spectrum of true lunate dislocation. The whole of the carpus dislocates posteriorly, leaving only the lunate in contact with the radius. The injury pattern may occur in combination with other fractures of the carpus, e.g. the scaphoid. The injury should be similarly treated as a true lunate dislocation, and **must** always be referred.

Scaphoid subluxations and dislocations

These are not common injuries, but should be recognized as their treatment is often operative. The most obvious abnormality is a widening of the space between the scaphoid and the lunate (the 'Terry Thomas' or 'missing tooth' sign, see Fig. 16.28). The injuries should be referred. Internal fixation may be required.

Other injuries of the carpus

Many other injuries of the carpus occur. They are recognized by the abnormal relationship of the carpal bones on x-ray. Their management is outside the scope of this book, other than to say that they should always be referred.

Carpal instability

This is a recently recognized phenomenon, and is gaining ground in explaining problematic wrists which have no obvious bony injury. The term denotes any ligamentous instability due to injury, and includes some of the injuries described above. A detailed description is not given here, but the idea is useful to understand.

The acutely painful wrist

A patient may present with an acutely painful wrist for a number of reasons. Other than trauma, dealt with in the other sections of this chapter, the wrist may be symptomatic in an 'emergency setting' for the following reasons, although the causes of any acutely painful joint may be responsible (see Chapter 2). No

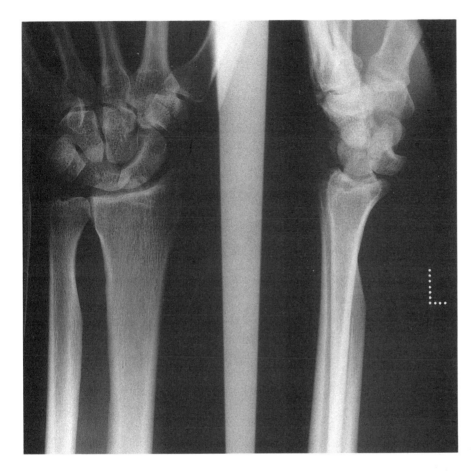

Figure 16.25 – Lunate dislocation – note that the lunate has displaced anteriorly and on the AP view is triangular in outline.

attempt is made to describe each condition in detail, but merely to give some differential diagnoses.

Rheumatoid arthritis

The wrist is a common site affected by rheumatoid arthritis, and an acutely swollen and painful joint may be a presenting symptom. The joint is affected by an inflammatory synovitis, which is warm, swollen, painful and stiff.

Carpal tunnel syndrome

This may present acutely, especially following prior trauma, e.g. Colles fracture. Symptoms are manifested according to the distribution of the median nerve.

Infection

All cases of a swollen painful wrist without antecedent trauma should have infection excluded as a cause. A predisposing factor may not always be present. The diagnosis is obtained from aspiration of the joint. Treatment should be as for any infected joint, with prompt exploration and debridement.

DeQuervain's synovitis

This may present as an 'emergency' with pain over the tendon sheath of extensor pollicis

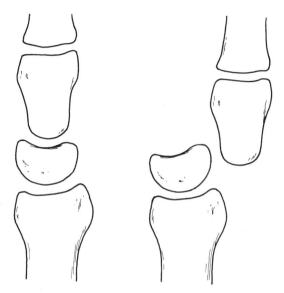

Figure 16.26 – Peri-lunate dislocation – compare normal (left) with peri-lunate dislocation in which the lunate remains in relationship with the radius, the carpus displacing dorsally.

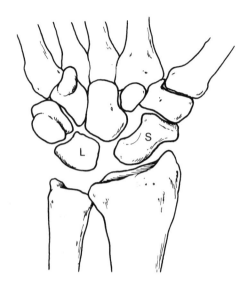

Figure 16.28 – Scapho-lunate disassociation – note the gap between lunate and scaphoid bones.

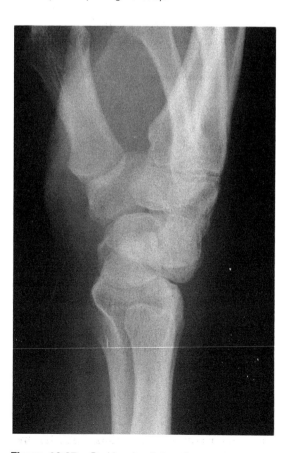

Figure 16.27 – Peri-lunate dislocation

brevis and abductor pollicis longus. Treatment consists of rest, anti-inflammatories, steroid injection and, ultimately, operative decompression.

Other

Examples of other causes of a painful wrist include:

- Cellulitis.
- Reflex sympathetic dystrophy following trauma (which may be only minor).
- Gout and pseudogout.

17
The hand

The hand – evaluation

Injuries to the hand make up a large volume of the Accident and Emergency workload. The normal functioning of this extremely complex tool can be interrupted in a number of different ways including fractures, tendon injuries, nerve injuries and infection. The optimal treatment of all hand injuries depends upon an accurate diagnosis, carefully determined management, meticulous surgery and appropriate aftercare. This is only possible if the doctor has a thorough understanding of the anatomy and function of the region.

History

The age, sex, occupation and hobbies of the patient should be recorded, and whether the patient is left- or right-handed. A full history of the injury should include when it occurred, the environment in which it occurred (e.g. was dirt, soil, glass etc. involved) and what exactly was the mechanism of injury? Was the hand fallen on, was it crushed or cut, were shearing forces involved etc.? What first aid measures have been applied?

Principles of examination and management

Rings should be removed and the hand elevated as soon as possible. Fingers stiffen very easily and both swelling and splintage contribute to this problem. A stiff, straight finger is useless and therefore every effort should be made to avoid it. The examination of even the most apparently minor injury should follow the formal assessment of hand function as described below. **Remember that fingers have names, not numbers**, i.e. thumb, index, middle, ring and little. It is helpful to record most hand injuries on a pictorial chart, and to note both positive and negative findings.

If splintage is required, this should be kept to a minimum and used for as short a time as possible. All uninjured joints should be kept free and the patient encouraged to mobilize these from day one. If the injured finger requires minimal splintage and immediate mobilization is desirable, **dynamic splinting** in the form of a garter or neighbour strapping is appropriate. Support is provided by the adjacent, uninjured finger and mobility possible at the metacarpophalangeal joints (MCPJs) and interphalangeal joints (IPJs).

If absolute immobility is required in the initial period, the 'safe' position of splintage **must** be used (see Fig. 17.1). The MCPJs should be flexed to as close to 90° as possible, and the IPJs fully extended. **The MCPJs must never be splinted in extension.** Available methods of achieving this immobilization include an aluminium splint, which should be applied to the volar aspect only and must not project beyond the fingertip (Fig. 17.2), or a plaster of paris volar slab with a finger extension.

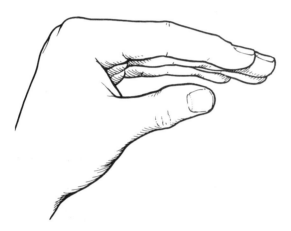

Figure 17.1 – 'Safe' position of splintage for the hand

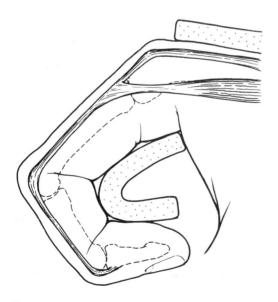

Figure 17.2 – Aluminium splint for phalangeal fractures

Assessment

Inspect the whole patient, their general state of health, physique and reaction to injury. Look at the general appearance of the hand, which may reveal chronic problems such as rheumatoid arthritis or signs of systemic disease such as clubbing or splinter haemorrhages. Look at the resting position of the hand as it may give clues of possible nerve or tendon injury.

Palpate gently, tell the patient what you are doing and ask them to tell you if they experience any pain or discomfort. Feel the temperature and moisture of the skin and assess for swelling, tenderness or crepitus. Assess sensation carefully (as described below).

Move: begin by asking the patient to make a fist and then extend their fingers, to gain a general impression of function. Ask them to flex, extend and oppose the thumb. It is then necessary to assess the function of individual tendons, especially **flexor digitorum profundus (FDP)** and **flexor digitorum superficialis (FDS)**. Testing of power as well as movement **is vital**, as with a 90% lacerated tendon movement is possible but power is decreased.

If the patient is unable to perform active movement, it is then necessary to assess passive movement to determine if pain is the limiting factor. If passive movement is full and pain free, then the assumption can be made that active movement is abnormal because of a nerve or tendon injury.

Functional anatomy of the hand

Nerve supply

The hand is innervated by the radial, median and ulnar nerves. All three nerves are involved in the control of the wrist, fingers and thumb.

Radial nerve

The radial nerve innervates only extrinsic muscles of the hand, not any of the intrinsic muscles. Its **motor** function is to innervate the forearm muscles that extend both the wrist and the MCPJs, and muscles that abduct and extend the thumb. A lesion of the radial nerve at or above the elbow, or of its main posterior interosseous branch, will produce a 'drop' wrist. Assess motor function of the radial nerve by asking the patient to actively extend the wrist against resistance (Fig. 17.3).

Sensation is supplied by the radial nerve to the radial three-quarters of the dorsum of the hand, the dorsum of the thumb and the dorsum of the index, middle and radial half of the ring finger to the level of the PIPJ. The best area to assess sensory function of the radial nerve is over the **dorsum of the first web space** (Fig. 17.4).

Median nerve

The median nerve enters the forearm through the pronator teres muscle. It is **motor** to flexor carpi radialis (FCR), palmaris longus (PL), FDS, the radial portion of FDP and flexor pollicis longus (FPL). Its thenar branch innervates abductor pollicis brevis (APB), opponens pollicis (OP) and the superficial belly of flexor pollicis brevis (FPB). The digital branch innervates the lumbricals of the index and middle fingers.

With a **proximal lesion** of the median nerve at the elbow there will be a loss of active flexion of the index finger. The commoner **distal lesion** at the level of the wrist will produce loss of abduction of the thumb. Assess by asking the patient to place the dorsum of their hand flat on a table, and point their thumb towards the ceiling against resistance (Fig. 17.5).

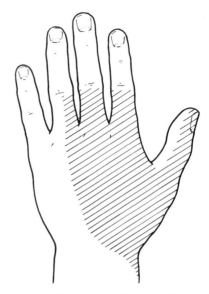

Figure 17.4 – Sensory distribution of the radial nerve in the hand

The median nerve supplies **sensation** to the palmar surface of the thumb, index, middle and radial half of the ring fingers, and the dorsal aspect of the index, middle and radial half of the ring fingers distal to the DIPJ (Fig. 17.6).

Occasionally, isolated motor median nerve loss can result if just the motor branch is lacerated, e.g. on glass.

Ulnar nerve

The ulnar nerve passes behind the medial epicondyle at the elbow. In the forearm it is

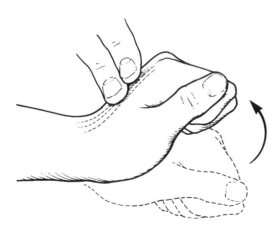

Figure 17.3 – Assessment of motor function of the radial nerve

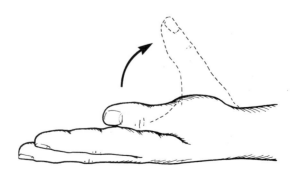

Figure 17.5 – Assessment of the motor function of the median nerve

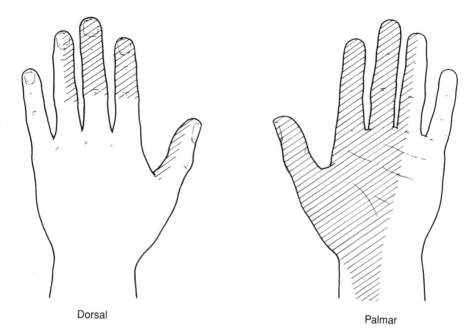

Dorsal   Palmar

Figure 17.6 – Sensory distribution of the median nerve in the hand

motor to flexor carpi ulnaris (FCU) and the ulnar part of FDP. It enters the hand through a tunnel in the wrist known as Guyon's canal. In the hand it innervates the interosseous muscles, the lumbricals to the ring and little fingers, the hypothenar muscles and adductor pollicis (AdP). Assess the motor function of the ulnar nerve by testing the power of abduction of the fingers. Ask the patient to spread their fingers wide apart and to hold them against resistance. The hand should be flat during this manoeuvre (Fig. 17.7).

Sensation is supplied to both the dorsal and volar aspects of the little and ulnar half of the ring fingers, and the ulnar quarter of the dorsum and palm of the hand (Fig. 17.8).

Sensory loss to the palmar aspect alone can result from blows with the heel of the hand against a hard object, or from lacerations affecting the superficial branch just distal to the pisiform. If the deep branch is cut in or distal to Guyon's canal, motor loss alone can result.

Assessment of nerve function in the fingers (the digital nerves) is described in the section on nerve injuries.

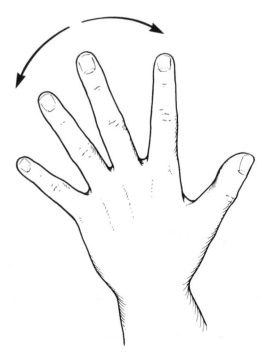

Figure 17.7 – Assessment of the motor function of the ulnar nerve

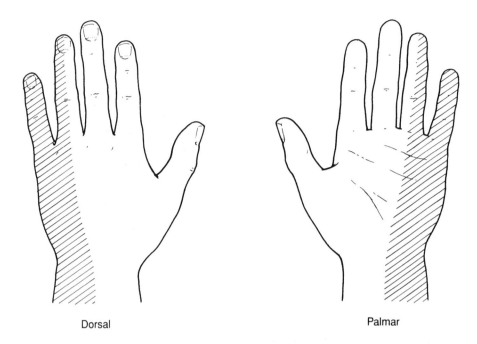

Dorsal   Palmar

Figure 17.8 – Sensory distribution of the ulnar nerve in the hand

The muscles and tendons of the hand
(Table 17.1)

The muscles and tendons of the hand are described as extrinsic or intrinsic. **Extrinsic** muscles have their belly in the forearm with the tendon insertion in the hand. **Intrinsic** muscles have both their origins and insertions in the hand.

Fractures and dislocations of the hand

Fractures of the hand are classified according to the nature and the site of the fracture. In an open fracture, management of the soft tissues is probably more important than that of the underlying fracture. On initial examination it may be obvious that a bony injury exists, but full radiographs must always be obtained. Rotational deformity must always be excluded.

Metacarpal head fractures

Closed metacarpal head fractures should be splinted with the joint in full flexion and

referred to the fracture clinic. Many of these fractures are open. Whenever a patient presents with a wound over the MCPJ, remember the possibility of a human bite (see bites), which have a high risk of infection. Patients with such injuries should be admitted.

Metacarpal neck fractures (Fig. 17.9)

The commonest metacarpal neck to be fractured is that of the little finger. The mechanism of injury is usually a punch with a clenched fist. The patient presents with pain and swelling over the fracture site, which is often palpable. The diagnosis is confirmed on radiography and the fracture is seen to be dorsally angulated.

In fractures of the ring or little finger metacarpal necks the angulation can largely be ignored unless it is gross (i.e., more than 45°), in which case manipulation under either local anaesthetic infiltration or an ulnar nerve block may be attempted. Fractures of the other metacarpals should be manipulated if the angulation is greater than 30°.

The fracture may either be splinted with neighbour strapping or held in a volar slab in

Table 17.1

Joint	Prime muscle	Nerve	Comment
1. The wrist			
Flexion	FCR	Median	Absence = weak wrist flexion
	PL	Median	
	FCU	Ulnar	
Extension	ECRL	Radial	Absence = wrist drop
	ECRB	Radial	Absence = wrist drop
Radial deviation	ECRL	Radial	
	FCR	Median	
Ulnar deviation	ECU	Radial	
	FCU	Ulnar	
2. Finger MCPJ			
Flexion	Interossei	Ulnar	Absence = claw hand
	Lumbricals	Median (index and middle fingers)	
	Lumbricals	Ulnar (ring and little fingers)	
Extension	EDC	Radial	Absence = MCP extension lag
	EIP	Radial	
Abduction	Dorsal interossei	Ulnar	
Adduction	Volar interossei	Ulnar	
3. Finger PIPJ			
Flexion	FDS	Median	Must block FDP to test
Extension	Interossei	Ulnar	
	Lumbricals	Median and ulnar	
	EDC, EIP, EDM	Radial	
4. Finger DIPJ			
Flexion	FDP	Median (index and middle fingers)	
		Ulnar (ring and little fingers)	
Extension	None	Strong DIPJ extension relies upon active PIPJ extension control	
5. Thumb CMCJ			
Flexion–adduction	AdP	Ulnar	
	Ulnar 1/2 FPB	Ulnar or Median	
	1st doral inteross.	Ulnar	
	FPL	Median	
Extension–abduction	EPL, EPB	Radial	
	APL	Radial	
	APB	Median	
Opposition	APB	Median	
	Radial 1/2 FPB	Median	
	OP	Median	
Supination	EPL	Radial	
6. Thumb MCPJ			
Flexion	FPL	Median	
	Hypothenar muscles	Ulnar	
Extension	EPB	Radial	
7. Thumb IPJ			
Flexion	FPL	Median	
Extension	EPL	Radial	

AdP, Adductor pollicis; APB, Abductor pollicis brevis; APL, Abductor pollicis longus; ECRB, Extensor carpi radialis brevis; ECRL, Extensor carpi radialis longus; ECU, Extensor carpi ulnaris; EDC, Extensor digitorum communis; EDM, Extensor digiti minimi; EIP, Extensor indicis proprius; EPB, Extensor pollicis brevis; EPL, Extensor pollicis longus; FCR, Flexor carpi radialis; FCU, Flexor carpi ulnaris; FDP, Flexor digitorum profundus; FDS, Flexor digitorum superficialis; FPB, Flexor pollicis brevis; FPL, Flexor pollicis longus; OP, Opponens pollicis; PL, Palmaris longus.

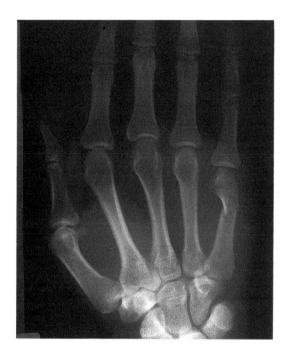

Figure 17.9 – Fracture of the metacarpal neck

Metacarpal shaft fractures (Fig. 17.11)

Fractures of the metacarpal shafts can be either transverse, oblique, spiral or comminuted. Transverse fractures usually result from a direct blow, whilst oblique or spiral fractures are due to a twisting force. The patient presents with pain, swelling and local deformity.

It is important on examination to look for **rotational deformity**; compare the plane of the nails of the partially closed hand – they should all lie on the same plane (Fig. 17.12). Another test is to look at the position of the fingers in a flexed position, they should all point towards the scaphoid. Any abnormality in either of these tests suggests a rotational deformity.

The commonest injury is an isolated, minimally displaced fracture, which requires no treatment other than neighbour strapping and

the Edinburgh position (Fig. 17.10), with a finger extension including the injured finger and its neighbour. The hand should be placed in a high arm sling and the patient referred to the fracture clinic. Fractures that are unstable following attempted reduction should be referred for consideration of internal fixation.

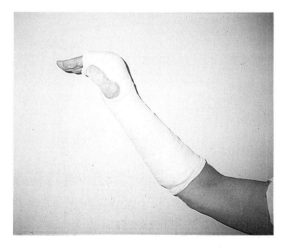

Figure 17.10 – The Edinburgh position – volar slab for metacarpal fractures

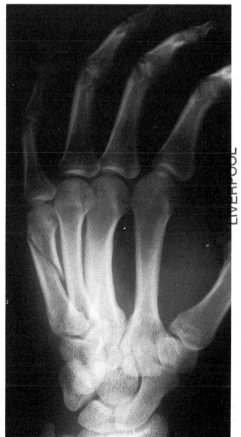

Figure 17.11 – Fracture of the metacarpal shaft

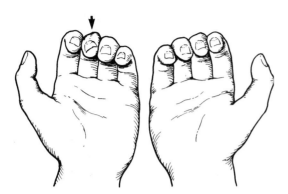

Figure 17.12 – Rotational deformity may be present in some metacarpal and proximal phalangeal fractures

a support bandage. A backslab extending to the metacarpal heads for comfort may be required. The hand should be elevated in a high arm sling and the patient referred to the fracture clinic.

Angulated fractures should be reduced by closed manipulation if the angulation is greater than 10° in the index and middle finger metacarpals, and 30° in the ring and little finger metacarpals. The position should be held in a slab. Transverse fractures with displacement should be referred for fixation. Patients with multiple metacarpal fractures or extensive soft tissue swelling must be admitted.

Fracture of the proximal and middle phalanges

The phalanx may be injured by direct violence, which usually results in transverse fractures, or by twisting forces which result in spiral fractures (Fig. 17.13). As described in the assessment of metacarpal fractures, it is **essential to exclude rotational deformities**.

Simple undisplaced fractures can be treated by neighbour strapping and early mobilization with review in the fracture clinic. Fractures with greater than 15° of angulation should be manipulated by pulling on the flexed finger with pressure on the fracture by the thumb to correct the angulation (Fig. 17.14).

The fracture requires a flexed position of the finger to maintain the reduction. This can be achieved either with a malleable splint, which can be incorporated into a plaster slab, or

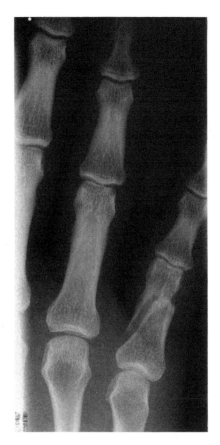

Figure 17.13 – Spiral fracture of the proximal phalanx

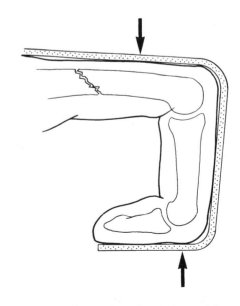

Figure 17.14 – Reduction of a phalangeal fracture

with the fingers flexed over a rolled bandage or with a plaster slab with a finger extension. To prevent rotation of the fracture, the injured finger should be strapped to its neighbour. The other fingers should be left free. The fingers should only be held in this flexed position **for a maximum of 10 days**.

Open fractures, multiple fractures and grossly unstable fractures must be referred for inpatient treatment.

Intra-articular fractures of the proximal or middle phalanges (Fig. 17.15) can be treated by neighbour strapping and mobilization unless the fragment is very large or grossly displaced, when the patient should be referred for internal fixation.

Fracture of the terminal phalanx (Fig. 17.16)

The priorities in treatment of terminal phalangeal fractures are the associated skin and soft tissue injuries, control of swelling and early mobilization, rather than the fracture itself. Exceptions to this include the Mallet type injury (described below), fractures of the epiphyseal plate (which require accurate reduction), and grossly angulated shaft fractures. The latter two injuries may require internal fixation if they are unstable.

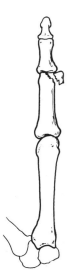

Figure 17.15 – Intra-articular fracture of the proximal phalanx

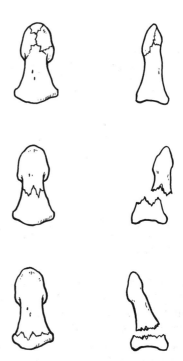

Figure 17.16 – Fractures of the terminal phalanx – tuft, shaft and base

Fractures of the base of the thumb metacarpal

A Bennett's fracture is a fracture subluxation of the base of thumb metacarpal. The particular features are:

1. The fracture line involves the trapezometacarpal joint, i.e. it is an intra-articular fracture.
2. The metacarpal is subluxed laterally.
3. The medial fragment maintains its normal relationship with the carpus.

This specific fracture should be distinguished from a simple fracture of the metacarpal base, as the management may differ (Fig. 17.17).

A Bennett's fracture must be referred for consideration of K wiring. Simple metacarpal base fractures that are either undisplaced or with minimal displacement or angulation may be treated in a plaster cast. All other fractures should be referred for probable open reduction and internal fixation.

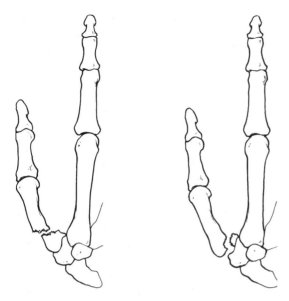

Figure 17.17 -- Fractures of the base of the thumb metacarpal – note the difference between the extra-articular fracture of the base of the metacarpal and the intra-articular Bennett's fracture

Dislocations of the MCPJ, PIPJ and DIPJ

These injuries commonly result from a hyperextension force, and are usually posterior dislocations. Although the diagnosis is usually obvious clinically, an x-ray must be taken to exclude accompanying fracture. Simple dislocations, or those with a tiny avulsion fracture, are usually reduced by traction and pressure in an anterior direction. After reduction, it is important to assess the stability of the joint to exclude a complete collateral ligament rupture. Occasionally, attempted reduction may fail in dislocations of the PIPJ, because the head of the phalanx has 'button-holed' through the volar plate. These patients require referral for open reduction.

Fracture-dislocations in which the fracture involves disruption of the joint surface should also be referred for open reduction.

Injuries to the collateral ligaments and volar plate

The collateral ligaments and volar plate form a U-shaped hood around the lateral and volar aspects of the IPJs and MCPJs. Following a hyperextension, abduction or adduction injury to the finger, the diagnosis of a simple sprain is often made, without appreciating the injury that has occurred to these structures. The PIPJ is the most commonly affected joint.

On examination, the patient usually presents with a fusiform, tender swelling around the joint. It is important to assess the stability of the joint by stressing in both lateral and hyperextension directions. This may be painful and require local anaesthesia to be performed correctly. The IPJs must be stressed in extension, and the MCPJs in flexion, as these are the positions in which the collateral ligaments are normally taut.

X-rays may show small accompanying avulsion fractures; these should not be confused with intra-articular fractures.

Complete disruption of both the collateral ligaments and the volar plate together will produce marked opening of the joint on stressing with no firm end point. These injuries should be referred as they may require surgical repair.

Much more commonly, the injury is less severe, and can be treated by splintage and early mobilization. This is usually dynamic splinting by neighbour strapping to the adjacent finger on the side of the injured ligament. Volar plate injuries may require initial splintage for a short time (maximum 2 weeks) in a padded aluminium splint followed by active mobilization.

The patient should be warned that the swelling may take several months to subside completely.

Ulnar collateral injury of the thumb

This injury, also known as gamekeeper's or skier's thumb, should be suspected in any patient who presents with an injury around the MCPJ of the thumb. Ligament rupture or avulsion may result in loss of the pincer ability of the thumb. The diagnosis is made by stressing the ligament by abducting the thumb on the metacarpal and comparing the amount of movement with the other side. This procedure can be very painful in the acutely-injured thumb, and local anaesthetic infiltration may be needed to assess the joint stability adequately.

On x-ray, a small avulsion fracture at the base of the proximal phalanx on the ulnar side may be present, which confirms the diagnosis (Fig. 17.18). If no fracture is present, stress films are required.

Management is either surgical or conservative. The age, occupation and hand dominance of the patient should be considered. Generally, if abduction at the MCPJ is greater than 20° beyond normal when compared to the uninjured thumb, surgical repair should be considered. If the angle is less than 20° and a firm end point is reached, the patient can be treated conservatively in a spica cast or splint for 3–6 weeks.

Hand wounds

Wounds of the hand can present to the Accident and Emergency Department in a variety of different forms, including clean lacerations, crush injuries, injections, burns and pulp injuries. The precise history of the injury is important, as the forces involved to produce the wound are related to the degree of tissue destruction; with more tissue destruction there is a higher risk of wound infection developing (Fig. 17.19). A wound that has been contaminated by soil will also have a higher potential for infection.

Much can be learnt about the extent of the injury by careful assessment of the hand rather than probing deep into the wound. As described above (assessment of the hand), **look**, **feel** and **move** in a structured manner in order not to miss an underlying injury. If the wound is bleeding profusely, lie the patient down, elevate the limb and apply direct pressure. **Do not clamp bleeding vessels** as nerves and tendons may inadvertently be damaged. All bleeding should eventually stop with pressure. Exclude a foreign body by x-ray if necessary. Glass, metal and some plastics will show up on x-ray, but it is important to specifically request a soft-tissue x-ray, and ask for a marker to be placed at the site of the wound.

The wound must be cleaned thoroughly. If the patient's hands are particularly dirty wash initially with simple soap and water and a degreasing agent if necessary. The wound itself should be cleaned with either saline or chlorhexidine. Hydrogen peroxide should **not** be used in cavities in the hand because the heat generated can produce pain and tissue damage.

Some wounds will require local anaesthesia to facilitate thorough cleaning. **The neurological status of the hand must be assessed prior to its use**. Lignocaine gel, local infiltration and nerve blocks can all be used, depending upon the site and extent of the injury. Carefully debride

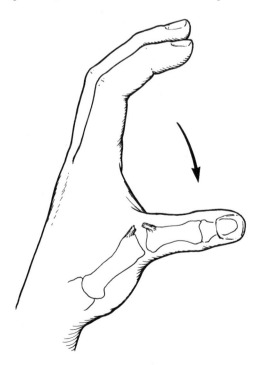

Figure 17.18 – Ulnar collateral ligament injury of the thumb

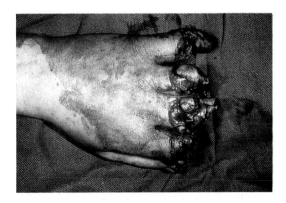

Figure 17.19 – Open hand injury

grossly contaminated or devitalized tissues, which will impair both wound healing and the ability to resist infection. **Care must be taken to remove no more tissue than is necessary**. If it is necessary to enlarge the wound for exploration, do not cross skin creases or web spaces. Do not be tempted to 'straighten' an irregular wound, this will increase tension across the wound and the patient may be left with a worse scar.

Closure of the wound can be with sutures, adhesive strips, histoacryl glue or dressings alone. Sutures should only be used if they can be placed without undue tension across the wound. They should also be avoided in wounds that are more than 8 hours old **and in any dirty injury**, e.g. foreign body stabbing injuries, bites (see below), crush injuries, penetrating garden injuries, and those wounds that will close naturally, e.g. superficial lacerations of the palm. Adhesive strips are very useful in the treatment of many hand wounds, especially fingertip injuries (see below). **Delayed primary suture must be used in wounds where there is a high risk of infection**.

Prophylactic antibiotics are rarely required as they are no substitute for thorough cleaning and careful debridement. If they are used, they ideally need to be given within 3 hours of the injury, and before wound treatment. Prophylactic antibiotics are given for some bites and open fractures. The choice of antibiotic should be governed by local hospital policy. **Remember to check the tetanus status of the patient**.

A particular wound to note is that sustained from the high pressure injection of oil or paint. Damage to tissues occurs as a result of both tension and the toxic effect of the substance involved. The degree of tissue destruction is usually considerably worse than suggested by the outer appearance of the wound. Patients with any of these injuries should be referred.

Tendon injuries in the hand

Extensor tendon injuries

Injuries of the extensor apparatus of the hand can be divided into three groups.

1. The dorsum of the hand.
2. Central slip injuries.
3. Mallet finger injuries.

Extensor apparatus injuries on the dorsum of the hand

Over the dorsum of the hand, the extensors work in mass action due to interconnecting bands which pass between them. This means that if only one or two tendons are cut, the ends do not retract and are therefore relatively easy to repair. This should be performed only with senior supervision using a non-absorbable monofilament suture. Tendon injuries due to crush forces or where there is a high risk of infection should undergo secondary repair.

Middle or central slip injuries (Fig. 17.20)

At the dorsal aspect of the proximal phalanx, the extensor mechanism divides into three parts: two lateral slips and a central slip. The lateral slips later rejoin and insert into the base of the terminal phalanx; the central slip inserts into the base of the middle phalanx.

Trauma to the dorsum of the PIPJ can lead to injury to the central slip at this point. The tendon may be lacerated, ruptured or contused. If this injury is not detected, the central slip becomes necrotic over the following 5–6 weeks. The lateral slips migrate sideways, allowing the PIPJ to button-hole through the defect in the extensor tendons, preventing the patient extending at the PIPJ. This is a **Boutonnière**

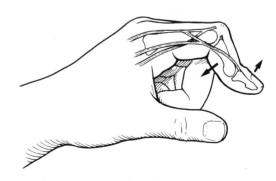

Figure 17.20 – Central slip rupture resulting in a Boutonnière deformity

deformity. Thus, detection of this injury is vital at initial presentation. Both function **and strength** must be assessed, as decreased power against resistance may be the only positive finding. Beware also the closed dislocation of the PIPJ which may have been reduced before the patient presents – there may be a central slip injury.

If a fragment of bone is avulsed or an open wound is present the patient should be referred for surgical repair. Closed injuries with no fracture can be treated with splintage; the PIPJ is splinted in extension for 6 weeks, leaving the DIPJ free to move.

Mallet finger injury (Fig. 17.21)

This common injury results from avulsion of the extensor tendon from its insertion at the base of the terminal phalanx. The tendon alone may be avulsed, or it may take a flake of bone with it. The mechanism of injury is usually forced flexion of the DIPJ from an extended position, e.g. in bed-making. The injury can also result from a 'stubbing' injury, e.g. catching a cricket ball, when the bone fragment may be larger.

Clinically the patient presents with drooping of the terminal phalanx, **with no active extension at the DIPJ** (Fig. 17.22). Most cases can be satisfactorily treated in a mallet splint for 6–8 weeks. The patient should be reviewed after 1–2 weeks, as a smaller splint may be required as the

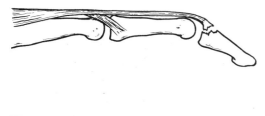

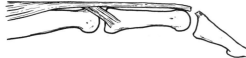

Figure 17.21 – Mallet finger injury – results from either an avulsion fracture or a 'pure' tendon rupture

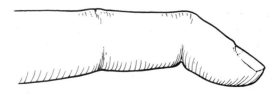

Figure 17.22 – Clinical appearance of a mallet finger – there is a loss of active extension at the DIP joint

swelling decreases. Full advice should be given regarding removal of the splint for washing whilst keeping the joint extended, and not to 'test' the function before the 6–8 weeks are up. They should also be warned of the possibility that the terminal phalanx may always have a slight 'droop'.

When the bone fragment involves more than one-third of the articular surface K wiring may be required to prevent volar subluxation of the terminal phalanx.

Flexor tendon injuries

The management of flexor tendon injuries in the Accident and Emergency Department consists of diagnosis and referral. When assessing function it is vital to assess both the function **and strength** of flexor digitorum profundus (FDP) and flexor digitorum superficialis (FDS) separately. It is often helpful to demonstrate to the patient what you are wanting them to do on an uninjured finger first.

To assess FDS, hold all three uninjured fingers in extension – this immobilizes the FDP of the injured finger. Ask the patient to flex the injured finger. Any active flexion must now be due to FDS (Fig. 17.23).

FDP can be assessed by holding the PIPJ of the injured finger in extension so that FDS cannot function. Ask the patient to flex the finger at the DIPJ; this movement is using FDP (Fig. 17.24).

Although lacerations are the commonest cause of flexor tendon injuries, FDP can occasionally be ruptured without skin injury by a sudden extensor strain against the flexed fingertip.

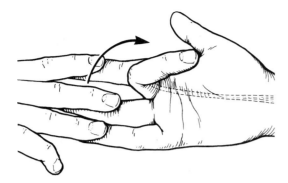

Figure 17.23 – Assessment of FDS function

All suspected flexor tendon injuries must be referred for specialist repair.

Nerve injuries in the hand

In any injury of the hand which may cause nerve damage, the sensory and motor function **must** be fully assessed. Injuries to nerves can be classified as:

1. **Neuropraxia** – blunt contusion.
2. **Axonotemesis** – this is more severe contusion which causes destruction of the nerve fibres but the myelin sheath is preserved.
3. **Neurotemesis** – complete transection of the nerve, and can only occur in penetrating trauma.

The hand is innervated by the median, radial and ulnar nerves, and **the sensory and motor modalities of each nerve should be assessed individually** (see Figs 17.3–17.8).

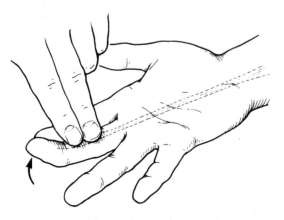

Figure 17.24 – Assessment of FDP function

The commonest nerve injury in the hand is complete or partial transection of a **digital nerve** complicating a laceration of a digit. If, on questioning, the patient complains of a subjective sense of numbness, **a partial nerve lesion must be present**, even if objective examination is normal. When assessing sensibility, 2-point discrimination is a more sensitive and helpful test than simple pinprick or soft touch testing. A bent paper clip is sufficient. If the patient is unable to distinguish 2 points more than 6 mm apart, this indicates nerve division or severe contusion.

Nerve division also causes loss of sympathetic innervation, and **the skin becomes dry** rather than its normal, slightly moist state. When dragging a ball point pen across normal skin, slight friction should be encountered; with nerve division the pen slides freely across the dry skin.

In children assessment of nerve injuries is often very difficult. A useful test is to immerse the hand in water for 5–10 minutes. Normally innervated glabrous skin will wrinkle, whereas denervated skin will not.

All open nerve injuries should be treated by exploration and repair, and therefore referred to the appropriate specialist.

Soft tissue injuries and infections of the hand

Hand infections

The management of hand infections starts with their prevention. Thorough wound cleaning and debridement, together with tetanus prophylaxis as required, is the mainstay of all hand wound management. However many patients do not present until infection is established. Common organisms involved are staphylococci, streptococci, occasionally *Escherichia coli* and mixed infection in 25% of cases.

When assessing the hand always remember the patient as a whole; certain conditions predispose to hand infections, including diabetes, ischaemia, some neurological conditions, steroids and intravenous drug abuse. General principles of management include rest, elevation, antibiotics and drainage of pus. **Always** ask for senior advice if unsure, as many hand infections require admission. The outcome of a mismanaged hand infection can be devastating.

Paronychia

This is an infection of the soft tissue around the finger nail, usually caused by a staphylococcal infection (Fig. 17.25). It requires incision and drainage either where the abscess points through the overlying skin, or under the eponychium along the lateral nail fold. If this is performed, routine antibiotics are not required.

Pulp space infection

The patient presents with a swollen, red, tender pulp which is extremely painful (Fig. 17.26). These infections, which are commonly caused by staphylococci, usually require drainage. An x-ray should be performed to exclude osteomyelitis of the distal phalanx (also consider tuberculous osteomyelitis). Drainage should be performed either over the site of maximal tenderness (usually mid-pulp), or via an anterolateral approach 5 mm beyond the distal digital crease, extending into the pulp space. The pulp should be curettaged and debrided. The incision **must not** be sutured afterwards.

Tendon sheath infections (purulent tenosynovitis)

Infections of the tendon sheath may be primary (from a wound) or secondary (from an adjacent focus). Staphylococci and streptococci are the

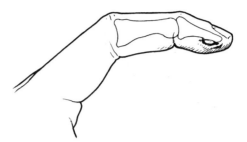

Figure 17.26 – Pulp space infection

commonest organisms involved. The patient presents with a swollen finger, held in a slightly flexed position, with tenderness over the flexor tendon sheath, and **pain on passive extension of the finger**. These findings are known collectively as **Kanavel's cardinal signs**.

Because of the anatomy of the tendon sheaths, an infection of the **thumb** or **little finger** may extend to the wrist, leading to the classic horse-shoe infection. Infections of the index, middle and ring finger can only extend to the palm (Fig. 17.27).

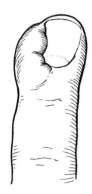

Figure 17.25 – Paronychia

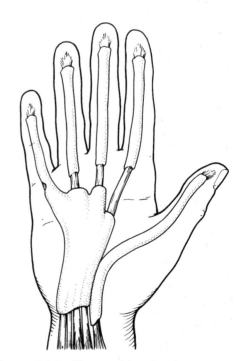

Figure 17.27 – Flexor tendon sheath anatomy. Note that infection of the tendon sheaths of the thumb and little finger may spread.

All tendon sheath infections must be referred for in-patient treatment, involving operative drainage, antibiotics and elevation.

Space infections

These uncommon infections can occur in the **thenar, web or palmar spaces** of the hand. Presentation may involve swelling actually over the dorsum of the hand, but maximal pain and tenderness will be elicited over the volar aspect. These serious infections must all be referred for surgical exploration.

Bites

Both human and animal bites are a common presentation to the Accident and Emergency Department. Human saliva contains staphylococci, streptococci, proteus species, anaerobes and other organisms. Dog and cat saliva also contains *Pasteurella multocida*. All these organisms can cause serious infection and destruction of local tissues. Human bites are frequently not reported as such, and careful history-taking is required.

All bites are potentially infected and should be thoroughly cleaned, irrigated and debrided as appropriate. Remove any tooth fragments in the wound. **The wound must not be sutured** but left to heal by secondary intention. If necessary, the wound can be closed 3 days later by delayed primary closure if no infection is present. Bites on the face may require primary suture to achieve an acceptable cosmetic appearance, and this should be the only exception to the rule concerning closure.

Patients with all but the most superficial wounds should be given prophylactic antibiotics according to local policy. **Remember to check tetanus status in all patients**. Beware the particular case of the human bite over the MCPJ, caused by a fist against an opponent's teeth. These wounds have a high risk of tendon, joint and cartilage injury, and of developing pyogenic arthritis or osteomyelitis. They **must** be referred to the specialist team for exploration and antibiotics.

Fingertip injuries

As fingertips and nails are constantly exposed, they are frequently injured and are a common presentation to Accident and Emergency departments. The aims of management are to provide:

- A useful, pain-free fingertip.
- Good sensation.
- An acceptable cosmetic appearance.
- Preservation of length if possible.
- A short morbidity with early return to normal activities.

Anatomy (Fig. 17.28)

The fingertip is that part of the finger distal to the insertion of the extensor and flexor tendons into the base of the distal phalanx. The pulp provides sensation and grip. The tuft of the distal phalanx is well padded by fat, with multiple fibrosepta tethering the skin to the underlying periosteum.

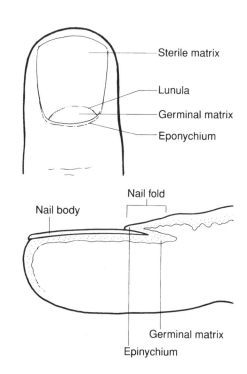

Figure 17.28 – The fingertip

The complex of the nail and its surrounding folds is known as the perionychium. It is important in providing additional stabilization to the pulp, and is also thought to enhance sensation of the tip. The nail body (or nail plate) is a keratinized structure arising from the germinal matrix in the nail fold. The cuticle is known as the eponychium, and bridges the nail body to the dorsal skin of the nail complex. The nail is firmly attached to the nail bed. The nail bed is comprised of proximal germinal matrix and distal sterile matrix. The lunula (moon) is the semi-circular division between the two. The nail is firmly adherent to the distal nail bed, but not adherent to the lunula, and only weakly adherent beneath the nail fold. This explains the pattern of injury seen with nail avulsions as described below.

Nail bed injuries (Fig. 17.29)

Lacerations and tears of the nail bed should be carefully repaired to avoid a permanently deformed nail. Avulsion of the nail from beneath the nail fold, whilst still adherent to the distal nail bed, is a common injury. This will be accompanied by a laceration in the nail bed, with or without a fracture of the distal phalanx. The nail needs to be removed in order to repair the nail bed. Most surgeons recommend careful repair of the bed with a fine absorbable suture, e.g. 6/0 nylon. The adjacent skin should also be repaired with a non-absorbable suture. There are some reports of good results by simple accurate replacement of the nail and holding it in place with adhesive strips.

The injury is sometimes accompanied by an angulated fracture of the distal phalanx. In adults, this will require a K wire to maintain a normal position after manipulation. In children, repair of the nail bed or adhesive strips may be sufficient to hold the position of the reduced fracture.

Once the nail bed is repaired, the nail can be replaced in situ once it has been gently cleaned. If the nail is too badly damaged to be used, some surgeons advocate a membrane of paraffin gauze to be placed between the nail fold and the nail bed to prevent the eponychium sticking to the nail bed. Others recommend simply dressing with non-adhesive paraffin gauze.

The whole finger should be dressed, elevated and reviewed in 3–7 days.

Finger tip amputation and tissue loss (Fig. 17.30)

The appropriate treatment depends upon the level and plane of the injury, the functional requirements of the patient, which digit is injured and the skill of the doctor. A number of different techniques exist, none of which is ideal. The simplest method appropriate for the situation should be chosen. Preserving the length of the finger is desirable, but not

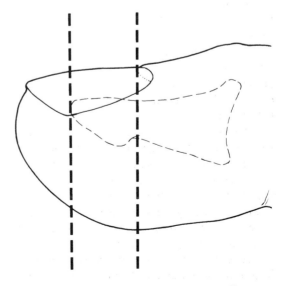

Figure 17.30 – Levels of finger tip amputations

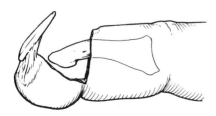

Figure 17.29 – Nail bed avulsion

essential. A pain-free pulp with good sensation is the desired result. However, preservation of length in the thumb is important, and if exposed bone cannot be covered easily the patient should be referred to the appropriate specialist.

Conservative management is most suitable for injuries to the pulp distal to the distal phalanx when bone is not exposed. The wound should be cleaned and a non-adherent paraffin gauze dressing applied. Regular review is required to ensure a pyogenic granuloma does not develop, every 2–5 days depending on the individual situation.

Larger defects with substantial loss of pulp skin and tissue (usually greater than 1cm diameter, although this will obviously depend on the size of the finger), and wounds with bone exposed **must** be discussed with senior colleagues. Elective shortening, primary suture, split-skin grafts, flap grafts or conservative management are all possible forms of treatment, depending upon the injury and the needs of the patient.

Fingertip injuries in children

The fingertips of children have remarkable powers of regeneration. Under 12 years of age, conservative management of injuries, even where bone is exposed, is the treatment of choice. This is with non-adherent dressings, which are periodically changed until healing is completed. The cosmetic results are usually excellent, and it is important to reassure the worried parents of this expected outcome. Good results with conservative management have been achieved even with amputation just proximal to the nail.

Part IV
The Lower Limb

18

Applied anatomy of the lower limb

The bones of the lower limb

The bones of the lower limb are shown in Figs 18.1–18.4.

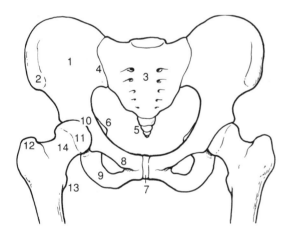

Figure 18.1 – AP of the pelvis
1. Ileum
2. Anterior superior iliac spine
3. Sacrum
4. Sacro-iliac joint
5. Coccyx
6. Pelvic brim
7. Pubic symphysis
8. Superior pubic ramus
9. Inferior pubic ramus
10. Acetabulum
11. Femoral head
12. Greater trochanter
13. Lesser trochanter
14. Femoral neck

The nerves of the lower limb

Space permits only an outline of the nerve supply of the lower limb.

The lumbo-sacral plexus

The lower limb derives its nerve supply from the segments L2–S2 via the lumbar and sacral plexaes. The lumbo-sacral plexus is situated on the posterior abdominal wall. Rarely it may be damaged in back and pelvic injuries.

The femoral nerve (L2,3,4)

The femoral nerve arises from the lumbar plexus and passes beneath the inguinal ligament to supply the anterior thigh. It is motor to the quadriceps muscle and sensory to the anterior thigh. It also gives off a sensory branch, the **saphenous nerve**, which supplies the skin on the medial aspect of the lower leg and foot.

The femoral nerve may be damaged by pelvic injuries and in particular anterior dislocation of the hip. The nerve can be assessed by active extension of the knee.

The obturator nerve (L2,3,4)

The obturator nerve is motor to the adductor muscles of the thigh and sensory to the medial aspect of the thigh. It is very rarely damaged in trauma. However, note that posterior abdominal and pelvic tumours may present with medial thigh pain via this nerve.

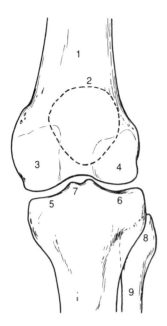

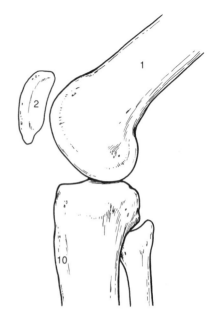

Figure 18.2 – AP and lateral views of the knee

1. **Shaft of femur**
2. Patella
3. Medial femoral condyle
4. Lateral femoral condyle
5. Medial tibial plateau

6. Lateral tibial plateau
7. Anterior and posterior tibial spines
8. Head of fibula
9. Neck of fibula
10. Tibial tuberosity

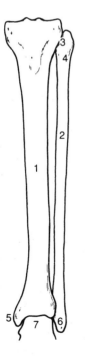

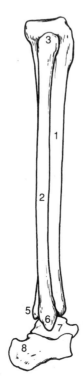

Figure 18.3 – AP and lateral views of tibia and fibula

1. Tibia
2. Fibula
3. Head of fibula
4. Neck of fibula
5. Medial malleolus
6. Lateral malleolus
7. Talus
8. Calcaneum

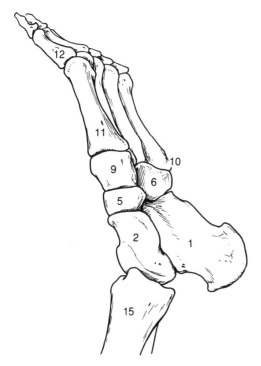

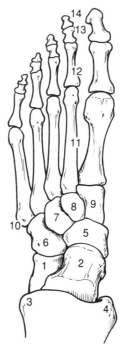

Figure 18.4 – AP and lateral views of the foot
1. Calcaneum
2. Talus
3. Medial malleolus
4. Lateral malleolus
5. Navicular
6. Cuboid
7. Lateral cuneiform
8. Intermediate cuneiform
9. Medial cuneiform
10. Base of fifth metatarsal
11. Metatarsal shafts
12. Proximal phalanx
13. Middle phalanx
14. Distal phalanx
15. Tibia

The lateral cutaneous nerve of the thigh (L2)

This nerve, a branch of the lumbar plexus, is sensory to a large strip of skin along the lateral thigh. Although rarely damaged by trauma, it may become irritated, producing troublesome thigh pain – this is termed **meralgia paraesthetica.**

The sciatic nerve (L4,5, S1,2,3)

The sciatic nerve supplies the rest of the lower limb not innervated by the femoral and obturator nerves. The main trunk supplies the hamstring muscles. It divides at around the level of the knee (variably) into two main trunks:

1. **The tibial nerve** – motor to the muscles of the popliteal fossa and calf, and sensory to the back of the calf and the sole of the foot.
2. **The common peroneal nerve** – motor to the extensor and peroneal muscles of the lower leg, and sensory to the shin area and dorsum of the foot.

The sciatic nerve itself is most commonly damaged in pelvic injuries, notably posterior dislocations of the hip. Other causes of damage include iatrogenic (surgical division, inadvertent buttock injections) and pelvic disease. A complete high sciatic nerve division will result in paralysis of the hamstrings and all the muscles of the lower leg (with a foot drop) in addition to a profound sensory loss in the foot.

The common peroneal nerve is commonly damaged in trauma. Causes include fractures and dislocations around the knee, direct trauma and iatrogenic injury from poorly applied casts and braces. The result is a footdrop and some sensory loss on the dorsum of the foot. Assess its function by the power of dorsiflexion.

The tibial nerve is rarely damaged in isolation as a result of trauma. The consequence is loss of the plantar-flexors of the ankle and sensory loss on the sole of the foot.

Segmental and peripheral sensory supply to the lower limb

The segmental sensory supply is summarized in Fig. 18.5 and that by peripheral nerves in Figs 18.6 and 18.7.

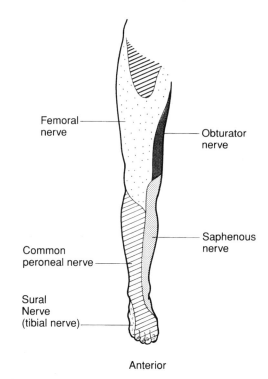

Figure 18.6 – Peripheral nerve sensory supply to the anterior aspect of the lower limb

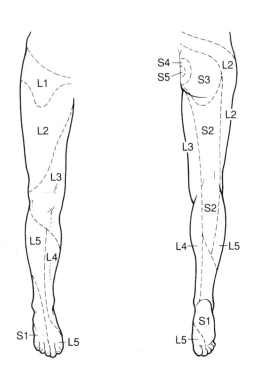

Figure 18.5 – Segmental sensory supply of the lower limb

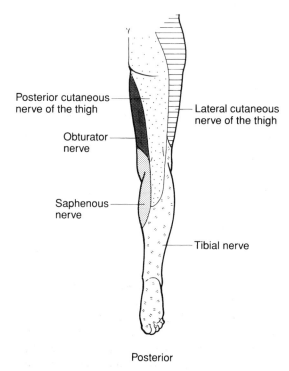

Figure 18.7 – Peripheral nerve sensory supply to the posterior aspect of the lower limb

19
Pelvic injuries

Pelvic fractures

Introduction and pathological anatomy

Pelvic fractures are an important group of injuries to diagnose and treat, both in terms of mortality and long-term morbidity. It is important to realize that the pelvis is not simply a bony structure – it contains many viscera and blood vessels etc., which may be damaged along with bony injury. It is also essential to understand that a patient may die from hypovolaemic shock simply through sustaining a pelvic injury; **pelvic injuries must be positively excluded in all major trauma**. In many cases, the bony fracture is not as important to the life of the patient as damage done to the viscera contained within it.

The visceral structures contained within the pelvis

Blood vessels

The single most important life-threatening complication from a pelvic injury is **haemorrhage** leading to **hypovolaemic shock**. The pelvis itself contains many large blood vessels (e.g. the iliac arteries and veins), which may be damaged as part of a pelvic injury. In addition, however, the bones and joints of the pelvis may bleed profusely when damaged, and this alone can result in death if untreated. Hence adequate fluid, and in particular blood, replacement is necessary in

many of these injuries (see Chapter 4 on the management of major trauma).

Urological structures

The bladder and urethra are at risk from anterior pelvic fractures, e.g. pubic rami fractures. In significant pelvic injuries it is therefore essential positively to exclude injuries to these structures.

1. The bladder may be torn, resulting in extraperitoneal or intraperitoneal extravasation of urine, depending upon the fullness of the bladder at the time of injury.
2. The membranous urethra may be torn, either partially or completely. The classical signs of urethral rupture are **blood at the urethral meatus, a high riding prostate gland on rectal examination, perineal bruising and rectal bleeding**. In such a patient it is **essential** to avoid retrograde urethral catheterization, lest a partial urethral tear be converted to a complete tear. If urethral injury is suspected, a urological surgeon should be summoned, so that a urethral injury can be excluded (e.g. by a retrograde urethrogram) and a suprapubic catheter inserted if necessary.
3. The penile portion of the urethra may be damaged by direct trauma, e.g. with falls astride objects.

Neurological structures

Some neurological structures (the sacral nerve roots and the lumbo-sacral trunk) may be damaged as part of a pelvic injury. Consequences include overflow incontinence and impotence. Whilst incontinence often resolves with time, impotence may be permanent.

Other structures

Any other structure within the pelvis may, more rarely, be damaged as part of a pelvic injury. The rectum is occasionally damaged, and rectal examination is **mandatory** in any pelvic injury. Gynaecological structures are also at risk. Collection of retroperitoneal blood may precipitate a **paralytic ileus**.

As many pelvic injuries imply a significant level of trauma to the patient, a full examination of the patient should be performed. A commonly missed associated injury, especially with vertical shear fractures of the hemipelvis (see below) is **rupture of the diaphragm**, usually on the left – this can be difficult to diagnose, but if suspected can be confirmed with chest radiographs and the passage of a nasogastric tube which may be seen within the thorax.

The concept of a pelvic ring

It is helpful to consider the bony structures of the pelvis as forming a ring (Fig 19.1). The ring consists of:

- the sacrum posteriorly, connected by –
- the sacroiliac ligaments (very strong) to –
- the hemipelvis, joined anteriorly by –
- the pubic symphysis.

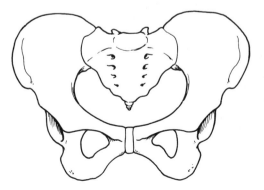

Figure 19.1 – The bony structures of the pelvis form a ring

As a principle, attempt to differentiate:

(a) isolated injuries of the pelvis in one place:
e.g. isolated pubic ramus fracture;
e.g. fracture of the wing of the ilium;

from

(b) a disruption of the ring in two places:
e.g. fracture of the pubic rami in association with 'opening' of the sacroiliac ligament.

In general terms, ring disruption implies a more significant injury, with a greater risk of instability, haemorrhage and visceral injury.

Pelvic fractures – classification and management

Classification of pelvic fractures

Many specialized classifications of pelvic fractures exist; however, they are not especially useful in the acute setting, and are more designed for decisions regarding reconstruction of the pelvis. A more simple designation of pelvic fractures is:

1. Avulsion fractures around the pelvis.
2. Isolated fractures of the pelvis, sacrum and coccyx.
3. Undisplaced disruptions of the pelvic ring.
4. Displaced disruptions of the pelvic ring.
5. Acetabular fractures including central dislocation of the hip.

Avulsion fractures around the pelvis

These are relatively common injuries, most often occurring in teenage athletic individuals with an immature skeleton. In these a small fragment of bone (usually epiphysis) is avulsed as a result of violent muscular action. Examples include:

1. Iliac crest – abdominal musculature (obliques etc.).
2. Ischial tuberosity – hamstring muscles.
3. Anterior superior iliac spine – sartorius.

4. Anterior inferior iliac spine – rectus femoris (Fig. 19.2).
5. Posterior superior iliac spine – back musculature.
6. Pubis – adductor muscles of the leg.

The symptoms can be treated conservatively with initial rest and analgesia, followed by physiotherapy if necessary.

Isolated fractures of the pelvis, sacrum and coccyx

These fractures are differentiated from pelvic ring disruptions both in their usual lesser level of causative violence and in their management. Examples include:

1. Pubic rami fractures (Fig. 19.3) – these are common, and may be single or double on the same side of the pelvis (NB: they may occur additionally as **part** of a pelvic disruption). They typically occur in osteoporotic bone, and it is essential to exclude them if there is pain in the pelvic region following a fall in the elderly (they are often missed in the absence of a fracture of the proximal femur).
2. Undisplaced fractures of the blade of the ilium.
3. Minimal displacement (sprain) of the sacroiliac joint (displacement denoting a ring disruption).
4. Fractures of the sacrum – most are of the isolated type, and may be transverse or vertical. Most are not complicated by neurological involvement, although this may occur.

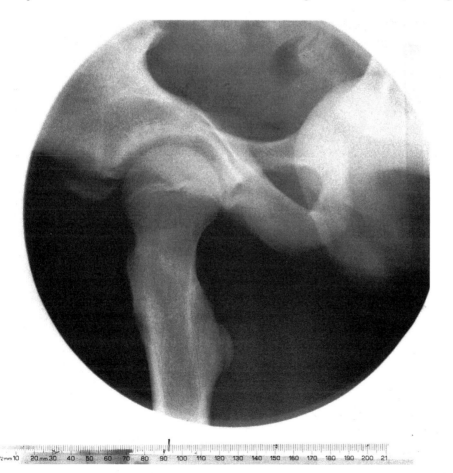

Figure 19.2 – Avulsion fracture of the anterior inferior iliac spine

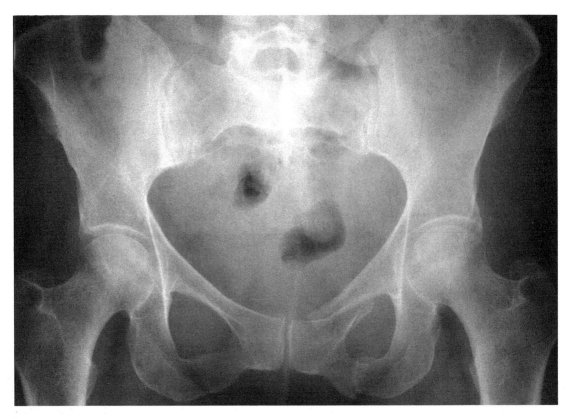

Figure 19.3 – Fractures of the superior and inferior pubic rami

Most are neuropraxias but some lesions may demand later exploration. Neurological involvement is denoted by **overflow incontinence, saddle anaesthesia and sacral nerve root involvement in the lower limbs.**
5. Coccygeal fractures – usually result from a fall onto the region, and many fracture patterns occur. They are not associated with significant neurological deficit, although they do have a troublesome tendency toward prolonged symptoms (**coccydynia**).

The vast majority of these isolated fractures are treated symptomatically, although admission may be warranted for analgesia, mobilization or social reasons.

Undisplaced disruptions of the pelvic ring

These are usually the result of a compressive force upon the pelvis, with the ring disrupted in two or more places. However, the fragments retain their approximate position with each other. Examples include:

1. Multiple pubic rami fractures on **both** sides of the pelvis (Fig. 19.4).

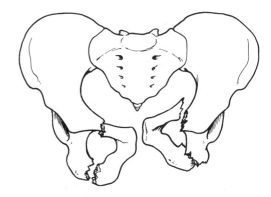

Figure 19.4 – Bilateral superior and inferior pubic rami, constituting a double break of the pelvic ring

2. Diastasis (i.e., separation) of the pubic symphysis in association with a pubic ramus fracture. (NB: note that an apparently isolated diastasis of the pubic symphysis is nearly always associated with damage to the posterior structures of the pelvis).

These injuries are often associated with damage to the pelvic viscera, notably the bladder and urethra. Although they may be severe, the orthopaedic aspects are usually managed conservatively with bed rest for 6–8 weeks.

Displaced disruptions of the pelvic ring

These are the most severe of pelvic injuries, and are again usually compressive in their aetiology. They include the classical 'open book' fracture where the blades of the ilium are literally forced apart by the compressive force. The incidence of visceral damage is high, as is the tendency to haemorrhage. Examples include:

1. Pubic rami fractures in association with disruption of the sacroiliac joint.
2. Pubic rami fractures in association with a sacral fracture.
3. Diastasis of the pubic symphysis in association with sacroiliac disruption (Fig. 19.5).
4. Vertical shear fracture of the sacroiliac joint in association with an injury elsewhere in the pelvic ring (Fig. 19.6).

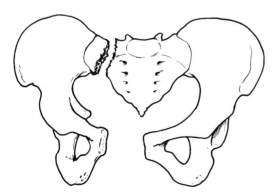

Figure 19.5 - Diastasis (separation) of the symphysis pubis in association with a sacral fracture

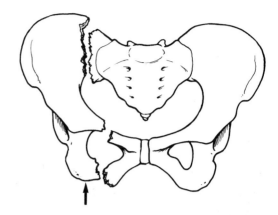

Figure 19.6 – Vertical shear fracture of the right hemipelvis

The management of these injuries **must** include a thorough general assessment of the patient, as over 50% are associated with significant injury in another area. Hypovolaemic shock should be anticipated, as large volumes of blood may be lost into the retroperitoneum (an average of 6 units of blood with sacroiliac disruption). **Early orthopaedic involvement is necessary**, as the fracture may need reduction using an external fixator (this can be life-saving by tamponading bleeding from the sacroiliac veins).

Acetabular fractures including central dislocation of the hip

These fractures result from the femoral head being driven through the acetabular floor, often by a force transmitted through the greater trochanter or vertically through the lower limb (Fig. 19.7). They may, as in all pelvic fractures, be associated with visceral damage. These fractures require careful orthopaedic assessment, as any significant incongruity of the acetabular articular surface inevitably results in secondary degenerative change.

Central dislocation of the hip may occur as part of an acetabular fracture. The leg is in a neutral position (contrast with anterior and posterior dislocations), and the hip may require traction for reduction. Visceral complications are common.

Acetabular fractures with no significant joint incongruency generally require bed rest with

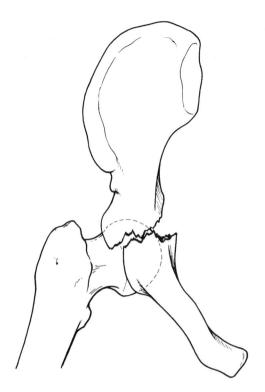

Figure 19.7 – Central dislocation of the hip; note the acetabular fracture

traction for 6 weeks; displaced fractures, especially in the younger person, may require surgical reconstruction.

Soft tissue injuries in the pelvic region

Injuries of the soft tissues around the pelvis are common, especially in the athletic individual. Many do not present in the acute setting, and are essentially overuse injuries, e.g. chronic adductor strain, sacroiliac strain. However, a number may present acutely, and these will be further discussed below. A thorough history and examination are essential in such cases.

Soft tissue injuries in the adolescent

These generally consist of traction injuries of the apophysis ('avulsion fractures'). A deforming force disrupts musculo-skeletal systems at the weakest point, and in the immature skeleton this is at the insertion of a tendon. In the skeletally mature the muscle itself tends to be affected.

Soft tissue injuries in the adult

Stress fractures

These are difficult to diagnose. Stress fractures may occur within the ischial or pubic rami, or more importantly, the femoral neck. The vital history is that of increasing exercise-induced pain in the region without a significant traumatic episode. The fracture site is generally tender, but radiographs are often negative for up to 6 weeks. If a stress fracture is suspected, a bone scan may be necessary. In general the treatment is conservative, but stress fractures of the femoral neck need very careful supervision lest they become complete fractures, and demand urgent referral in the first instance.

'Groin strain'

This is a very common complaint in young athletes, e.g. soccer players. The adductor muscles are usually responsible.

In the adult the most common cause is a strain of the tendinous origin of **adductor longus**, a tendon which may easily be felt as it arises from the inferior pubic ramus. Tenderness is noted over the tendon, with pain on passive abduction and resisted adduction. The treatment is conservative. The adductor longus muscle itself may, more rarely, rupture; unless the patient is a high-class athlete, the treatment is again conservative (repair is feasible in certain cases).

Another common injury pattern is a strain of the **ilio-psoas** as it inserts into the lesser trochanter of the femur. The tendon is painful anteriorly over the hip joint, with pain on passive flexion and resisted extension of the hip joint. Treatment is again conservative.

Many other injury patterns may occur, e.g. gluteal strain in forced hip flexion, and are treated on conservative lines.

Meralgia paraesthetica

This constitutes entrapment of the lateral cutaneous nerve of the thigh as it passes beneath the lateral portion of the inguinal ligament. It may present acutely, although it usually manifests in a more chronic setting. Paraesthesiae are present along the anterolateral aspect of the thigh. Treatment is usually conservative, although a number of refractory cases may need to undergo decompression of the nerve.

20

The hip joint and proximal femur

Traumatic dislocation of the non-prosthetic hip joint

Introduction and classification

Traumatic dislocation of the (non-prosthetic) hip joint is a very significant injury. It demands early diagnosis and treatment, so that its complications (including subsequent avascular necrosis of the femoral head) can be avoided. It is notoriously easy to miss in the presence of other injuries in multiple trauma – it is **essential** to exclude a dislocated hip in any significant lower limb trauma, but especially so in:

1. Fractures of the shaft of the femur.
2. Fractures of the patella.
3. Fractures of the calcaneum following a fall from a height.

In all hip dislocations, it is **mandatory** to establish the integrity of the sciatic nerve both before and after reduction – up to 10% of dislocated hips are associated with sciatic nerve palsy.

Hip dislocations can be classified as:

1. Posterior.
2. Anterior.
3. Central.

Posterior dislocation of the hip

Posterior dislocations are by far the most common form of hip dislocation, and are generally caused by a severe force transmitted through the shaft of the femur or via the greater trochanter. There is a frequent association with other lower limb injuries.

The dislocation may be a 'pure' type, or may be associated with a fracture of a portion of the acetabular rim. (Acetabular fractures offer a worse prognosis, as they give the hip less stability, often need surgery, increase the risk of degenerative arthritis, and are associated with an increased incidence of sciatic nerve injury). In addition, femoral head and neck fractures may be associated with the dislocation.

The clinical picture is that of a patient in **significant pain**, often said to be the worst pain experienced from a single injury. Other fractures may be present. **The lower limb is short, adducted, flexed and internally rotated** (internal rotation being the 'hallmark' of posterior dislocation, Fig. 20.1). The **sciatic nerve** may be compromised, and its integrity should therefore be established and documented in writing. (A quick examination of the sciatic nerve's integrity can be done by checking dorsiflexion at the ankle and sensation in the sole of the foot).

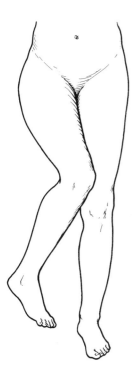

Figure 20.1 – Posterior dislocation of the hip – note that the limb is short, adducted and internally rotated

The diagnosis is usually apparent clinically, but should be confirmed by radiography (this is one of the types of dislocation where the doctrine of 'relocation before radiography' can be set aside). It is essential that both an anteroposterior and lateral x-ray is taken where a dislocation is suspected. In view of the risk of avascular necrosis (see below), arrangements for x-ray should be immediate.

Reduction of posterior dislocation

Dislocation of the hip is a **surgical emergency**, and reduction should be carried out without delay, as if the hip is left dislocated for more than 6 hours, the risk of avascular necrosis of the femoral head is classically said to be increased. Reduction should be performed by experienced orthopaedic surgeons, but it is essential to have knowledge of reduction technique in case senior cover is unavailable.

The procedure is best done under general anaesthetic, but circumstances may dictate the procedure to be performed under sedation in the Accident and Emergency Department. In either case, adequate **muscle relaxation** is necessary to overcome the very large muscle groups around the hip. It is often easier to perform the reduction with the patient brought down to floor level, as a better mechanical advantage can be achieved. A little muscle power is necessary!

There are a number of reduction techniques available.

1. The most satisfactory method is the 'reduction by opposing forces' technique:

- The patient's pelvis must be securely fixed by an assistant pushing down on both anterior superior iliac spines.
- The knee and hip are flexed to 90°. ⎫
- The internal rotation of the thigh is corrected. ⎬ these steps correcting the hip position to neutral
- The adduction of the thigh is corrected. ⎭
- The hip is then pulled back into its acetabulum by direct traction (Fig. 20.2) in the line of the femur (and this is where adequate muscle relaxation is useful).

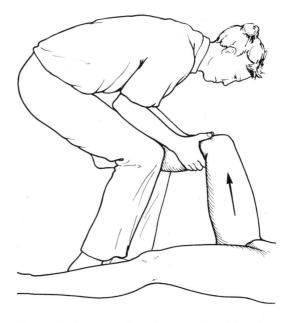

Figure 20.2 – Reduction of a posterior dislocation of the hip

- The hip should reduce with a definite 'clunk'; if it does not, it implies an element of instability, usually due to an acetabular rim fracture.
- **Check the sciatic nerve!**

2. The 'Allis' method may be used: the limb, after correction back to neutral as above, is held over the surgeon's shoulder, this allowing a greater mechanical advantage. This is only of real use where the patient, for whatever reason, cannot be placed on to the floor and effective counter-traction by an assistant is not possible.

3. The hip can also be reduced with the patient prone; the pelvis is placed over the edge of the operating table, allowing direct traction of the limb with gravity. This can be useful if there is an associated femoral shaft fracture. This method is only used with an intubated patient in view of the prone position.

In uncommon cases, the hip may not reduce. This may be because of:

- Inadequate technique.
- Inadequate muscle relaxation.
- A fragment within the joint preventing reduction.
- A rim fracture or acetabular labrum flap preventing a stable reduction.

In such cases, the patient must undergo urgent open reduction of the hip, supplemented by acetabular reconstruction if necessary.

Reduction should always be checked by radiography, again with both an anteroposterior and a lateral x-ray. An acetabular rim fracture may be more obvious at this stage. It is also important to ensure that the joint line is congruous, as a fragment left in situ often leads to degenerative change.

Following successful reduction, the patient is admitted, and is usually kept non-weight-bearing for a period of approximately 6 weeks, often on traction.

Anterior dislocation of the hip

Anterior dislocation of the hip is caused by a different mechanism from posterior dislocations, with the hip in abduction at the time of injury rather than adducted and flexed. However, it also can be complicated by avascular necrosis, and demands early reduction. In addition, the dislocated femoral head may put pressure on the femoral neurovascular structures in the groin, and their viability should always be checked.

The position of the limb is characteristic, in that the limb is **short, abducted and externally rotated** (Fig. 20.3). (Compare this to posterior dislocation in which the limb is internally rotated.)

The reduction technique is slightly modified for an anterior dislocation. The best method is to convert the dislocation into a posterior dislocation by:

- Flexing the hip.

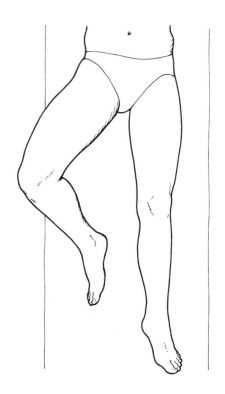

Figure 20.3 – Anterior dislocation of the hip – note that the limb is short, abducted and externally rotated

- Correcting the abduction and external rotation deformities.
- Proceed as for a posterior dislocation by traction on the limb etc.

Central dislocation of the hip

This occurs when a force is transmitted via the femoral head from the greater trochanter, with resulting displacement of the head through the acetabular floor (see Fig. 19.7). It is a very significant insult to the pelvis, and associated injuries should be positively excluded (e.g. pelvic organ damage).

The orientation of the limb is variable, but it is usually in neutral (cf. anterior and posterior dislocations). The limb is usually shortened.

The reduction of the hip is not as urgent as with anterior and posterior dislocations. The limb is put on skeletal or skin traction, with a gradual reduction. Attention is then paid to the fracture of the acetabular floor; in the younger patient reconstruction may be necessary to minimize the risks of degenerative change as a result of joint incongruency.

Complications of dislocation of the hip

There are a number of complications of hip dislocation, and a large proportion will be minimized by prompt appropriate treatment.

1. **Avascular necrosis** This is a cause of much morbidity following hip dislocation. The overall rate is around 10–20%, but is said to be over 50% if the hip remains dislocated for longer than 6 hours. The problem is due to disturbance of the capsular blood supply to the femoral head. The inevitable sequel to avascular necrosis is degenerative change within the hip.

2. **Sciatic nerve palsy** This is particularly associated with posterior dislocations, and especially if there is an accompanying acetabular fracture. It is essential to monitor and document the integrity of the nerve before and after reduction of the dislocation.

3. Other complications include myositis ossificans, secondary degenerative change with or without avascular necrosis, recurrent dislocation and missed dislocation.

Fractures of the proximal femur

Introduction and classification

A large proportion of fractures of the proximal femur occur in the middle-aged and elderly; those occurring in children and young adults should be considered as a separate problem. The incidence of these fractures is increasing in epidemic proportions, and now accounts for a large part of every orthopaedic unit's workload. The initial management of these fractures is important in determining the ultimate prognosis.

In the elderly population, proximal femoral fractures occur in five times as many women as men; this is due in part to the increased longevity of the female population, and partly due to their higher incidence of osteoporosis. Unfortunately, the fracture can be regarded as a pre-terminal event in many patients. Mortality rates vary widely, but the 6-month mortality rate approaches 40%.

Elderly people tolerate prolonged periods of immobilization in bed on traction extremely poorly. Complications include thromboembolism, pressure area breakdown, bronchopneumonia, urinary tract infections and ultimately death on an almost inevitable basis. For this reason it is important to operate on these fractures relatively promptly and mobilize the patients soon afterwards.

Fractures of the proximal femur are classified as follows (Fig. 20.4):

A **Intracapsular fractures**
1. Subcapital fractures of the neck of the femur.
2. Transcervical fractures of the neck of the femur.
B **Extracapsular fractures**
3. Basicervical fractures of the neck of the femur.
4. Intertrochanteric fractures of the proximal femur.
5. Subtrochanteric fractures of the proximal femur.

(NB: In the younger age groups, many basicervical fractures are intracapsular.)

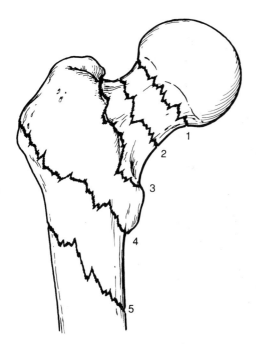

Figure 20.4 – Fractures of the proximal femur
1. Subcapital
2. Transcervical
3. Basicervical
4. Intertrochanteric
5. Subtrochanteric

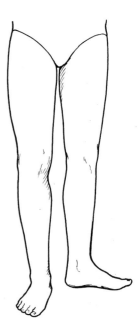

Figure 20.5 – The position of the limb in displaced fractures of the proximal femur – short, adducted and externally rotated

Clinical features

The history is variable, most of the patients having a history of a fall with subsequent pain in the groin. Some, however, have no clear history of trauma or a fall, and the fracture must be positively sought if suspected. There may have been a pre-fracture medical event (e.g. myocardial infarction, cerebrovascular accident) and this may need investigation and treatment. Always radiograph the hip if a proximal femoral fracture is suspected.

In displaced fractures, especially so in inter-trochanteric fractures, the limb is **short, externally rotated and adducted** (Fig. 20.5). The is due to the lack of ilio-psoas action upon the distal limb. Note however that impacted and undisplaced fractures may not show any limb deformity, and the patient may even be able to weight-bear. An undisplaced fracture, if undiagnosed, may go on to become a displaced fracture when sent home, a progression with a worse prognosis and of some medico-legal implication.

Radiographic examination is mandatory and **must** include both anteroposterior and lateral radiographs of the proximal femur. Some fractures are difficult to establish on an anteroposterior X-ray, and the fracture line may be more clearly seen on the lateral view. Care should be taken with impacted fractures as they are easily missed (Fig. 20.6); follow the contours of the neck into the femoral head. **If in doubt, the patient should be referred and admitted.** If necessary the patient can undergo bone scanning after one day to confirm the diagnosis.

An interesting feature is that only rarely does an osteoarthritic hip joint sustain a proximal femoral fracture. It is also worth noting that the differential diagnosis of a proximal femoral fracture includes a **fracture of one or more of the pubic rami**, and this should be positively excluded in the absence of an obvious femoral fracture.

Initial medical management of proximal femoral fractures

The medical management of elderly patients with proximal femoral fractures is probably of more importance than the surgical treatment,

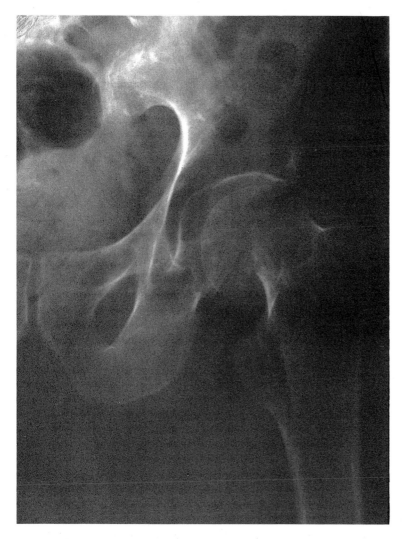

Figure 20.6 – Impacted subcapital fracture of the neck of the femur

and this includes the initial management within the Accident and Emergency Department. The management of the patient includes:

1. Nursing care and physiotherapy of the highest standard.
2. Any underlying medical disorders should be diagnosed; they may have been responsible for the fall that resulted in the fracture.
3. The patient should be transferred to the ward as soon as possible. A hard trolley in the Accident and Emergency Department is

not suitable for long periods, and pressure area breakdown can occur within 6 hours.
4. The patient may be dehydrated, having been without food and drink for a considerable period prior to admission. An intravenous fluid line is often needed, but avoid fluid overload if the patient has an element of cardiac failure.
5. If there is any suspicion of urinary or respiratory infection, appropriate investigations should be carried out and antibiotics commenced if appropriate. Chest physiotherapy preoperatively is often needed, and is

usually more important than administration of antibiotics.

6. Chest x-ray and ECG if appropriate (many units now have protocols for such screening investigations).

7. Blood analysis according to the unit's protocol. This may include full blood count, serum electrolytes including glucose, and cross-match.

8. Prophylactic antibiotics are usually given prior to surgery.

9. Prophylaxis against thromboembolism. Proximal femoral fracture surgery carries a high risk of thromboembolism. As well as mechanical methods, many units prescribe low-dose heparin or its analogues on admission.

10. Traction. In the past, skin traction prior to surgery was routine, with the aim of minimizing fracture displacement and providing analgesia. However, these benefits are now disputed, and traction may cause problems with pressure care areas and prevent efficient respiratory movements. It is still, nevertheless, widely used.

11. Analgesia. The patient must be given adequate appropriate analgesia.

Intracapsular fractures of the proximal femur

Blood supply to the head of the femur

The blood supply to the head of the femur is derived from two main sources (Fig. 20.7).

1. Vessels from the femoral circumflex arteries, that pass from the subtrochanteric region up the neck of the femur towards the head. The vessels pass through the cervical region within and around the capsule of the hip joint, which extends down the neck to a large extent.

2. Vessels passing within the ligamentum teres. Although these are significant in youth, by adulthood, their contribution is negligible.

As a consequence, in the adult, the blood supply of the head of the femur is largely dependent

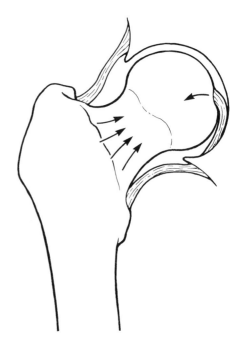

Figure 20.7 – Blood supply to the head of the femur

upon the integrity of the capsule surrounding the femoral neck. Interruption of the blood supply inevitably leads to **avascular necrosis** of the head, with subsequent collapse and secondary degenerative change. Hence intracapsular femoral neck fractures may prejudice the blood supply of the head, and the greater the displacement of the fracture, the greater is this risk.

Subcapital fractures of the neck of the femur

These common fractures have been classified according to the **Garden classification** (Fig. 20.8).

Garden 1

- Impacted fractures with an incomplete fracture line.
- Trabeculae through fracture angulated as the head is abducted.

Garden 2

- Impacted fracture with a complete fracture line.

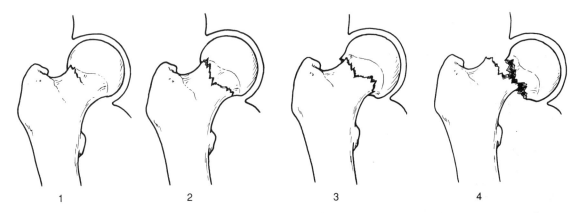

Figure 20.8 – Garden Classification of subcapital fractures

- The trabeculae appear interrupted but not angulated.

Garden 3

- Femoral head is displaced.
- The trabeculae are interrupted and angulated.

Garden 4

- Femoral head is more displaced ('fallen off').
- Trabeculae may appear parallel as the head may not be abducted.

This classification system corresponds with increasing insult to the blood supply of the femoral head. Grades 1 and 2 are relatively undisplaced fractures, with a lower risk of avascular necrosis than the more displaced Grades 3 and 4. The system also allows a treatment strategy (see below).

Subcapital fractures are prone, in addition to other complications associated with all femoral neck fractures, to two particular problems:

(a) **avascular necrosis of the femoral head** – this is unpredictable, but generally the prognosis is worse with greater displacement and with proximal fractures; and
(b) **non-union** of the fracture.

The treatment of these fractures is controversial. Many centres now adopt the following protocol:

1. All young patients undergo internal fixation **as a surgical emergency** in an attempt to reduce the fracture, decompress the intracapsular haematoma and fix the fragments. Subsequent avascular necrosis or non-union is treated on its merits, often with a total hip replacement. (Primary total hip replacement as an emergency treatment is regarded by many to have an unacceptable complication rate, although this policy is adopted by some).
2. In older patients:
   Garden 1 and 2 fractures are internally fixed.
   Garden 3 and 4 fractures are assumed to have a high risk of complication with internal fixation, and so as to avoid multiple operations, undergo a **hemiarthroplasty**, replacing the head of the femur whilst leaving the acetabulum intact (Fig. 20.9). A risk of hemiarthroplasty is that the metallic femoral head may 'bore' its way into the acetabulum, causing pain and erosion. For this reason, with their softer bone, hemiarthroplasty should be avoided in patients with rheumatoid arthritis.
3. In the very old or frail patient, all femoral neck fractures are recommended to undergo hemiarthroplasty.

It is important to know the protocol of the unit in which you practise. Especially, it is vital to realize that internal fixation of a femoral

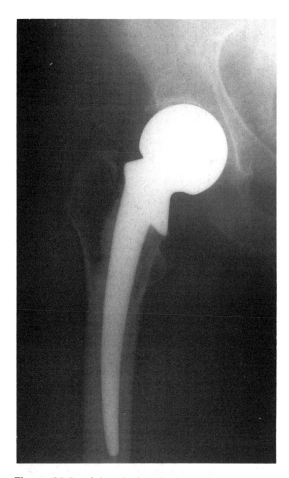

Figure 20.9 – A hemiarthroplasty

neck fracture (e.g. by cannulated screw fixation) in a young patient should be regarded as a **surgical emergency**. Many authorities feel that early decompression of the fracture haematoma and prompt reduction may reduce the risk of avascular necrosis; **the admitting orthopaedic surgeon should be immediately notified** so that theatre facilities etc. can be arranged.

Transcervical fractures of the neck of the femur

These fractures are largely treated as per subcapital fractures. They tend to have a lesser risk of avascular necrosis and non-union than subcapital fractures. Note that Garden's classification, strictly, does not apply to these fractures.

Extracapsular fractures of the proximal femur

Despite the term 'fractured neck of femur' often being used to include extracapsular fractures of the proximal femur, they are not fractures of the neck and are thus incorrectly labelled. For many purposes, however, the term is useful as the general management plan of extracapsular fractures is similar to true fractures of the neck.

As opposed to intracapsular fractures, most extracapsular fractures unite satisfactorily without fixation, with a low risk of avascular necrosis of the femoral head. However, because most of the patients sustaining this injury are elderly, it is important to mobilize them as soon as possible. For this reason nearly all extracapsular fractures undergo surgery. The most commonly used fixation device is the **dynamic hip screw** (Fig. 20.10), but in some cases other devices

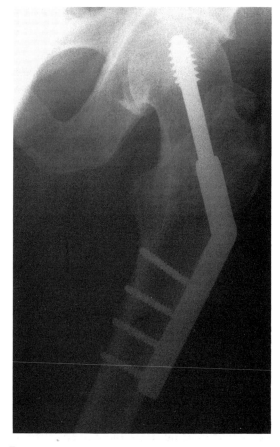

Figure 20.10 – A dynamic hip screw

are needed, e.g. reconstruction nails, 'Gamma' nails, and a 'reversed' dynamic condylar screw.

Basicervical fractures of the neck of the femur

The vast majority of these fractures in the elderly are extracapsular, and, if there is no involvement of the trochanteric region, are treated with a hemiarthroplasty. Any involvement of the trochanteric region, however, demands the use of a dynamic hip screw, and some would use the hip screw with all basicervical fractures.

Great care should be taken with basicervical fractures in children and younger adults. Great force is required to produce the fracture in this age group. As well as excluding other injuries, there may be an element of intracapsular involvement as the capsule extends further down the neck in the younger age groups. The fracture may need **urgent** decompression and fixation with, for example, cannulated screws.

Intertrochanteric fractures of the proximal femur

These are very common fractures in the elderly age group and are entirely extracapsular (Fig. 20.11). They are often associated with poor bone quality due to osteoporosis, osteomalacia etc. The fracture may be highly comminuted, and the fracture fragments may be described as 2-part, 3-part and 4-part. The majority require fixation with a dynamic hip screw.

Subtrochanteric fractures of the proximal femur

These are less common fractures, but are important in that they are often pathological fractures, the subtrochanteric region being a common site for skeletal metastasis. A full history and examination of the patient is of obvious importance, and radiographs of the entire femur are necessary. Many fractures may be internally fixed with a long-plate version of dynamic hip screw, but often reconstruction nails etc. are needed.

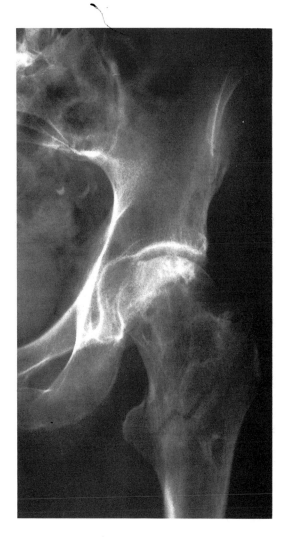

Figure 20.11 – Intertrochanteric fracture

Fractures of the femoral neck in children

These uncommon fractures are either secondary to an underlying pathology within the femoral neck (e.g. cyst, tumour, osteogenesis imperfecta etc.) or are due to great violence. They can be classified as:

1. **Subcapital**   These are essentially a fracture-dislocation of the proximal femoral epiphysis, and are associated with a high risk of avascular necrosis.
2. **Transcervical.**
3. **Basicervical**   These are **intracapsular** fractures (cf. elderly patients).
4. **Intertrochanteric fractures.**

All displaced fractures demand **urgent** decompression, reduction and internal fixation. The treatment of non-displaced fractures is controversial, as fixation is associated with complications. There is, however, an increasing tendency to fixation rather than treatment with traction and bed rest.

The acutely painful hip in patients with hip prostheses

As more and more patients are given hip prostheses or have internal fixation of fractures, the more commonly they will present to the Accident and Emergency Department with complications associated with that device.

The two main prosthesis types that are seen are:

1. **Hemiarthroplasty** Replacement of the femoral head with a metallic component with preservation of the acetabulum. The diameter of the femoral head is similar to that of the original (see Fig. 20.9).
2. **Total hip replacement** Replacement of both the femoral head and the acetabulum. The diameter of the femoral head is considerably less than the original, and the acetabular cup often has a metallic ring within it (Fig. 20.12).

In addition, complications may be seen with internal fixation devices, e.g. the commonly used **dynamic hip screw**, as used for intertrochanteric fractures of the proximal femur (see Fig. 20.10).

Dislocation of a prosthesis

This is becoming a more common problem, and may typically present to the Accident and Emergency Department. Although the dislocation rate is less for total hip replacement than hemiarthroplasty, the former is seen more often in the emergency setting – this is because most hemiarthroplasties that dislocate do so soon after operation and before the patient is discharged home. A total hip replacement may dislocate at any

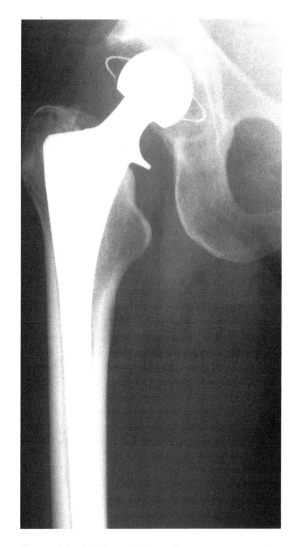

Figure 20.12 – A total hip replacement

time, although far more commonly in the period following operation.

An important point in the history is to determine whether the dislocation is acute, in which case successful reduction can be anticipated, or chronic, where surgical reconstruction may be necessary. In the acute event, the patient gives a clear history of a 'giving way' of the hip during a movement usually involving **adduction** of the hip, a movement patients are told to avoid! Immediate agonizing pain is experienced within the hip with shortening of the limb. More specifically:

- If the limb is short, adducted and **internally rotated**, then the hip prosthesis has dislocated **posteriorly**.
- If the limb is short, abducted and **externally rotated**, then the hip has dislocated **anteriorly**.

Neurovascular examination of the limb is **mandatory**. Specifically check the integrity of the sciatic nerve in posterior dislocations and the femoral vessels and nerve in anterior dislocations.

The diagnosis is confirmed on radiography, with anteroposterior and lateral views, although the diagnosis is usually obvious on a single view (Fig. 20.13).

Reduction should be performed by orthopaedic personnel. This can be achieved under intravenous sedation, but in some cases may need a general anaesthetic with muscle relaxation. Recurrent dislocations are generally easier to reduce. It is important not to exert large amounts of force in attempting to reduce the hip; the bone is often porotic around the prosthesis, and large 'stress risers' below the

femoral stem may induce a fracture. An image intensifier is useful to confirm reduction and to diagnose any mechanical problems predisposing to a further dislocation. The surgeon should always comment upon the stability of the reduced hip, and note the range of movement of the hip with the prosthesis in socket.

Reduction techniques are as for the dislocated non-prosthetic hip (see above), although the force required is usually less. It is essential, for this reason, to establish clinically whether the prosthesis is dislocated anteriorly or posteriorly. Some prostheses will not reduce by closed methods, and may require open reduction and/or revision of the prosthesis. Following reduction, it is again **mandatory** to check and document the integrity of the neurovascular structures.

Many centres adopt a period of skin traction with the hip in abduction following reduction, prior to mobilization. This helps the soft tissues to 'scar up' around the hip, affording further stability. Antibiotics are sometimes given prophylactically to prevent a tendency to infection in the tissues around the prosthesis following dislocation.

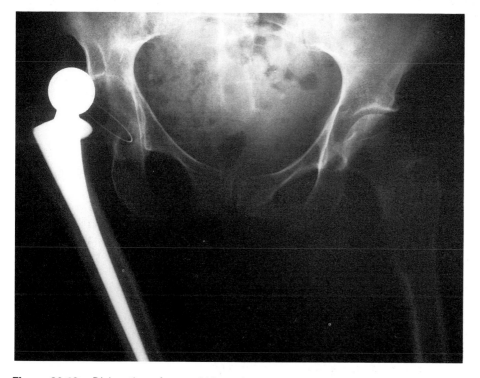

Figure 20.13 – Dislocation of at total hip replacement

Fracture of the shaft of the femur around femoral prosthetic stems

Insertion of a femoral prosthetic stem, for a number of biomechanical reasons, causes stress shielding and osteopenic change in the femoral shaft around the prosthesis. A common result is a fracture of the stem just distal to the tip of the prosthesis. This can be a difficult problem to manage. In the immediate setting, the neurovascular status of the limb should be verified, and on a radiograph dislocation of the hip prosthesis must be excluded. The patient may be placed on skin traction to allow fracture reduction and analgesia. If the prosthesis is loose it will have to be revised. If the prosthesis is well fixed, the fracture can be treated on its merits.

Fracture of the prosthetic stem

As inevitable mechanical loosening occurs around a prosthetic femoral stem, stress forces may induce a fracture of the prosthesis itself. This is becoming less common with better prosthetic materials. The radiograph may appear alarming. The patient need not necessarily be admitted, but should be referred for urgent assessment in the orthopaedic clinic, as a revision will probably be necessary.

Problems associated with fixation around the greater trochanter

Some surgeons insert a hip prosthesis via an osteotomy of the greater trochanter. The trochanter is then fixed with wire. A common problem is malunion or non-union of the osteotomy, and this may lead to an abnormal radiograph. Most of these patients are followed routinely in the orthopaedic clinic until union of the osteotomy site occurs, but if this is not the case, an orthopaedic outpatient referral is appropriate.

Heterotopic ossification

An alarming sight for the uninitiated is the abundance of calcification and new bone formation that is sometimes seen around a prosthetic hip joint. This can almost be regarded as a variant of normal, and need not be referred unless a patient with a recently inserted hip complains of great pain in the region (heterotopic ossification is rarely painful more than one year after prosthesis insertion).

Osteolysis around a prosthetic hip

This is rarely seen as a primary problem in the emergency setting, as the process is chronic. Patients may, however, present with concurrent problems, and osteolytic change may be noted around the acetabular or femoral component of the arthroplasty. Severe osteolysis may present at a later stage with fracture or gross loss of bone stock, and therefore out-patient referral may be appropriate; some osteolytic changes are not symptomatic until a late stage, at which time revision is more difficult.

Problems associated with internal fixation devices

A number of complications may occur with internal fixation devices around the hip joint. Probably the commonest is 'cut out' of the screw of the dynamic hip screw device used for intertrochanteric fractures of the proximal femur. This may occur with or without union of the fracture, and may present a considerable time after the time of fixation. If the screw head is abutting the acetabular floor, its removal is usually required.

The acutely painful hip in adults

The cause of an acutely painful hip in the adult can be difficult to diagnose. As well as local pathology, pain in the hip region may be referred from other sites. The two most important referral patterns are:

1. Pain referred from the back.
2. Pain referred from the posterior abdominal wall causing irritation of the psoas muscle.

It is therefore important to examine the abdomen and back when a patient presents with hip pain.

The following is a checklist of some of the conditions that may cause pain in the hip region.

1. A fracture or dislocation of the acetabulum or proximal femur.
2. Soft tissue injuries around the hip (see Chapter 19, p. 184).
3. Infection within the hip joint.
4. Connective tissue disorders. Hip involvement is a common presenting feature of rheumatoid arthritis, and may also occur in ankylosing spondylitis. A reactive arthropathy (e.g. Reiter's syndrome with eye and urethral symptoms) may also present with monoarticular hip pain.
5. Deterioration of primary or secondary osteoarthritis of the hip.
6. Presentation of a benign or malignant tumour within the acetabulum or proximal femur (osteoid osteoma classically occurs within the femoral neck).
7. Lumbo-sacral region pathology, e.g. prolapsed intervertebral disc with referred pain.
8. Psoas abscess with hip irritation and limitation of hip extension.

The acutely painful hip in children (the limping child)

Pathology

The limping child with an acutely painful hip is a common diagnostic problem that often presents in the emergency setting. The vast majority of cases are treated conservatively, but it is of vital importance to diagnose cases with specific pathologies that may, if untreated, lead to long-term morbidity.

A useful guide to the age ranges for hip pathology is as follows:

1. **Septic arthritis** may occur at any age, but is more common in infancy. The infection may be acute (e.g. staphylococcal) or chronic (e.g. tuberculosis).

2. **Transient synovitis** may also occur at any age, and is a common differential diagnosis. Other pathologies **must** be excluded before this diagnosis is made.
3. **Perthes disease** most often presents in the 4–10 age group.
4. **A slipped proximal femoral epiphysis** tends to occur in the young adolescent (10–15).
4. **Other,** e.g. monoarticular rheumatoid arthritis, at any age.

Management

As always, a full history is important. A recent history of a viral infection (e.g. upper respiratory tract infection) is common prior to transient synovitis. Acute suppurative infection within the hip usually has no obvious primary cause, although a history of septicaemia is significant. There is commonly a history of minor trauma that may be misleading. It is of supreme importance to realize that the child may complain of **pain in the knee** as a presenting feature of hip pathology – many an unfortunate case has been diagnosed late because the knee has been examined in isolation.

Examination may be difficult in an uncooperative child. The limp may be obvious. The general condition of the child is important. A toxic pyrexial child who looks unwell is almost sure to have septic arthritis in this setting. The demonstration of a fixed flexion deformity by Thomas' test (flexion of the normal hip abolishing any lumbo-sacral curvature, thereby revealing any loss of extension in the abnormal hip) is indicative of hip pathology. The range of movement of the hips should be carefully examined and documented. In most hip pathology, **abduction in flexion** and **internal rotation** are the movements to be restricted first.

Special investigations include:

1. **X-ray** Usually unremarkable in the acute setting, although vital in the diagnosis of a slipped upper femoral epiphysis and may be useful in Perthes disease.
2. **Ultrasound of the hip** This may demonstrate fluid within the joint as a confirmation of pathology, but may not be of much use in

obtaining a specific diagnosis. The technique may allow ultrasound-directed aspiration of fluid to allow analysis.

3. **Serum parameters** These include erythrocyte sedimentation rate, C-reactive protein and white cell count. A high WCC may indicate infection and a raised ESR and CRP often indicates significant pathology. Values in transient synovitis are usually unremarkable. However, over-reliance on these investigations can be misleading, and many cases of significant suppurative infection have normal indices.

4. **Blood cultures** may be positive in acute suppuration.

The child with a painless limp

This is not a common presentation in the emergency setting, and is not discussed in this book. However, causes include **congenital dislocation of the hip**, polio and developmental coxa vara.

Acute suppurative septic arthritis of the hip joint

Acute suppurative infection within the hip joint is usually due to the organism *Staphylococcus aureus*. The hip joint is prone to sepsis as the proximal metaphysis of the femur is intracapsular, allowing direct spread of an osteomyelitis from the bone into the joint. The consequences are serious as the femoral head may be destroyed very quickly, allowing dislocation and permanent deformity of the joint.

The disease is most common in infancy, and may be an occult focus of infection in a septicaemic neonate. There is an association with umbilical infection and invasive procedures such as umbilical artery or femoral vessel catheterization. However, septic arthritis may occur at any age during childhood, and should always be considered in the differential diagnosis of an acutely painful hip. The infant or child is usually toxic, pyrexial and dehydrated. The diagnosis is usually clinical but may be confirmed by raised ESR and CRP, positive blood cultures and aspiration of pus from the joint. X-rays are usually unhelpful in the acute

stage, although in more advanced cases they may show destruction.

Treatment involves intravenous antibiotics and open drainage of the joint. This is a **surgical emergency**: the famous surgical quote 'never let the sun set on undrained pus' is relevant here!

Tuberculosis of the hip joint

In developed countries this is less commonly seen than in the past. However, it may resurge due to the increasing numbers with immunodeficiency, and may also be seen in immigrants where endogenous tuberculosis is common. The problem may arise from tuberculous synovitis or by direct spread from an osteomyelitic segment of bone in the area. The onset of symptoms is less acute than with acute suppuration, with a gradual increase in pain and significantly **night pain.** Radiographic changes are slow to develop and include general rarefaction of the bone ultimately resulting in destruction and dislocation. The diagnosis may be difficult if not thought of! Diagnosis may be confirmed by joint aspiration and treatment largely consists of chemotherapy.

Transient synovitis

This is a relatively common condition, which is not clearly understood, but may represent a viral infection of the synovium within the joint or a reactive synovitis. The condition is certainly more common following a viral upper respiratory tract infection. The child presents with a painful hip in association with a limp. A history of minor trauma is common. The child is well systemically, unlike sepsis. There is a restricted range of movement, typically internal rotation but also abduction in flexion. X-rays are normal but an ultrasound scan may show an effusion.

Management is now controversial. In the past all cases were routinely admitted for bed rest and traction. More commonly, cases are seen in the emergency setting and investigations performed, including full blood count, ESR and CRP. If these are normal and the child clinically has no features of sepsis or other pathology detailed below, the patient may be allowed home. However, follow-up is mandatory, in particular to check that the range of movement of the hip returns to normal (see Perthes disease). All cases should be discussed with senior orthopaedic personnel prior to being allowed home with a follow-up appointment.

Perthes disease

Perthes disease is a poorly understood condition in which the developing femoral head undergoes partial or 'whole head' avascular necrosis. The cause of this process is not clear, but may represent a vascular phenomenon. It most commonly presents in the 4–10 age range.

The patient, usually male (80% male to 20% female), presents with a painful limp which gradually settles. The condition may be bilateral. In the early stage, where the presentation is typically to the Accident and Emergency Department, the hip joint is irritable with a decreased range of movement in abduction in flexion and internal rotation. The x-ray may be normal at this stage – hence the importance of follow-up of painful hips until resolution of symptoms and with the hip back to a full range of movement. As the disease progresses, pain often subsides. The radiological features are increased density of the head (partial or 'whole head' involvement), an increase in the joint space and widening of the metaphysis. Later the femoral head becomes distorted and flattened.

The long-term treatment is outside the scope of this book. The majority of cases however may be treated conservatively, and most cases presenting under the age of 7 have a reasonable prognosis. Surgery to 'contain' the femoral head by osteotomy etc. may be needed if the condition progresses.

Slipped upper femoral epiphysis

This is a condition which every doctor dealing with Accident and Emergency presentations should be aware of, as the consequences of missing the diagnosis may be unfavourable. It is also known as **slipped capital femoral epiphysis**, where the proximal femoral epiphysis displaces from the metaphysis as a form of Salter–Harris type I lesion. The process may be sudden or gradual. Boys are affected slightly more often than girls. The condition typically occurs in two phenotypes and in the adolescent age group:

1. The short, fat, sexually underdeveloped child (more common).
2. The tall, thin normally developed child.

There may be a history of trauma and symptoms may be bilateral. A limp with pain in the groin **with radiation to the thigh and knee** is typical. Knee pain may be the sole presenting feature – **hence the importance of always examining the hip joint in all cases of knee pain.** Examination may reveal true leg shortening, a decreased range of movement (with loss of abduction in flexion and internal rotation), and a Trendelenberg gait.

Radiological assessment is **mandatory** in such a presentation. An anteroposterior view of the hip is not sufficient as an early slip may not be obvious. **Always ask for a lateral view of the hip;** a slip is usually more obvious on this x-ray. Signs include (Fig. 20.14):

- A widened and patchy growth plate.
- Trethowan's sign: normally a line drawn up the femoral neck enters a portion of the femoral head. In a slip, the femoral head is below this line.
- The head may be easily seen to have 'slipped'.

Treatment includes a semi-urgent fixation with a pin or screw system, e.g. cannulated screws. The slip may in some cases be reduced. The condition may be bilateral and some advocate prophylactic pinning, although this is far from universal practice. Consequences of a 'missed' slip include avascular necrosis, chondrolysis of the femoral head, coxa vara and subsequent secondary degenerative change within the hip joint.

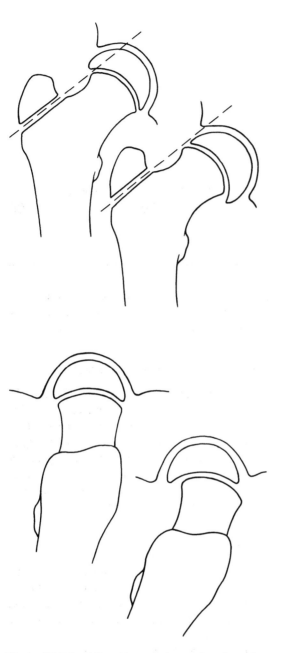

Figure 20.14 – AP and lateral views of a slipped upper femoral epiphysis – note, on the AP view, Trethowan's line (illustrated) which normally passes through the femoral head.

21
The femur

Fractures of the femoral shaft in adults

A great deal of energy is required to break a normal femur in the adult. In general terms, fractures of the shaft of the femur are of two types:

1. Fractures caused by a large amount of energy and violence in a normal femur (Fig. 21.1).
2. Fractures caused by a low level of energy in an abnormal femur, often secondary to metastatic deposits, and usually in the elderly (Fig. 21.2).

Femoral shaft fractures therefore should always alert you to the possibility of other problems – either the coexistent injuries of severe trauma or an underlying malignancy.

General effects of femoral shaft fracture

Isolated closed fracture of a femoral shaft, especially in the younger adult patient, may allow the loss of 2–3 units of blood from the intravascular space into the soft tissues. An open fracture may double the blood loss. Therefore a femoral shaft fracture alone may cause hypovolaemia, but in association with other injuries, often produces haemorrhagic shock. Adequate fluid and/or blood replacement should be estimated quickly. Adequate reduction and splin-

tage of the fracture at the scene of trauma or early in the Accident and Emergency Department may reduce the blood loss.

Description of femoral shaft fractures

Fracture may occur in any portion of the shaft. Those in the supracondylar and intercondylar regions are described separately. The fracture pattern may be **spiral** from a twisting type force or **transverse** from a direct or angulatory force. Pathological fractures are usually transverse. The fracture may also have a **butterfly fragment** or may be **segmental** (Fig. 21.3).

Diagnosis

The diagnosis is usually obvious. The history may indicate the degree of violence involved in the trauma. The neurovascular status must be checked before and after any reduction of the fracture.

The fracture should be confirmed on x-rays. As with all fractures, the joints above and below the fracture must be visualized. In particular a **dislocation of the hip** and a **patellar fracture** should be excluded, as they often accompany femoral shaft fractures.

Treatment

The vast majority of closed femoral shaft fractures are now treated by intramedullary locked

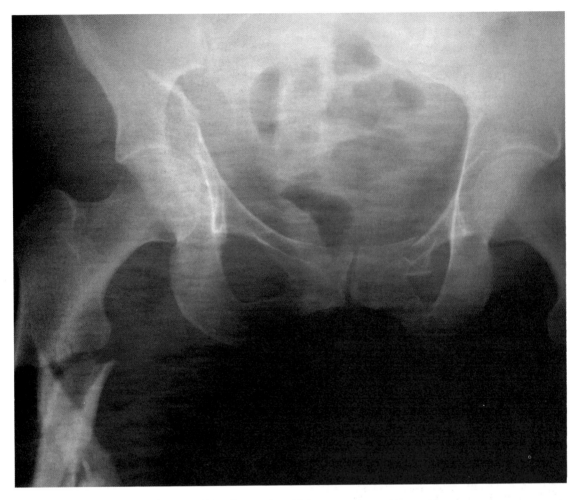

Figure 21.1 – High energy fracture of the femur. In addition, note the pubic rami fractures.

nailing. In addition, most centres nail open femoral fractures. Other possibilities include conservative treatment on traction, external fixation and internal fixation with plates and screws. In pathological fractures of the femoral shaft, most centres now fix the femur with a reconstruction-type nail so as to obviate further treatment should a second deposit develop in the bone, e.g. at the level of the femoral neck.

The initial treatment involves:

1. The haemodynamic stabilization of the patient.
2. The exclusion of other injuries or malignancy (see above).

3. The application of temporary traction prior to (if any) definitive surgical treatment. This may be skin traction or skeletal traction.

Note that in the multiply-injured patient, it has been clearly shown that early fracture stabilization reduces the risk of complications such as fat embolism and the adult respiratory distress syndrome (ARDS or 'shock lung').

Skin traction

Skin traction is a satisfactory temporary form of traction, and offers gradual fracture reduction and analgesia. It is particularly useful in

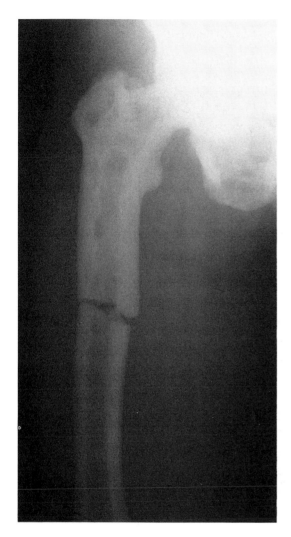

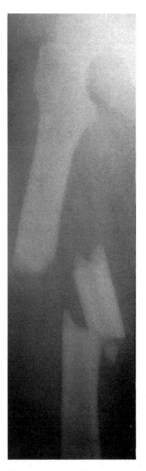

Figure 21.3 – Segmental fracture of the femur

Figure 21.2 – Pathological fracture of the femur – a transverse fracture of the shaft of any long bone raises the suspicion of an underlying pathology, in this case Paget's disease.

the elderly, but has a restricted use in muscular adults, in whom the dynamics may not be sufficient. Complications include skin blistering and breakdown.

Standard skin traction sets are now available. Strapping is placed around the lower leg, but should not extend laterally above the knee as the common peroneal nerve may be compressed, often as the traction is applied.

Skeletal traction

Skeletal traction is useful in those patients needing longer-term traction, and in the young and more muscular patient. It is also needed prior to intramedullary nailing. In the elderly with more osteoporotic bone, the pin may be inserted under local anaesthetic. However, in the harder bone of the young adult, this may not be possible, and a general anaesthetic may be needed simply to insert a traction pin. A Steinman (plain) or Denham (threaded) pin may be used. Remember that even in the busy Accident and Emergency Department, a sterile technique is important – the pin may have to be in site for a considerable period. Pin tract infections are a distressing complication for a patient on traction.

The usual site for pin insertion is the proximal tibia, with the entry site 2 cm distal and posterior to the tibial tubercle. The common peroneal nerve must be avoided. It is easier to insert the pin from lateral to medial. The area is prepared aseptically. Local anaesthetic is infiltrated both into the skin and the underlying periosteum, as these are the areas that cause pain during pin insertion. A cruciate incision is made into the skin, allowing egress of subsequent secretions and helping to prevent pin tract infections. The pin must be inserted at 90° to the long axis of the limb. As the pin is exiting, local anaesthetic and a further cruciate incision are needed on the medial side of the limb. Aseptic spray is then applied to the pin sites and gauze dressing covers the area. Traction may then be applied.

Should the proximal tibia be an unsuitable site for traction (e.g. where there is a coexisting knee injury), the pin may be placed through the femoral condyles by a similar technique.

Fractures of the femoral shaft in children

Femoral shaft fractures in children tend to occur with a lesser degree of violence than in the adult and can be considered separately in terms of treatment. The vast majority are treated conservatively because they unite relatively quickly and without complication.

Treatment

Most femoral shaft fractures in children are spiral type. Transverse fractures are unusual and raise the suspicion of a pathological fracture.

Children under the age of 2 years are treated on **Gallows traction**. Skin traction apparatus is applied to each leg and overhead traction applied, with the limbs in abduction and moderate external rotation. The force should just raise the child's sacrum from the bed surface. This method should not be used in older children as there is a risk of circulatory insufficiency.

In older children, more conventional longitudinal balanced traction is applied. Both limbs may need to be put on traction to prevent the child from pulling itself from the bed.

Supracondylar and intercondylar fractures of the femur

Supracondylar and intercondylar fractures in the middle-aged and elderly

These fractures form a difficult group of injuries, usually occurring in the osteoporotic bone of the elderly (Fig. 21.4). Because they are difficult to treat, there are a number of advocated managements, none of which is entirely satisfactory.

Pure supracondylar fractures can be given immediate reduction and analgesia by skin or skeletal traction. They can be definitively managed by:

1. **Conservative management** This is not ideal for a number of reasons, including the

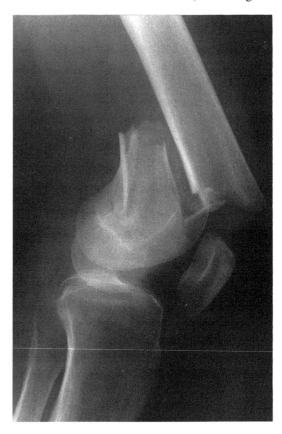

Figure 21.4 – Supracondylar fracture of the femur

long period required on traction and the tendency for the distal fragment to angulate and rotate due to the local muscular forces. However, in some cases, it may be necessary.

2. **Internal fixation** The most common internal fixation device is the **dynamic condylar screw**. Whilst this is satisfactory in the middle-aged patient with reasonable bone stock, it has a high failure rate in osteoporotic bone.

3. **Total knee replacement** A simple hinge type knee replacement may be appropriate.

4. **Amputation** Although rarely performed as a primary procedure, this is unfortunately an all too common sequel to this fracture following failure of other methods.

Supracondylar fractures with intercondylar extensions, or pure intercondylar and condylar fractures, are even more difficult to treat. In the younger patient with good bone quality, internal fixation may be possible. In the osteoporotic patient, internal fixation is often not possible, total knee replacement being needed. A high failure rate is again seen.

Intercondylar and condylar fractures in the young adult

These are generally high energy fractures. Where there is a significant intra-articular component, there may be an associated osteochondral fracture, meniscal injury or other intra-articular pathology. Accurate open reduction and internal fixation is required to maintain adequate knee function and prevent secondary degenerative change.

It is essential to document the integrity of the neurovascular structures in fractures of this type. Fractures may need to be urgently reduced in the Accident and Emergency Department if there is any deficit – this can be effected by longitudinal traction with skin or skeletal traction. In addition, as with any fracture, always x-ray the entire femur, including joints above and below – there is an association with hip injury and patellar fracture.

Fracture-separation of the distal femoral epiphysis

This injury may occur in the adolescent skeleton. Forced abduction of the straight knee may cause the distal femoral epiphysis to slip laterally. Similarly a hyperextension injury may cause the epiphysis to slip forwards.

Examination reveals a tense haemarthrosis, and the diagnosis is made on x-ray. Careful examination of the neurovascular structures is essential as the popliteal artery may become trapped by the fracture, in which case urgent closed reduction of the fracture is necessary. Open reduction is sometimes necessary; internal fixation is avoided if at all possible, although temporary strong K wire fixation may be necessary.

22
The knee joint

Applied anatomy and functional examination of the knee joint

The knee consists of two main portions:

1. The tibio-femoral joint.
2. The patello-femoral joint.

The two joints should be considered separately when attempting to diagnose knee pathology. When assessing pathology within the knee joint, it is useful to consider the main intra-articular and extra-articular structures of the knee joint. These are:

1. The menisci – medial and lateral.
2. The anterior cruciate ligament.
3. The posterior cruciate ligament.
4. The collateral ligaments – medial and lateral.
5. The extensor mechanism of the knee joint, comprising quadriceps tendon and muscle, the patella, the patellar tendon and its insertion into the tibial tuberosity.
6. The synovium of the knee joint.
7. Bursae around the knee.

Always remember that knee pain may be referred from the hip. In all cases of knee pain exclude hip pathology.

Symptoms associated with knee pathology

Despite the knee joint being a complicated anatomical and functional structure, symptoms due to pathology within it are surprisingly few.

1. **Pain** This may be localized, as in injury to the collateral ligaments, or diffuse, as with an effusion due to synovitis.
2. **Swelling** of the knee This may be localized, as in pre-patellar bursitis, or diffuse, as in effusion, haemarthrosis and pyarthrosis.
3. **Giving way** This is an important symptom which should always be sought. It is non-specific and suggests instability of the knee, whether due to anterior cruciate insufficiency, meniscal tears, loose bodies or extensor mechanism disorders.
4. **Locking** True locking in a medical sense is **an inability to fully straighten the knee**. Many patients use the term loosely to describe stiffness or incomplete flexion of the knee, which is technically incorrect. True locking suggests a mechanical block

within the knee, e.g. a meniscal tear, loose bodies etc. **Sudden unlocking** is an even more reliable symptom of a mechanical problem, the fragment suddenly moving out from the tibio-femoral articulation. (When patients talk of 'locking' the cause is frequently to be found in the patello-femoral joint where subluxation or pain causes muscle spasm which 'locks' the knee in flexion).

Demonstration of an effusion at the knee joint

This can often cause difficulty. An effusion indicates the presence of synovial fluid within the joint (whilst a haemarthrosis implies blood and pyarthrosis implies pus). An effusion may be demonstrated in a number of ways, depending upon its severity.

1. For large quantities of fluid, the knee exhibits **cross-fluctuation**. Fluid thrill is transmitted from top to bottom and side to side of the knee.
2. For moderate effusions, the knee has a **patellar tap**. Compress the suprapatellar pouch whilst pushing the patella backwards. In the presence of an effusion, the patella strikes and bounces off the femur. (This is a good sign in chronic swellings; in acute effusions, however, the sign elicits pain and is usually impossible to demonstrate).
3. For small effusions, the **bulge test** may be positive. Stroke fluid away from the medial side of the knee where there is usually a dimple. Sweeping the examining hand proximally over the lateral side will cause the medial side to refill.

Functional examination of the knee with respect to structure

The menisci

The menisci are attached to the intra-articular surface of the tibia, and stay with it on tibio-femoral movement (Fig. 22.1). The most common disorder of a meniscus in the acute setting is a tear.

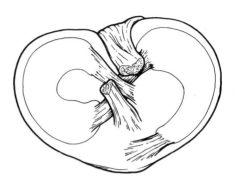

Figure 22.1 – The menisci

- The typical mechanism of injury is **rotational stress upon the flexed weight-bearing knee**.
- Symptoms may include **pain, swelling** of the knee, limp and **locking and unlocking** of the knee.
- Signs include **effusion, a locked knee, joint line tenderness and pain on rotational testing** (see Meniscal Injuries below).

Note that none of these symptoms or signs may be present.

The anterior cruciate ligament

The anterior cruciate ligament (ACL) runs from the interspinous area of the tibia towards the inner surface of the lateral femoral condyle. Its primary role is in preventing forward translation of the tibia upon the femur.

- As with meniscal injuries, the typical mechanism of injury is **rotational stress upon the flexed weight-bearing knee**, particularly when there is an additional valgus force (hence many ACL and meniscal injuries often coexist). **Hyperextension injuries** may also cause rupture of the ACL.
- Early symptoms of ACL rupture are **immediate swelling** of the knee, an **inability to continue sport etc. after injury**, a history of hearing a **'pop'** as the ligament ruptures and a **'two-fisted'** action by the patient to describe the injury. Later symptoms are of **giving way** of the knee.
- Early signs are of **haemarthrosis, and seldom little else as the patient is in too much pain to**

permit functional testing. Remember that haemarthrosis in the adult, in the absence of a radiological fracture, implies a rupture of the ACL in over 90% of cases. Later signs are of increased tibial rotational instability, namely **anterior draw, Lachman and pivot shift tests** (see Anterior Cruciate Ligament Injuries below).

The posterior cruciate ligament

The posterior cruciate ligament (PCL) extends from the tibial spine and posterior surface of the tibia towards the inner surface of the medial femoral condyle. Its primary role is in preventing posterior translation of the tibia upon the femur.

- The typical mechanism of injury is **a posteriorly directed force upon the tibia** as in dashboard injuries. Note that this is different from the rotational forces in ACL injuries.
- Signs are of **increased posterior translation of the tibia, i.e. a posterior sag, posterior draw and reverse pivot shift test** (see Posterior Cruciate Ligament Injuries below).

The collateral ligaments

The collateral ligaments are extracapsular structures running along the medial and lateral aspects of the knee, connecting the femur to the tibia and fibula (Fig. 22.2). The role of the medial ligament is in preventing valgus deformation of the knee, whilst the lateral ligament prevents varus deformation.

- The typical method of injury of the medial ligament is an **excessive valgus strain upon the knee**, but realize that this may be caused by a lateral force upon the fixed weight-bearing knee.
- The lateral ligament is damaged by an excessive varus force.
- Symptoms are of localized **swelling** and **pain** along the ligament. A sensation of **instability** is also common.
- Signs include localized **swelling and bruising** along the ligament, the absence of an effusion (in pure collateral injuries), **localized ten-**

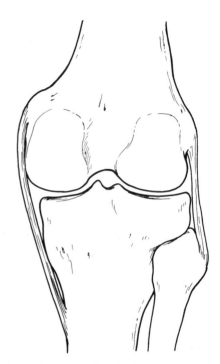

Figure 22.2 – The collateral ligaments

derness along the ligament (maximal at the point of rupture) and **abnormal stress tests** (see Collateral Ligament Injuries below).

The extensor mechanism

When examining the knee, especially following trauma, it is essential to ensure that the extensor mechansim is functioning. This may be done by the **straight leg raise**. However, be careful, as in some cases the hamstrings may be able to lift an extended leg into the air with an absent extensor mechanism. Always check, in addition, that the patient can actively **extend the lower leg from a flexed position against gravity**.

Bursae

See discussion of bursae (pp. 224–25) below.

Acute traumatic haemarthrosis and effusion

Seldom does a knee injury present itself with a clear-cut diagnosis such as cruciate injury, meniscal injury etc. The doctor in the Accident and Emergency Department must deduce from the history, examination and limited special investigations a logical diagnosis. Many traumatic knee injuries present with a haemarthrosis or an effusion, and it is therefore important to be able to make a differential diagnosis from the clinical findings.

Acute haemarthrosis

Haemarthrosis denotes blood within a joint. The presence of blood within the knee joint is very important to recognize, as a considerable degree of damage is needed to effect it. Most traumatic haemarthroses develop soon after injury (cf. traumatic effusions). The knee has a tense and 'boggy' nature on palpation. Note that whilst a tense haemarthrosis implies a large amount of intra-articular blood, a mild haemarthrosis does not necessarily denote a less significant injury – a capsular tear may allow dissipation of blood into the soft tissues.

The differential diagnosis of the cause of traumatic haemarthrosis is:

1. An intra-articular fracture (the blood usually containing fat globules from bone marrow).
2. **Rupture of the anterior cruciate ligament.**
3. Rupture of the posterior cruciate ligament.
4. Dislocation of the patella.
5. Osteochondral fractures (that may not be obvious on x-ray).
6. Peripheral tear of the menisci (**not** central tears, which are within an avascular zone).
7. **Some** collateral ligament ruptures associated with capsular tears (in isolation, *per se*, they do not result in a haemarthrosis).

In the absence of a fracture seen on x-ray, 90% of acute haemarthroses in adults are due to rupture of the anterior cruciate ligament.

The management of an acute haemarthrosis is made more difficult because the patient is in great discomfort, and therefore dynamic testing of the knee is often impossible. Delayed examination is needed, often under anaesthesia, to make an accurate diagnosis. Opinion varies as to whether the knee should be aspirated. In favour of this, aspiration makes the patient more comfortable. However, aspiration carries the risk of introducing infection to the joint. If aspiration is to be performed, it **must be performed under strict aseptic conditions**.

Acute traumatic effusions

Commonly, the knee joint may develop an effusion following injury. The differential diagnosis is less specific than with haemarthroses, and includes:

1. **Traumatic synovitis** This is a common non-specific condition of the synovium whereby it produces fluid as a result of injury. It may or may not be associated with intra-articular structural pathology. The effusion may become persistent and require prolonged quadriceps physiotherapy.
2. **Meniscal injuries** Most commonly central tears within the avascular zone.
3. **Infection** (more accurately termed a **pyarthrosis**) Usually resulting from an iatrogenic cause, e.g. introduction of a needle for aspiration. (Be careful to differentiate an effusion, which is generalized swelling of the knee, from a localized swelling around the knee, e.g. pre-patellar bursitis).

Anterior cruciate ligament lesions and associated injuries

The anterior cruciate ligament (ACL) is an intracapsular structure of the knee, which plays an important part in the dynamics of the knee. It consists of two main bundles which run from the interspinous area of the tibia to the postero-medial aspect of the lateral femoral condyle (Fig. 22.3).

Ruptures of the anterior cruciate ligament are common in the young adult, and are under-diagnosed in the acute setting. The acute presentation is very different from the problems resulting from chronic anterior cruciate insufficiency. If left untreated, there is increased risk of chronic knee instability, meniscal tears and degenerative change. Also the acute and chronic ACL rupture commonly coexists with a second

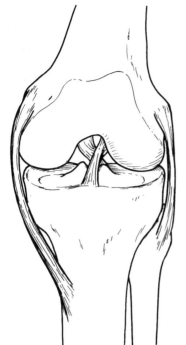

Figure 22.3 – The anterior and posterior cruciate ligaments

pathology, e.g. meniscal tears. Ruptures of the ACL cannot be primarily repaired; some form of reconstruction is necessary.

Avulsion fracture of the anterior tibial spine also results in anterior cruciate insufficiency, and these injuries are also dealt with in this section.

Presentation of acute tears of the ACL

Rupture of the ACL classically occurs as part of **rotational force upon the flexed weight-bearing knee**; typically this occurs in contact sports and skiing. **Hyperextension injuries** may also be responsible. The history is often given of the above mechanism of action, a definite 'pop' heard by the patient, a 'two-fisted' action by the patient to describe the injury, and early swelling of the knee. Patients often cannot continue with the activity in which they injured the knee, although this is variable.

Examination of the knee is often difficult. A **haemarthrosis** is present, giving the knee a 'doughy' feel. However, if there is a capsular tear in addition, much of the blood may be dissipated into the surrounding tissues. Note that in approximately 90% of cases, an acute haemarthrosis in adults is indicative of a rupture of the ACL – a haemarthrosis is therefore a very significant finding. Specific diagnostic tests of joint laxity are very difficult in the acute stage, and certainly the anterior draw, Lachman and pivot shift tests are indeterminate and painful (see Chronic ACL lesions below).

Radiographic findings, other than demonstrating a haemarthrosis, are usually unhelpful. However, look carefully for an avulsion fracture of the anterior tibial spine, the bone to which the ACL is attached (Fig. 22.4, see below).

Management of acute ACL tears

Different protocols exist from unit to unit as to managing acute ACL tears (see discussion of the management of haemarthroses, p. 210). The initial step in the Accident and Emergency Department is aspiration of the joint. Aspiration can relieve the pressure within the capsule and provide effective analgesia. This should be done under **strictly aseptic conditions**; blood is a very good culture medium for microorganisms, and in addition, reconstruction may be needed at a later stage, which will be hampered by the presence of intra-articular infection. The knee should be partially immobilized in a brace with a range of motion from 30°–90°.

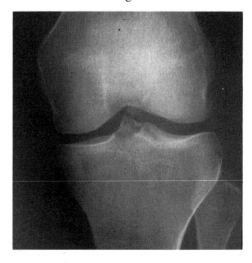

Figure 22.4 – Avulsion fracture of the tibial spine

If a brace is not available, give the patient some crutches with which to mobilize and advice as to cooling of the knee with ice packs, frozen peas etc.

Many units, in the presence of an acute haemarthrosis, arrange an emergency or semi-elective examination under anaesthetic and arthroscopy to wash out the haemarthrosis, confirm the diagnosis and exclude any coexistent intra-articular pathology, e.g. a meniscal tear. Following this, a decision can be made regarding reconstructive surgery, which can be carried out after a minimum of 3–6 weeks.

Avulsion fracture of the anterior tibial spine

The ACL arises from the region of the anterior tibial spine. An avulsion fracture may result from a twisting weight-bearing injury, as with pure ACL tears, but may also occur as a result of a hyperextension force, especially in younger patients. A similar clinical picture to ACL rupture ensues, with an acute haemarthrosis. The diagnosis is made on x-ray – the spine may be non-displaced or displaced (see Fig. 22.4).

The diagnosis is an important one, as the management differs from a 'pure' ACL tear. If the fracture is undisplaced, the knee should be immobilized in plaster for 4–6 weeks. Should the fracture be displaced, it is essential that open reduction and internal fixation is performed – this may be done arthroscopically or at an open arthrotomy. Such cases should therefore be admitted or referred for urgent fracture clinic assessment.

Chronic anterior cruciate insufficiency

A total rupture of the ACL, if left untreated, almost inevitably results in a chronic cruciate deficiency state. In the acute stage, the secondary restraints of the knee may be enough to provide stability for the knee. However, as these become compromised with time, the knee becomes chronically unstable, **with the principal symptom of giving way**. As many acute ACL ruptures are not diagnosed at the time of injury, chronic cruciate insufficiency is relatively common.

The patient with chronic ACL insufficiency does not present *per se* in the emergency setting and is usually dealt with on an elective basis. **Such patients may present, however, following an episode of instability with an acutely swollen knee** – a further intra-articular injury having occurred, e.g. a meniscal tear, traumatic synovitis etc. This is surprisingly common.

The chronic ACL-deficient knee may have the following features on examination, the degree of which depends on the integrity of the 'secondary restraints' of the knee, i.e., collaterals, quadriceps tone etc. (Fig. 22.5).

1. An **anterior draw sign**: the patient has the knee flexed at 90°, and the examiner sits on the

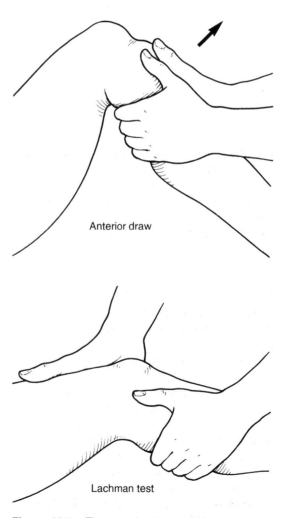

Anterior draw

Lachman test

Figure 22.5 – The anterior draw and Lachman tests

foot. The hamstrings must be relaxed. The tibia is pulled forwards upon the femur; normally there is a firm endpoint with minimal displacement, and this can be compared with the opposite leg. The displacement can be graded as:

    1 + = 0.5 cm anterior translation
    2 + = 0.5–1.0 cm anterior translation
    3 + = more than 1.0 cm anterior translation.

Ensure that at 90° the knee does not 'sag' – if so, it may indicate a posterior cruciate rather than an ACL injury.

2. A positive **Lachman test**: this is the most sensitive test for ACL deficiency. Anterior translation of the tibia upon the femur is assessed at 15–30° of flexion. A firm endpoint should normally be obtained. A similar grading scheme as for the anterior draw sign can be used.

3. A positive **pivot shift test**: this is the best method of determining instability from ACL deficiency. The knee is given a valgus stress in 10–20° of flexion. In the symptomatic ACL-deficient knee, as the knee is flexed, the lateral tibial plateau subluxes forward and reduces again as the knee is flexed under continuous valgus strain. The test is often uncomfortable for patients, and cannot be obtained if the hamstrings are tensed. It is essentially a test of **anterolateral rotatory instability** of the knee. It not only demonstrates the sign of ACL instability, it also reproduces the symptoms which the patient can confirm.

Note that these tests can be modified by a second pathology, e.g. a collateral tear. Note also that there is a great deal of individual variation in the tests, and examination of the opposite limb is invaluable. Many units do not grade displacements in the anterior draw and Lachman tests so accurately, as the tests depend somewhat on the strength of the examiner and the muscular build of the patient. 'Lax' and 'very lax' are good alternatives.

The patient presenting with a swollen knee, who on examination has signs of ACL insufficiency, can be regarded to have a chronic lesion with a second recent pathology. This is most often a meniscal tear or traumatic synovitis. If the knee is locked (i.e. with a block to full

extension) the patient should be admitted or referred for an early fracture clinic assessment – it is highly likely that an arthroscopic assessment will be required. In the absence of locking, a referral should be made noting the ACL insufficiency – a reconstruction may be needed as well as correction of the recent pathology.

Posterior cruciate ligament injuries

The posterior cruciate ligament (PCL) extends from the posterior tibial spine region and the back of the tibia to the lateral aspect of the medial femoral condyle (see Fig. 22.3). Its main mechanical function is in preventing posterior displacement of the tibia upon the femur. It is injured less frequently than the anterior cruciate ligament. Avulsion fractures of the PCL tibial attachment are also dealt with in this section.

Clinical features of posterior cruciate ligament rupture

The main deforming force in PCL ruptures is a **posteriorly directed force** upon the proximal tibia, as in dashboard injuries. **Hyperextension injuries** of the knee sometimes rupture the PCL. This is in contrast to anterior cruciate ruptures, where there is a predominantly rotational force. Isolated injury is uncommon, collateral ligament and meniscal lesions often coexisting.

As with anterior cruciate ruptures, there is a haemarthrosis. However, as there is often a capsular tear in PCL ruptures, this may be dissipated. Acute examination may be difficult. Formal examination may only be possible under anaesthetic – this may demonstrate the following features.

1. **Posterior sag sign**: with the knee flexed at 90° the tibia may be seen to sublux backwards upon the femur (Fig. 22.6, compare with the opposite side).

2. **Posterior draw test**: this is similar to the anterior draw sign, but in reverse. With the knee at 90°, the tibial excursion with a posteriorly directed force is increased. **Care must be taken, as many PCL ruptures are incorrectly**

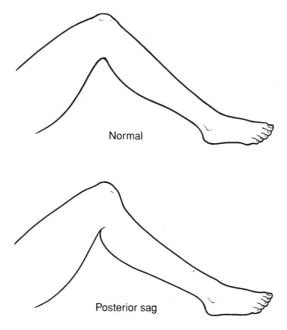

Normal

Posterior sag

Figure 22.6 – The posterior sag sign

described as **ACL ruptures** (the 'false-positive anterior draw sign'). This is because the knee sometimes subluxes ('sags') in PCL injury – no further posterior motion is possible but the tibia can be pulled forwards into its anatomical position.

3. **Reverse pivot shift test**: this is similar to the pivot shift test used in ACL injuries. The knee is flexed to 90° in valgus. In PCL ruptures, as the knee is extended, the lateral tibial plateau reduces from its subluxed position.

Radiographs are usually normal other than demonstrating a haemarthrosis. Look out for an avulsion fracture of the PCL tibial attachment (see below).

In the acute setting of the Accident and Emergency Department, it is difficult to diagnose a PCL rupture confidently. However, the history of a posteriorly directed force upon the tibia is suggestive. As with haemarthroses due to ACL rupture, admission or urgent fracture clinic referral is appropriate. The knee should be immobilized in a plaster slab or a flexion-restricting brace. Aspiration of the knee under aseptic conditions may relieve pain and be helpful.

Untreated PCL ruptures may lead to chronic instability and degenerative change. Acute surgical repair may be indicated.

Avulsion fractures of the posterior tibial spine

These are similar in their nature to PCL ruptures. They are diagnosed from the x-ray. If the fragment is undisplaced, the knee should be immobilized in a plaster. If the fragment is displaced, the patient should be admitted for open reduction and internal fixation of the fragment.

Meniscal injuries

Meniscal injuries are a common cause of morbidity and often present in the acute setting. The medial meniscus, as a result of its more fixed attachments, is more liable to tears than the lateral meniscus. Conversely, congenital and other abnormalities of the lateral meniscus (e.g. discoid meniscus) are more common, and these predispose to tears. The diagnosis of a torn meniscus can often be made clinically – special tests such as MRI and diagnostic arthroscopy are largely used to confirm the diagnosis.

An important symptom associated with meniscal injuries is **locking**. Locking of the knee implies an inability to straighten the knee fully, and on examination there is a springy lock to full extension. This is largely due to the fact that a portion of displaced meniscus is lying within the joint preventing full extension. Locking is a somewhat non-specific symptom for meniscal tears, also being caused by loose bodies; however sudden **unlocking** is a very specific symptom, occurring with reduction of the displaced meniscal tear. Note that the layman's term of locking is not that used in orthopaedics – it is often used to imply a loss of flexion of the knee.

Meniscal anatomy

The blood supply of the menisci somewhat dictates the treatment of tears. Although the peripheral portion of the meniscus has a blood supply, the central area is avascular – thus central or radial tears cannot effectively repair whilst peripheral tears may do so (Fig. 22.7). There is a watershed area between the two zones where repair possibly may occur. In view of this, central and radial meniscal tears are treated by partial meniscectomy whilst meniscal repair may be contemplated in peripheral tears. Obviously, an early diagnosis of a peripheral tear aids the prognosis for meniscal repair.

Meniscal tears in adolescents and young adults

Meniscal tears in the young adult classically result from a **rotational stress upon the flexed weight-bearing knee** (Fig. 22.8). Note the similarity with the mechanism of injury of anterior cruciate ligament (ACL) ruptures; indeed ACL and meniscal injuries often coexist.

A meniscal tear may present acutely following a rotational weight-bearing injury.

1. There is usually **delayed swelling** (around 6 hours), consisting of an effusion, due to synovial reaction. This is in contrast to a haemarthrosis where there is immediate swelling. (Some peripheral tears occur in the vascular zone of the meniscus and can cause a haemarthrosis).

2. If the knee is **locked** the diagnosis is obvious; the patient should be admitted or referred urgently to the fracture clinic – an arthroscopic meniscectomy is usually required.

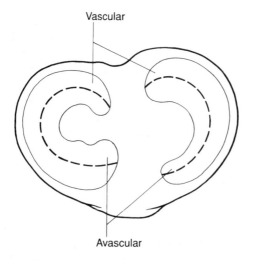

Figure 22.7 – Blood supply of the menisci – as the peripheral portions are vascular, meniscal repair is possible. The central portions are avascular.

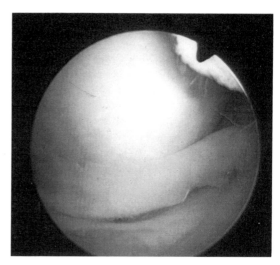

Figure 22.8 – A meniscal tear

3. If the knee has a full range of movement, the diagnosis is more difficult to make. In the presence of an effusion with a history of recent injury, a meniscal tear is a differential diagnosis. **Tenderness along the respective joint line** is usually present. **Rotation** of the flexed knee may cause symptoms on the side of the tear, and a click may be felt along the joint line. **McMurray's test** is one of these rotational tests, used to diagnose a medial meniscal tear – lateral rotation of the abducted knee in varying degrees of flexion precipitating symptoms. The **grinding test** may be positive – with the patient prone the flexed knee is rotated and force applied to the tibia longitudinally; symptoms may be reproduced on the side of the lesion. X-rays, other than demonstrating an effusion, are usually normal. Referral to the fracture clinic should be made where further assessment can be arranged. MRI or diagnostic arthroscopy may be required to confirm the diagnosis.

A meniscal tear may also present in the chronic setting. The patient may give a history of a twisting weight-bearing injury. Symptoms may be ill-defined, including clicking, locking and unlocking, medial or lateral joint line pain and recurrent swelling. Pain on turning or twisting is significant. On examination there may be an effusion, joint line tenderness and rotational stressing may provoke symptoms.

Degenerate meniscal tears

With advancing age, the menisci become more brittle and immobile. As a consequence, minor trauma may cause tears of the menisci. This is common in middle age and beyond. The patient may not easily be able to recollect one particular traumatic episode. An effusion may be present, and the joint line is often tender. Rotational tests may be positive. These **degenerate tears** may settle with conservative treatment – if symptoms are prolonged partial meniscectomy may be required.

Meniscal cysts

These are more common in the lateral meniscus. They are associated with degenerative changes within the meniscus. The cyst itself may cause ill-defined symptoms with joint line tenderness and the patient may notice a lump on the side of the knee that reduces spontaneously. Clinically the cysts are most obvious when the knee is flexed to 30°, tending to disappear in full flexion or extension. The cyst also predisposes to meniscal tears. Meniscal cysts (along with discoid menisci) should be suspected in younger patients presenting with meniscal pathology.

Collateral ligament injuries of the knee

The collateral ligaments, medial and lateral, run along the sides of the knee, and play an essential role in maintaining the stability of the knee (see Fig. 22.2). They are largely extracapsular structures, although collateral injuries may coexist with capsular tears and intracapsular damage. As with many ligament ruptures, partial tears may be more painful than complete tears; complete tears may be missed unless careful examination is undertaken.

Anatomy and biomechanics of the collateral ligaments

The **medial collateral ligament** (MCL) is made up of two main bands, superficial and deep. The composition of the ligament is complex, including the muscles that form the pes anserinus; however, it essentially runs from the medial aspect of the femur to the medial aspect of the tibia. The ligament is very closely related to the medial capsule of the knee. The function of the medial ligament complex is to provide stability to valgus stress – its role differs at varying degrees of flexion of the knee. At 30° of flexion it acts as the primary stabilizer, whilst in full extension it acts as a secondary stabilizer, with the anterior cruciate ligament and the postero-medial capsule acting primarily. (This different stabilization role has relevance in examination of the knee – see below).

The **lateral collateral ligament** (LCL) is a complex structure, running alongside the lateral aspect of the knee in conjunction with the biceps tendon and the ilio-tibial band of the fascia lata. It connects the lateral aspect of the femur to the tibia, fibula and patella. Its function is to act as a primary restraint to varus stress upon the knee – it acts in this primary role in full extension of the knee up to 25° of flexion.

Medial collateral ligament injury

Clinical features

Injury to the medial collateral ligament can be due to direct or rotational forces. A rotational force may cause a combination of injuries, and classically starts with the MCL, and with further force damages the medial meniscus and ACL (hence the importance of examining these structures in MCL injuries). A direct injury causing MCL injury is one which produces a valgus stress upon the knee – however, this is most commonly due to a lateral force applied to the fixed knee, resulting in valgus stress to the medial structures.

In isolated injuries of the MCL, as most of the structure is extracapsular, there is usually no haemarthrosis or effusion. Bruising may be seen on the medial aspect of the knee, although this is unusual and may take several days to develop. Tenderness is often elicited along the line of the ligament, especially towards the attachments and insertions. Dynamic stress tests of valgus instability are useful in grading the severity of the injury but they are best done under anaesthesia as pain may prevent accurate assessment. It is important when functionally assessing the MCL to do so in both full extension (where the MCL acts as a secondary stabilizer) and at 30° of flexion (when it acts as the primary restraint) – if only examined in extension, a more severe rupture of the MCL may not be diagnosed. A grading system can be used:

Grade 1: <0.5 cm opening up of the joint on valgus stress (mild)
Grade 2: 0.5–1.0 cm   opening   up (moderate)
Grade 3: >1.5 cm opening up (severe)

(Note that many MCL tears are associated with haemarthroses and effusions in reality; this is due to the coexistence of capsular tears and intra-articular damage.)

Radiological tests are not usually helpful. On plain films medial soft tissue swelling may be seen. An avulsion fracture may also be noted. Chronic MCL lesions may be diagnosed by the presence of calcification within the proximal medial ligament, a condition termed as **Pelligrini–Steida disease**. Stress radiographs may be helpful in grading the severity of damage. In unclear cases, MRI can accurately assess the anatomical damage.

Treatment

The vast majority of isolated MCL tears can be treated conservatively. Grade 1 tears can be treated with a Tubigrip and exercises. Grade 2–3 tears should be immobilized in a plaster cylinder for 4–6 weeks with the knee at 30° of flexion. Brace protection and physiotherapy may be needed after this. Operative treatment of isolated MCL ruptures is now seldom indicated.

Severe MCL ruptures usually occur in conjunction with other knee injuries, e.g. ACL and medial meniscal tears, there may be a case for repair of the ligament in association with other surgery.

The complications of untreated medial collateral ruptures include persistent valgus instability and subsequent rotatory instability. There is usually an associated ACL injury in such cases.

Lateral collateral ligament injury

Clinical features

The clinical features of LCL injury are similar to those of MCL injury. Injury is usually due to a direct force resulting in abnormal varus stress upon the knee. Rotational forces may also be responsible. Examination findings are similar to those of the MCL, with point tenderness over a portion of the ligament being a common feature. The LCL acts as a primary stabilizer to varus stress in full extension (cf. MCL). A similar grading scheme is used. It is **essential** to establish and document the integrity of the common peroneal nerve (dorsiflexion of the foot and sensation over the dorsum of the foot) in injuries of this type. Radiography may demonstrate an avulsion fracture of the head of the fibula.

Treatment

Treatment is much as for MCL injuries. Grade 1 sprains are treated symptomatically. Grade 2 injuries are treated in plaster with the knee in full extension. Grade 3 injuries are usually associated with intra-articular pathology, and may require surgery. When there is an avulsion fracture of the fibula, it should be stabilized by internal fixation.

Injuries to the extensor mechanism of the knee

General aspects

The extensor mechanism of the knee consists of all the elements needed to extend the knee, namely:

1. The quadriceps muscle.
2. The quadriceps tendon.
3. The patella.
4. The patellar tendon.
5. The tibial tubercle, into which the patellar tendon inserts.

It is impossible to walk normally with a deficient extensor mechanism. Therefore it is **essential** in all cases of knee injury to ensure that there is an effective **straight leg raise** – if it is not present the extensor mechanism is compromised. In most cases where there is an inadequate straight leg raise surgical intervention will be required.

Any part of the extensor mechanism may be damaged at any age, but the common patterns of injury are as follows (Fig. 22.9).

1. The quadriceps muscle and tendon are damaged in the middle-aged and elderly.
2. The young and middle-aged sustain patellar fractures.
3. All ages may rupture the patellar tendon.
4. The young avulse the tibial tuberosity. Partial avulsion of the tibial apophysis is common in active children – Osgood–Schlatter's disease (see below).

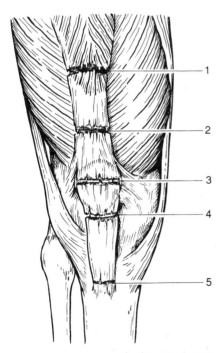

Figure 22.9 – The extensor mechanism of the knee. The extensor mechanism may be disrupted at a number of levels ; 1. The quadriceps muscle, 2. The quadriceps tendon, 3. The patella, 4. The patellar tendon, 5. The tibial tuberosity

Ruptures of the quadriceps muscle and tendon

The quadriceps muscle

Quadriceps muscle tears are relatively common, especially in the young athlete, but are rarely complete. The commonest tear is within the rectus femoris portion. The history is usually clear, and on examination the proximal muscle belly may be seen and palpated, especially upon stress testing. Indeed, the commonest clinical problem with these tears is in differentiating an old tear from a tumour. The treatment is conservative, with initial rest and subsequent physiotherapy.

Ruptures of the quadriceps tendon

This is an important injury which is easy to miss if not specifically sought. Rupture occurs generally in the degenerate tendon of the middle-aged and elderly. The history is often of a stumble or fall, usually of a minor nature. The patient is unable to walk properly afterwards, and is in considerable pain. Examination may reveal a haemarthrosis, and **there is an inability to straighten the leg**. On attempting to straighten the leg, a palpable gap is found in the area, representing the area of the tear. Radiographs may show soft tissue swelling in the area of the tendon, fluid within the knee joint, and the patella may be situated abnormally low on the lateral view.

The treatment in nearly all of these cases is **operative**. Unless an adequate surgical repair of the tendon is performed, the extensor mechanism is seriously compromised, and the patient will be unable to walk properly. All such cases should therefore be referred and admitted immediately. Plaster immobilization may be required postoperatively.

Fractures of the patella

Mechanisms of patellar fracture

The patella may be fractured by:

1. Direct violence – by a direct blow upon the front of the knee or as in a dashboard injury.

2. Indirect violence – by sudden resisted extension of the knee.

In direct-type injuries, the fracture may be of any orientation, whilst indirect injuries tend to be of a transverse pattern. In addition, direct blows to the knee may cause soft-tissue injury to the area anterior to the patella – this may have a bearing upon the management. Injury to the hip joint may occur in direct injuries to the patella and the hip should be examined carefully to exclude this possibility.

Clinical features of patellar fracture

The history is often as above. The patient, often young, has a great deal of pain and holds the knee in flexion. There is an obvious haemarthrosis, which may be quite tense. Two patterns of patellar fractures are possible, and it is important to distinguish between them in the early management of these injuries:

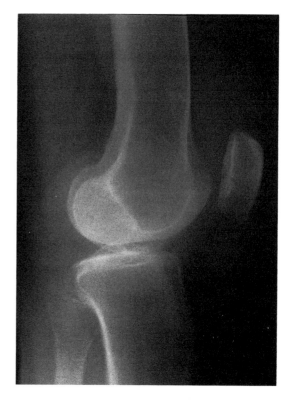

Figure 22.10 – Undisplaced fracture of the patella

1. In patients with some undisplaced (Fig. 22.10) and comminuted fractures, **there is the ability to straight leg raise** – these fractures therefore **may** be treated conservatively providing the articular surface of the patella has not been compromised. For there to be extension, the retinacular fibres around the patella must be intact.

2. Some patients with patellar fractures, especially those with displaced fractures (Fig. 22.11), **have an inability to straight leg raise** – these patients must **not** be treated conservatively as the extensor mechanism has been compromised.

The injury is accurately diagnosed on radiography, with anteroposterior and lateral x-rays.

Management

Undisplaced transverse fractures **with a straight leg raise** may be treated conservatively in a long leg plaster with 10–20° of flexion. If the patient is uncomfortable and there is a tense haemar-

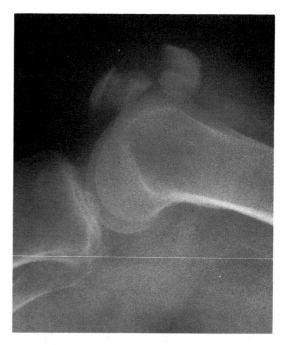

Figure 22.11 – Displaced fracture of the patella

throsis, the knee may be aspirated under strict aseptic conditions (remember that the blood within the knee is a good culture medium for micro-organisms). Check x-rays 1 and 2 weeks post fracture are needed to ensure that the fracture has not displaced.

Displaced transverse fractures, and all transverse fractures with an inability to straight leg raise require open reduction and internal fixation of the fracture. The knee may be aspirated and a temporary backslab applied. The fractures are usually fixed using the tension band wiring technique.

Longitudinal fractures are often initially missed as they are not clearly seen on the lateral x-ray. As they are usually undisplaced, they can be treated conservatively in plaster. (These fractures are not uncommon in patients with total knee replacements and can be best seen on skyline radiographs).

Comminuted fractures are difficult to manage. Surgical reconstruction may be impossible. Partial or complete patellectomy may be required. Chronic stiffness and anterior knee pain is a common result.

When interpreting x-rays, take care with the relatively common **bipartite patella**. This is a congenital variant of normal, whereby the patella is not completely fused. The line seen on x-ray is usually in the upper-outer quadrant of the patella. If doubt exists, a fracture usually hurts when palpated, the condition is usually bilateral and the 'line' seen on x-ray is rounded in bipartite patella, unlike a typical fracture. Tripartite patella is rare but occasionally seen.

Dislocation of the patella

Dislocation of the patella is a common and rather confusing injury. Many patients describe 'the knee dislocating' when in fact there has been some other intra-articular injury. Except in rare circumstances, a patella dislocates laterally, implying tearing of the medial retinacular fibres. Because many dislocations reduce prior to attendance in hospital, unless there is a clear history of a laterally displaced patella, regard the term 'dislocated patella' with suspicion. The management of recurrent dislocation of the patella is outside the scope of this book, and the reader is advised to consult larger texts.

Dislocation of the patella for the first time

In the first episode of dislocation of a patella, there is usually a clear history of trauma, often of a sudden muscular contraction during sport. Females are more liable to sustain dislocation, but the dislocations with more extensive soft tissue damage are seen in males.

A dislocation that has not reduced is very obvious. There is medial retinacular tenderness (where the fibres are torn to allow the patella to dislocate laterally). As long as the clinical situation is seen and documented, an x-ray is not necessary, although one taken in dislocated position can be useful in future management. Reduction is easy providing the knee is extended, and does not require a general anaesthetic. Intravenous sedation with Entonox supplementation may be required. It is important to radiograph the knee following reduction to exclude a second injury – up to 10% of traumatic dislocations are associated with an osteochondral fracture or other injury. The knee may require aspiration under strict aseptic conditions to relieve the pain of the haemarthrosis. Where facilities for immediate physiotherapy exist they should be used to start instant quadriceps rehabilitation and cooling to reduce swelling. A supporting bandage should be applied. Alternatively a plaster cylinder could be applied with the knee in extension. A referral should be arranged for the fracture clinic.

A common clinical problem is the patient who has sustained a 'dislocated kneecap' on the sporting field, and who has had some form of manipulation prior to reaching hospital. The history of the injury and of a laterally displaced patella is important to obtain, as well as some description of the mechanism of reduction. A haemarthrosis should be present. Tenderness over the medial retinacular fibres should be seen acutely; if not present, it is unlikely that a dislocation has occurred. If confirmed, the knee should be treated as above.

Recurrent dislocation of the patella

All too often, a patella may recurrently dislocate, often with trivial trauma. If this is a recurring pathology associated with generalized joint laxity and patellar malalignment, for which the patient is being assessed, there is little point in referring acutely nor in immobilizing. It is important, though, to exclude a second pathology. If no treatment is arranged already, a fracture clinic appointment with physiotherapy referral is appropriate. Elective surgical correction may be necessary in the persistent case.

Rupture of the patellar tendon

The patellar tendon connects the inferior pole of the patella to the tibial tuberosity, forming part of the extensor mechanism of the knee. Rupture of the patellar tendon usually occurs in the degenerate tendon of the middle-aged or elderly (with minimal trauma), but may also occur following sporting injury in the young.

The diagnosis, as with ruptures of the quadriceps tendon, is easy to miss if not specifically sought. The patient is unable to walk. A haemarthrosis is present. **There is an inability to straight leg raise**. On attempted knee extension, there may be a palpable gap within the tendon. X-ray demonstrates a haemarthrosis and the patella may lie 'high' on the lateral view.

Treatment for a complete rupture is **invariably surgical**, with **no** place for conservative management. If the tendon is not repaired, the patient will not be able to walk effectively and will have a permanent limp.

Avulsion fracture of the inferior border of the patella

This injury pattern may occur at any age. Unless it is a chronic avulsion (see below) it should be managed by internal fixation and surgical repair.

A more chronic injury pattern that may be seen is **Sinding–Larsen–Johansson syndrome**, where there is a traction apophysitis of the inferior pole of the patella. Treatment is conservative.

Avulsion fracture of the tibial tuberosity

The patellar tendon inserts into the tibial tuberosity as the last component of the extensor mechanism of the knee. The injury pattern is as for indirect-type patellar fractures, with a sudden muscular contraction resulting in the patellar tendon avulsing a portion of the tibial tuberosity. The injury tends to occur in the adolescent or young adult. The avulsion may be quite extensive when the epiphysis is still open.

Clinical features are of an inability to walk. A haemarthrosis is not usually present unless the joint surface is involved. There is tenderness localized to the area of the tibial tuberosity. There may be an inability to straight leg raise. The lateral x-ray view of the knee is the most useful (Fig. 22.12). If the fracture is undisplaced, the knee should be immobilized in a plaster cylinder for 4–6 weeks. If the fracture is displaced it requires internal fixation. However, in the younger adolescent, internal

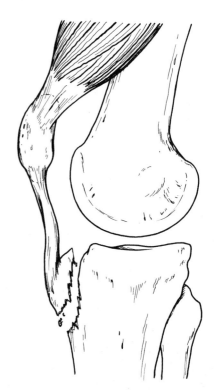

Figure 22.12 – Avulsion fracture of the tibial tuberosity

fixation has the risk of premature epiphyseal fusion, so it is best avoided if possible.

A common subacute and chronic problem is **Osgood–Schlatter's syndrome**, which represents a traction apophysitis of the tibial tuberosity. It typically occurs in adolescent males. Pain, tenderness and swelling are localized to the area. Lateral x-ray demonstrates fragmentation of the epiphysis. This condition is largely self-limiting and can be treated conservatively.

Dislocations around the knee

Dislocation of the knee joint

Dislocation of the knee joint is fortunately a rare injury that follows a considerable degree of violence, and has a high complication rate. The tibia may displace in any direction in relation to the femur, most commonly anteriorly. The fact that the knee has dislocated implies at least damage to the collateral and cruciate ligaments of the knee, as well as to other intra-articular and vital extra-articular structures (Fig. 22.13).

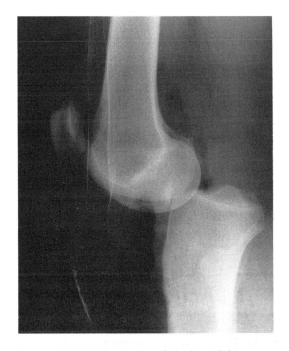

Figure 22.13 – Dislocation of the knee joint

Clinical features are of a grossly deformed and swollen knee joint. As with most dislocations, do **NOT** take an x-ray of a dislocated joint – reduce it first and then assess it radiologically. Both before and after reduction, establish the integrity of the distal neurovascular status of the limb – common peroneal nerve injury and popliteal artery/vein damage are common. Reduction is effected by longitudinal traction on the limb, and is usually relatively easy as many of the ligamentous structures are damaged. If it is not easily reduced, it is most often due to rupture of the medial collateral ligament, and may require an urgent open reduction. Radiological assessment, in particular, may demonstrate tibial spine avulsions (implying cruciate ligament rupture) and collateral ligament avulsions.

The patient must be admitted with regular checks of the distal neurovascular status of the limb – there is a high incidence of **compartment syndrome** following dislocation of the knee. If there is any suggestion of vascular injury, urgent arteriography is required. Neurovascular complications increase with time following dislocation of the knee and unreduced dislocations of over 8 hours inevitably result in amputation. Skeletal traction may be necessary for several days within a split plaster backslab.

Dislocation of the proximal tibio-fibular joint

This is an uncommon injury, most often caused by twisting of the weight-bearing flexed knee. It requires a considerable degree of violence and is associated with parachute jumping and horse riding. Other injuries must be excluded.

On examination there is lateral tenderness over the proximal tibio-fibular joint. The integrity of the common peroneal nerve (dorsiflexion of the foot and sensation on the dorsum of the foot) must be verified, as the nerve passes close to the joint. The diagnosis should be suspected clinically, as it is difficult to see it on x-ray. Movement of the ankle tends to cause pain in the knee. Comparison with the other side is helpful.

The dislocation can be reduced, under intra-venous sedation or general anaesthetic if necessary. Reduction is effected by pressure over the fibular head with the knee flexed. The knee should be immobilized in an above-knee plaster non-weight-bearing for 4–6 weeks.

The acutely painful knee

The acutely painful knee can be a difficult diagnostic problem. Consider the following causes:

1. Fractures and acute ligament injuries

- see previous relevant sections

2. Internal derangement of the knee

- e.g. **meniscal tears**
- e.g. **loose bodies** (the main causes of loose bodies within the knee are fractures, osteochondral fractures, bucket-handle tears of the meniscus, osteochondritis dissecans, synovial chondromatosis and osteoarthritic osteophytes).

3. Underlying osseo-cartilagenous pathology

- e.g. **osteochondritis dissecans**, where lesions develop in the femoral condyles resulting in pain and loose body development. The craters can be seen on x-ray.
- e.g. **benign or malignant tumour of bone and cartilage** – these can be difficult to diagnose, and are easily missed on x-ray, especially if suspecting a fracture! Night pain is a conspicuous feature of tumours.

4. Rheumatological and 'medical' conditions

- e.g. **rheumatoid arthritis** – rheumatoid arthritis may, not uncommonly, first develop within the knee, and be part of monoarticular disease. The initial features are of a synovitis with effusion. The presentation may be far from typical, however, and therefore in all cases of unexpected knee pain it is worth-while performing a serological screen for rheumatoid and other connective tissue disorders.
- e.g. **reactive arthropathy** – this is an ill-defined group of disorders, whereby an arthropathy may develop due to stimulus by an organism or other antigen. One form is termed **Reiter's disease**, a combination of arthropathy, conjunctivitis and non-specific urethritis.
- e.g. **ankylosing spondylitis**
- e.g. **gout and pseudogout (pyrophosphate arthropathy)** – see Chapter 2
- e.g. **acute exacerbation of osteoarthritis**
- e.g. **villo-nodular synovitis**

5. Infection within the knee

This may take acute and chronic forms.

Acute infection of the knee (**septic arthritis)** is a devastating illness, and if left undiagnosed may result in joint destruction and even death. In children, the condition is usually the consequence of intracapsular osteomyelitis. In a normal adult, it is usually the result of an inoculation of micro-organisms, either by injury or iatrogenically, e.g. steroid injection, aspiration of the knee. Gonococcal or chlamydial septic arthritis can occur following genito-urinary infections. It may also occur endogenously in an immunocompromised patient.

The patient is **very ill, toxic, pyrexial and dehydrated**. There is a **pyarthrosis**. On attempted movement of the joint, **there is hardly any movement at all, active or passive**. The condition is a **surgical emergency** – rehydration and early surgical washout are necessary. Antibiotics should be withheld if surgery is anticipated in a short period so as to obtain accurate microbiological sensitivities. Beware the rheumatoid patient on steroids in this context as there may be fewer symptoms!

Chronic infection is largely **tuberculous**, and is currently seldom seen in the UK, although its incidence is now increasing.

6. Bursae around the knee joint

There are many bursae around the knee – some are independent structures, whilst many communicate with the knee joint. It is important to distinguish swelling of a bursa from generalized swelling of the knee (i.e., an effusion), or an incorrect diagnostic path will be followed.

Popliteal bursae

These are common structures, with no clear-cut anatomical definition. Most intercommunicate with the knee. The most common are:

- **Semimembranosus bursa** This is a bursa lying between the medial head of gastrocnemius and the semimembranosus. A fluctuant lump is present in the area of the popliteal fossa. The bursa does communicate with the knee joint but in most cases the fluid within the cyst cannot be compressed into the knee because of the valvular nature of the communication. The bursa may present acutely with 'bursitis' – treatment is by rest, aspiration and anti-inflammatories. If symptoms are prolonged the bursa can be excised, although there is a high risk of recurrence.
- **'Baker's cyst'** This term is used to describe a pathological popliteal bursa that communicates with the knee joint. The knee is usually osteoarthritic (in some cases rheumatoid), resulting in synovial herniation and rupture. The cyst itself does not usually cause problems, but it may rupture into the calf musculature causing pain and tenderness. The condition is an important differential diagnosis of a deep venous thrombosis.

(With all popliteal lumps, it is essential to exclude a **popliteal aneurysm**, which is pulsatile **and** expansile, and which may interfere with the distal vasculature).

Bursae at the front of the knee

There are two common anterior bursae, often caused by repetitive kneeling.

- **Prepatellar bursa** A bursa normally exists between the patella and skin, which can become abnormally enlarged by constant friction, when it is colloquially termed as **housemaid's knee**. In some cases the localized swelling may become inflamed or infected with surrounding cellulitis – there may be a need for admission with intravenous antibiotics and surgical drainage. There may be an associated condition such as gout or rheumatoid arthritis.
- **Infrapatellar bursa** A bursa also exists between the infrapatellar ligament and the skin, which may also enlarge and become inflamed (**'clergyman's knee'**).

7. Hip pathology

Never forget to examine the hip in cases presenting with knee pain. It is remarkably easy to be caught out!

8. Overuse syndromes

- e.g. chondromalacia patellae and other variants of anterior knee pain
- e.g. stress fractures of the femur
- e.g. quadriceps tendinitis
- e.g. hamstring tendinitis
- e.g. stress fractures of the tibia
- e.g. patellar tendinitis ('jumper's knee')
- e.g. Sinding–Larsen–Johannson syndrome and Osgood–Schlatter's syndrome (see Extensor Mechanism section above).

23
The lower leg

Fractures of the proximal tibia

Tibial plateau fractures

Tibial plateau fractures are generally caused by a fall upon the extended knee. The majority are lateral tibial plateau fractures, with the knee in valgus at the time of the fall, i.e. they are compression-type fractures, the tibial plateau crushed by the femoral condyle. The most common classification is that of **Schatzker** into six types (Fig. 23.1).

Type 1 Wedge fracture of the lateral tibial plateau.
Type 2 Wedge fracture of the lateral plateau with depression of the adjacent plateau.

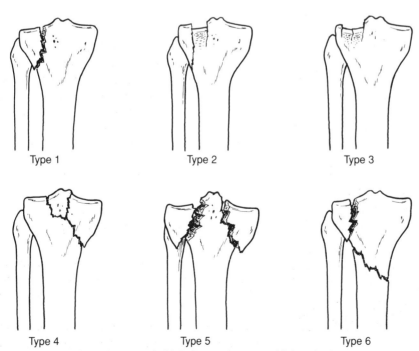

Type 1   Type 2   Type 3

Type 4   Type 5   Type 6
Figure 23.1 – Classification of tibial plateau fractures (Schatzker)

Type 3 Central depression of the articular surface of the lateral plateau without a wedge fragment.

Type 4 Fracture of the medial tibial plateau.

Type 5 Bicondylar fracture.

Type 6 Tibial plateau fracture with separation of metaphysis from diaphysis.

As well as the fracture, a common pattern is for the opposing collateral ligament to be sprained or ruptured, e.g. the medial collateral ligament with lateral plateau fractures.

As the fractures are intra-articular, the patient presents with a **haemarthrosis**. There may be extensive bruising, and the opposing collateral ligament may be damaged. Clinical testing may be difficult in the acute situation, although under anaesthesia the collateral ligaments may be unstable. The diagnosis is accurately made on radiography (Fig. 23.2), although tomograms may be needed to fully identify the fracture type.

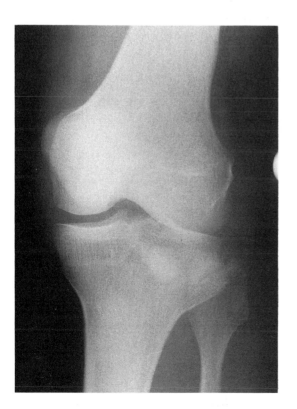

Figure 23.2 – Lateral tibial plateau fracture

All fractures should be referred immediately for assessment. Tomograms or CT scanning will determine the fracture pattern and, importantly, any associated depression of the articular surface. An examination under anaesthesia may also be required to determine the stability of the knee. Fractures without significant fracture displacement and articular depression may be treated conservatively. However, most require accurate open reduction and internal fixation to restore the congruity of the articular surface; the collateral ligament may also need to be repaired. Note, in addition, that there is a high incidence of meniscal tears with these injuries.

Proximal tibial epiphyseal injuries

These fractures in children correspond to tibial plateau fractures in adults. The mechanism is resisted extension of the knee, usually during sport. Two grades of injury occur:

1. Smaller forces result in an avulsion fracture of the tibial tuberosity.
2. Greater forces result in avulsion and displacement of the entire proximal tibial epipyhsis.

The fractures present with a **haemarthrosis**, and on lateral x-ray the tibial epiphysis can be seen to have displaced anteriorly. The distal neurovasculature should be checked as there is a small incidence of popliteal vessel entrapment. The injury should be immediately referred. Closed reduction is preferable to avoid surgery on the epiphysis, but open reduction with K wire fixation is sometimes necessary.

Fractures of the tibial shaft

Fractures of the tibia are a relatively common injury. They may occur as isolated injuries, but also occur in the multiply-injured patient. The open tibial fracture continues to be a difficult management problem, and the initial treatment in the Accident and Emergency Department can make a large difference to the outcome of the injury. It is essential in all tibial fractures to make an assessment of the soft tissues, as they have an important role to play in the healing of the fracture. This is because the tibia is relatively avascular, and so depends on the surrounding soft tissues for its blood supply.

Always check the distal neurovasculature, and monitor for the development of a **compartment syndrome**, which occurs especially with proximal tibial fractures.

Tibial fractures may be sustained from direct or indirect violence. Direct injuries occur most commonly in sport, and may be isolated with no fibular fracture (Fig. 23.3). Indirect fractures usually involve fracture of both tibia and fibula (Fig. 23.4), and may be due to torsional force or vertical stress, as in falls from a height. The

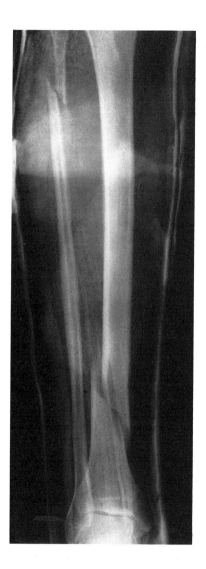

Figure 23.4 – Fracture of the tibia and fibula

fracture may be oblique (usually from torsional forces) or transverse. As with all long bone fractures, it is mandatory to assess the whole length of the bone, including the joint above and below, i.e. the ankle and knee joints **must** be seen on x-ray!

A problem with tibial fractures, in addition to their long union times, is their tendency to slip from a satisfactory position. When planning treatment for an individual fracture, contemplate how stable the fracture is – long spiral fractures may easily slip and angulate whilst transverse fractures are more stable. This is

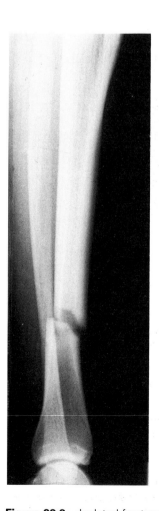

Figure 23.3 – Isolated fracture of the tibia

one of the many reasons that locked intramedullary nailing of tibial fractures has become more common in recent years. If plaster treatment is indicated, **never put a fresh tibial fracture in a below-knee plaster – an above-knee plaster should always be used.** This is because a below-knee plaster will not be able to control the fracture.

As the tibia is a relatively superficial structure, open fractures are common. The management of these fractures has changed enormously in recent years. Non-operative treatment is now avoided if possible, with early debridement and fixation. Although there is a risk of chronic infection with early internal fixation, most authorities are of the view that an infected stable fracture is preferable to an unstable infected fracture. Always remember, as with all open fractures, **never primarily suture an open wound!**

Undisplaced tibial fractures in the adult

Undisplaced tibial fractures generally have an intact periosteum (Fig. 23.5), so that there is less risk of displacement of the fracture. An assessment of the soft tissues is mandatory. Opinion varies as to whether all tibial fractures should be admitted for 1–2 days for elevation and observation of the soft tissues and circulation, and it is worthwhile checking the policy of your unit.

The initial plaster should be an **above-knee backslab**, with mobilization non-weight-bearing on crutches. Once the swelling has settled this is converted to a full plaster. Regular radiological checks are necessary. Although a fracture may appear stable, it may angulate, and varus angulation is to be avoided if at all possible. A general plan is that the limb should be non-weight bearing for 4–6 weeks with a further 4–6 weeks weight-bearing; the above-knee plaster can be converted to a Sarmiento or below-knee plaster once the fracture is stable, usually half-way along the treatment plan. (A Sarmiento plaster is a form of below-knee plaster that is moulded around the patellar ligament, and offers more control than a conventional below-knee plaster).

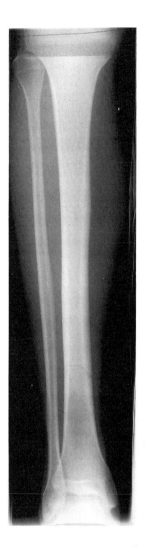

Figure 23.5 – Undisplaced fracture of the tibia

Displaced fractures and potentially unstable fractures of the tibia

Unfortunately, most tibial fractures are unstable, or at least potentially unstable. Their management is influenced by the protocol of your orthopaedic unit. There is an increasing tendency to perform **locked intramedullary nailing** on tibial fractures of this nature – it allows early mobilization, avoidance of plaster and ensures stability. However, the operation does carry some risk, and some surgeons believe conservative treatment to be a safer option.

Whatever management plan is followed, all the patients should be admitted for elevation and observation etc. Monitor for **compartment syndrome**. A calcaneal traction pin should be inserted, either under local anaesthetic in the Accident and Emergency Department or under general anaesthetic. If conservative treatment is planned, a moulded plaster can be applied after a few days. Alternative treatment options, in selected cases, include plating of the tibia and external fixation, although, in most cases, intramedullary nailing is the treatment of choice.

Open fractures of the tibia

Open fractures of the tibia are **a surgical emergency**. There has been a recent change in the management of these fractures. The British Orthopaedic Association has stated that these fractures are optimally managed by cooperation between orthopaedic and plastic surgeons. A management plan is as follows:

1. Before assessing the limb, assess the patient. Resuscitate if necessary.
2. Assess the limb, checking for integrity of the distal neurovasculature. Inspect the wound and grade the fracture as compound grade 1–3, as according to the Gustillo grading (see Chapter 3). If the fracture is grossly displaced, reduce it immediately.
3. Photograph the limb, as this is important documentation of the severity of the injury.
4. Give intravenous antibiotics, and add anaerobic cover if any soil etc., is present.
5. Check the tetanus status of the patient, and treat appropriately.
6. Apply an antiseptic-soaked swab on the wound, and temporarily splint the limb.
7. **Then** obtain necessary x-rays. An open tibial fracture is very apparent, and x-rays are not needed immediately. They can wait until the patient has been stabilized.
8. The patient **must** undergo surgery as soon as possible, and certainly within 6 hours. The wound should be assessed, debrided and cleaned. Current opinion is that the fracture should be stabilized if possible, using either intramedullary nailing, external fixation or internal fixation. It has been clearly shown that the skeleton must be stabilized for the soft tissues to heal, and this certainly applies to any grafts placed on the wound. There is a risk of infection with introduction of foreign materials, but it is now accepted that the majority of open fractures fare better with aggressive primary management.
9. **Never, no matter how tempting, primarily close the wound!**

Undisplaced tibial fractures in children

Greenstick tibial fractures are relatively common in children. If they are undisplaced, the fractures can be immobilized in an **above-knee backslab**. The plaster should be well padded. The child can usually be allowed home as long as there is not a great deal of soft tissue swelling. The child should be seen within one week in the fracture clinic for completion of plaster and a radiological check. Weight-bearing may commence once callus appears. In general terms, union can be expected in weeks corresponding to the age of the child, i.e. 4 weeks in a 4-year-old, 8 weeks in an 8-year-old, up to 12 weeks from 12 years to adulthood.

A problem in the very young child is that a plaster, once applied, tends to be kicked off! If this happens, it is acceptable to allow the limb to be free, as most children will not attempt to weight-bear on a fracture that has not united.

Angulated and displaced tibial fractures in children

Fractures of this type may be associated with soft tissue swelling, and it is therefore safest to admit the child. Rest in an above-knee backslab with elevation and ice is advisable. After a few days, a full plaster can be applied under general anaesthetic with correction of the deformity. Skeletal traction is not usually required. Internal fixation is avoided if at all possible, and is not often needed. Careful monitoring of the fracture is required until callus appears, as there is a high incidence of slippage and shortening of the fracture.

Open tibial fractures in children

Because there is more subcutaneous tissue in front of the tibia in children, and their periosteum is thicker and stronger, open tibial fractures are less common than in adults, and therefore require a violent causative force. The initial management is as for adults, but intramedullary nailing is avoided as it interferes with the tibial epiphyses.

Isolated fractures of the fibula

Beware the isolated fibular fracture!

Fibular fractures may be due to:

1. Direct forces, e.g. a kick direct onto the lateral aspect of the leg.
2. Indirect forces, i.e. due to rotational stress.

In direct force to the fibula, an isolated fracture of the fibula may exist as such. However, if the force is indirect, **a fibula fracture must be associated with either a fracture of the tibia/ankle or a ligamentous rupture at the ankle.** It is therefore **essential** both to examine and to x-ray the entire lower leg when an isolated fibular fracture is seen.

Isolated fractures of the fibula associated with direct injury

Isolated fibular fractures are usually transverse. (Suspect an indirect injury pattern if the fracture is spiral). As the fibula does not play an important role in the weight-bearing dynamics of the limb, this fracture can be treated conservatively. A below-knee backslab may be applied initially (an above-knee is not necessary as with tibial fractures), later converted to a full plaster. Mobilization should be initially non-weight-bearing, with weight allowed after 3–4 weeks. The limb should be immobilized for a total of 6 weeks.

Fracture of the fibula associated with indirect injury

Most indirect-type fibular fractures are spiral. The fibular fracture may be associated with:

1. **A fracture of the shaft of the tibia** In such a case, treat the tibial fracture on its merits.

2. **A fracture of the ankle** This is dealt with fully in the section on ankle fractures. However, it is important to realize that should a spiral fracture of the fibula exist above an ankle fracture, the interosseous membrane must have ruptured in the interval between the two sites, producing a potential **diastasis** (Chapter 24).

3. **A rupture of the medial ligament of the ankle** This is also dealt with in Chapter 24 on the ankle. However, it is the fracture pattern in the lower limb that is most commonly missed. The non-weight-bearing x-ray of the ankle may be normal, but it is essential to realize that there may be a **diastasis** in that the interosseous membrane has ruptured between the two sites (Fig. 23.6). The patient must therefore be carefully clinically examined. If there is medial ligament tenderness, the patient should be admitted for examination under anaesthetic and consideration of

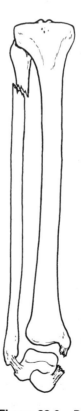

Figure 23.6 – Diastasis. Note that this high fibular fracture is associated with a rupture of the medial ligament of the ankle. The interosseous membrane is ruptured between the two sites (Maisonneuve's fracture).

placement of a diastasis screw between fibula and tibia. **If the patient with such an injury is allowed home in a plaster, with subsequent weight-bearing, a permanent diastasis may result with disastrous consequences for the ankle and for you medico-legally.**

Gastrocnemius tears and rupture of the achilles tendon

Pathology associated with the mechanism for plantarflexion of the ankle is common. Two main systems plantarflex the ankle:

1. The gastrocnemius–soleus muscular unit, connecting to the calcaneum via the achilles tendon.
2. The long flexors of the foot, which although they bypass the ankle on their way to the forefoot, have an influence on plantarflexion of the ankle. It is important to realize, therefore, that **active plantarflexion of the ankle is possible when the achilles tendon has ruptured**, of relevance in examination of suspected injury.

Gastrocnemius-soleus tears

Partial **muscular** tears of the gastrocnemius–soleus complex are relatively common. The tear is often specifically related to an injury, which may be minor. Intense pain and bruising is noted in the upper calf. There is pain on palpation of the calf. Importantly, no palpable gap can be felt in the lower leg in the region of the achilles tendon and Simmond's test (see below) is negative. Treatment is conservative. The injury is very painful, so plaster immobilization in a below-knee weight-bearing cast is helpful. Physiotherapy may be needed subsequently. Important differential diagnoses of the condition are deep venous thrombosis and rupture of a popliteal cyst – the history is therefore of great value.

Rupture of the achilles tendon

This is a common condition that unfortunately is often missed in the acute setting. It is an important diagnosis to make as an untreated rupture inevitably results in a chronic limp.

The history is often distinctive. The injury most commonly occurs in middle age when the tendon becomes degenerate, and follows sudden muscular activity. The patient complains that 'I felt that I was kicked in the back of the calf', a statement almost pathognomonic of the condition; in addition, there is an inability to walk normally and stand upon the toes. Steroid injections into the achilles tendon sheath for tendinitis predispose to rupture.

Examination reveals a palpable gap in the achilles tendon, most commonly 4–6 cm above the ankle. There is weakness of plantarflexion of the ankle, **but active plantarflexion does not exclude an achilles tendon rupture**, as the long flexors also act in this respect. **Simmond's test** is positive – this is carried out by compressing the calf of the prone patient who has the foot hanging over the edge of the bed (Fig. 23.7). Compression normally causes passive plantarflexion of the ankle, whilst in rupture this is not so. The test is remarkably accurate. **In all cases of calf pain Simmond's test should be performed and the result documented in the medical records.**

Treatment of achilles tendon ruptures is, at present, controversial. The injury can be treated conservatively in a below-knee plaster, initially in full plantarflexion so as to approximate the ends of the tendon. Over the next 6–10 weeks

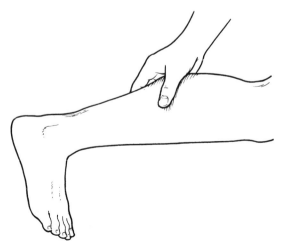

Figure 23.7 – Simmond's test for rupture of the achilles tendon

the plaster is changed several times in progressively more dorsiflexion until the ankle is neutral. Operative treatment is also possible, whereby the tendon is surgically repaired with subsequent plaster immobilization. Operative treatment offers better results in terms of strength and a lower re-rupture rate, but there is a significant risk of wound breakdown following the procedure. The decision as to management rests with the protocol of your orthopaedic unit – the patient should be referred immediately.

The acutely painful lower leg

The acutely painful lower leg can be arbitrarily divided into anterior and posterior categories.

Acute anterior lower limb pain

The following diagnoses should be considered.

1. Traumatic injury to bone, ligament or muscle.
2. **Stress fracture of the tibia** These fractures can be difficult to diagnose. The key history is of repetitive injury, e.g. in sport, pain on weight-bearing and of very localized tibial pain on palpation. X-rays are often normal acutely, with later films demonstrating periosteal reaction and callus at the fracture site. If the injury is suspected, the limb may be temporarily immobilized whilst a bone scan is arranged, which is the definitive investigation.
3. Anterior tibial **compartment syndrome** This is a rare but very serious condition. It is usually precipitated by fracture, but trauma to the soft tissues alone may cause it. Prolonged athletic activity without trauma has been known to result in the syndrome occasionally There is intense, agonizing pain, unrelieved by analgesics. On examination the anterior compartment is tense and there is **pain on passive flexion** of the toes. The condition is a **surgical emergency** as without a prompt decompressive fasciotomy, the muscle of the compartment undergoes ischaemic necrosis with resultant contracture.

4. 'Shin splints' This is a relatively common sporting condition encompassing a number of clinical conditions including stress fractures, periostitis of the tibia, muscle hernias and a form of chronic compartment syndrome on repeated activity. The full description of these disorders is outside the scope of this book.
5. **Acute osteitis of the tibia** This is an infectious condition of the tibia predominantly occurring in children where intense pain and tenderness develops over the metaphyseal regions of the tibia. There may be a preceding history of infectious illness. The child is systemically unwell with pyrexia, tachycardia etc. The diagnosis is a clinical one as initial x-rays are normal. The child should be admitted for rest, elevation and intravenous antibiotics. Medical treatment usually suffices, although occasionally drainage is necessary. Antibiotics should be continued for at least 6 weeks.
6. Undiagnosed primary or secondary bone tumour.
7. The neurological manifestations of syphilitic disease (tabes dorsalis) may cause anterior leg pain, as may herpes zoster, the tell-tale rash developing shortly after the pain.

Acute posterior lower limb pain

The following diagnoses should be considered.

1. Rupture of the gastrocnemius-soleus complex.
2. Rupture of the achilles tendon.
3. Deep venous thrombosis.
4. Rupture of a popliteal cyst.
5. Popliteal artery aneurysm.
6. Spinal stenosis with neurogenic claudication.
7. Intermittent claudication due to vascular disease.
8. Sciatica from lumbo-sacral nerve root entrapment or irritation.
9. Superficial thrombo-phlebitis.
10. Herpes zoster.

24
The ankle joint

Functional anatomy and diagnosis of ankle injuries

The ankle joint consists of two major articulations:

    1. The ankle joint *proper*, the articulation between the distal tibia and fibula with the talus.
    2. The inferior tibio-fibular joint.

The integrity of the ankle joint complex is vitally dependent upon the ligamentous structures of the region; significant disruption of any of the ligaments may lead to considerable dysfunction.

The ligaments around the ankle joint (Fig. 24.1)

    1. The **medial ligament (deltoid ligament),** a very strong ligament that extends from the medial malleolus to the medial surface of the talus and other tarsal bones.
    2. The **lateral ligament**, which extends from the lateral malleolus to the lateral aspects of the talus and calcaneum.
    3. The **anterior and posterior inferior tibio-fibular ligaments**, which connect the inferior portions of the tibia and fibula.
    4. **The interosseous membrane**, extending between tibia and fibula throughout their length. It has some mechanical properties. Its disruption, along with the inferior tibio-

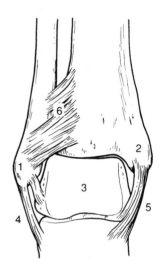

Figure 24.1 – The normal ankle; 1. Lateral malleolus, 2. Medial malleolus, 3. Talus, 4. Lateral ligament, 5. Medial (deltoid) ligament, 6. Inferior tibio-fibular ligament.

fibular ligaments, produces a potential **diastasis** (see Fig. 23.6).

Clinical diagnosis of ankle fractures

It is not acceptable to x-ray an ankle injury before taking a history and examining the patient. Not only is it bad practice, but incorrect x-rays may be taken and fracture patterns missed.

    Although the classification of ankle injuries has not been given in this text according to the mechanism of injury, it is nevertheless useful to establish the history of the event. As a minimum, an **inversion injury** should be distinguished from an **eversion injury**. Note also that inversion injury is associated with lateral ligament sprain and fifth metatarsal fractures, implying that those areas should be carefully examined. In addition, if there has not been a clear history of an injury, an underlying pathology may be responsible for the patient's symptoms (see The Acutely Painful Ankle below).

It is **mandatory** to examine the patient with a painful ankle before radiography. **If the ankle is clinically dislocated or subluxed, reduce it immediately.** Areas to examine specifically are:

1. The medial ligament (deltoid ligament) of the ankle – there may be a rupture of the ligament that is not obvious on x-ray. The examination findings should be documented.
2. The anterior inferior tibio-fibular ligament.
3. The lateral ligament.
4. **The entire length of the fibula** – do not be caught out by the **Dupuytren's fracture** (medial ligament injury with intermediate level fibular fracture) or **Maisonneuve's fracture** (medial ligament rupture with a high fibular fracture, see Fig. 23.6).
5. The foot, especially the fifth metatarsal. Remember that standard ankle x-rays to do not visualize the base of the fifth metatarsal,

so the fracture will be missed unless you look for it.

Radiological diagnosis of ankle fractures

Radiological diagnosis is essential in ankle injuries. Look for the fracture patterns as described below, but the x-ray must be interpreted in conjunction with the clinical findings. If in doubt, go back and examine the patient!

Two important terms used when discussing ankle injuries are:

1. **The ankle mortise** This describes the congruent fit of the tibial and fibular articular surfaces with that of the talus. Radiologically, this is best seen on an anteroposterior x-ray with 20° of internal rotation. There should be an even gap around the talus. The treatment of ankle fractures is primarily based on whether there is a disturbance of the ankle mortise. Establish whether there is any **talar tilt** or **talar shift** within the mortise, good indicators of an unstable fracture (Fig. 24.2).
2. **Diastasis** This denotes that the talus has, **or may potentially be,** forced superiorly between the tibia and the fibula, implying rupture of the inferior tibio-fibular ligaments and a portion of the interosseous membrane

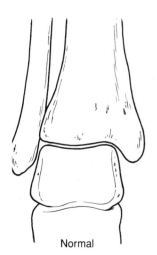
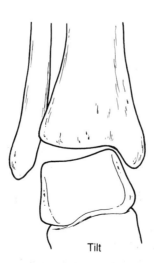
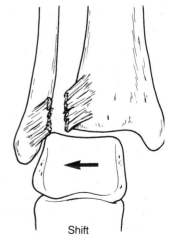

Normal   Tilt   Shift

Figure 24.2 – The ankle mortise – talar tilt and shift

(Fig. 24.3) (or more simply, the **syndesmosis).** A diastasis implies that there is, **or the potential for**, abnormally wide separation of the distal tibia and fibula.

(A term not to use if possible is *Pott's fracture* – the term can be used to describe almost any ankle fracture, and is so non-specific as to be useless). Note also, when assessing ankle injuries radiologically, that the x-ray has usually been taken with the leg supine and non-weight-bearing. **Potential instability must be suspected on fracture patterns** on the x-ray, as the bones may not be significantly displaced on the x-ray.

Take care in x-ray interpretation with the following:

1. The epiphyseal line of the distal fibula in adolescents, especially in the lateral view, can look remarkably like a fracture. If unsure, re-examine the patient as a fracture usually hurts!
2. There are a number of accessory bones in the region, the most common being the **os trigonum** behind the talus. Accessory bones have a clearly defined rounded margin, but may be mistaken for an avulsion fracture.
3. 'Footballer's ankle': in a seasoned footballer, repeated episodes of trauma around the ankle may cause osteophytes and old avulsion fragments may be present. The

abnormalities may be confused for new fractures unless the area is carefully examined.

Classification of ankle injuries

There are a number of classification systems used to describe ankle injuries. The fact that so many exist implies that no one system is perfect. Many are difficult to understand and remember. A simple classification system **based upon whether the ankle needs referral for reduction or operative treatment** is described in the section on ankle fracture management. A list of the other common systems is given below, which the reader may consult if necessary.

1. Henderson's classification – classifies fractures into uni-, bi- or trimalleolar fractures.
2. Lauge–Hansen classification – classifies injuries in terms of the mechanism of injury.
3. Danis–Weber system – this is probably the most widely used system in current use, and is based upon the level of the fibular fracture.
4. The AO classification – similar to the Danis–Weber system.

Ankle fractures in adults

Management considerations

The decision as to whether an ankle fracture requires operative fixation can be difficult for the doctor in Accident and Emergency, and is made more so by the wide variance in protocols between units. The conservative management of 'unstable' ankle fractures is no longer widely practised, for the method is less reliable and requires greater skill and judgement than open fixation. Most units now advocate open fixation of most unstable fractures, with conservative treatment only for stable fracture configurations.

Another difficulty with ankle fractures are those occurring in the elderly with osteoporotic bone – operative fixation can prove difficult in these patients, and therefore there is a greater

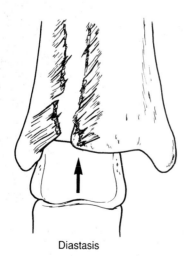

Diastasis

Figure 24.3 – Diastasis

tendency to allow conservative treatment in this group. However, operative treatment should not be denied solely on the basis of age.

The early management of ankle fractures in the Accident and Emergency Department plays an important part in determining the prognosis for an ankle fracture. If a fracture is not optimally managed, prolonged swelling, fracture blisters etc. may form, delaying operative treatment with resultant prolonged stiffness. Many fractures may initially be part of a **subluxation** or a **dislocation**. **Remember never to leave an ankle dislocation or subluxation unreduced whilst waiting for an x-ray – reduce it first as an emergency, place the limb into a splint or backslab and then take the film.** Once reduced, the fracture(s) can be treated on its merits, bearing in mind that significant force is needed for the subluxation/dislocation to occur.

Conservative treatment of ankle fractures

No specific details of conservative treatment of **unstable** ankle fractures are given as this is now rarely performed and is outside the scope of this book. The patient should be referred for more expert management. However, the basic principles of plaster fixation and moulding etc. apply to ankle fractures as much as to all fractures.

When applying a plaster for a **stable** ankle fracture in a patient planned for discharge without admission, bear the following points in mind.

1. **Always** ensure that the ankle is at 90° and not plantarflexed – residual stiffness with loss of movement is almost inevitable if the foot is kept plantarflexed for a long period.
2. It is permissible to apply a backslab initially for a stable fracture – a full plaster can subsequently be applied after a few days once the swelling has settled when the patient is seen in the fracture clinic.

Open reduction and internal fixation of ankle fractures

Many fractures will need referral for open fixation. However, the initial management must

still be performed in the Accident and Emergency Department.

1. **Never place an unreduced ankle fracture into a plaster and send the patient to the ward** – this is a recipe for disaster. Even if the fracture is to undergo surgery (which may have to wait, for many reasons, for several days), ensure that it is satisfactorily reduced (Fig. 24.4).
2. A plaster backslab is useful for a patient undergoing surgery as it gives pain relief and keeps the foot dorsiflexed. Ensure that it is well padded. A good backslab is one with both a dorsal slab and a U slab of plaster. **Always dorsiflex the foot to 90° when applying a backslab.**
3. Inform the orthopaedic team if there is gross swelling or any blistering of the skin (due to underlying soft tissue pressure) as this may affect their management strategy.

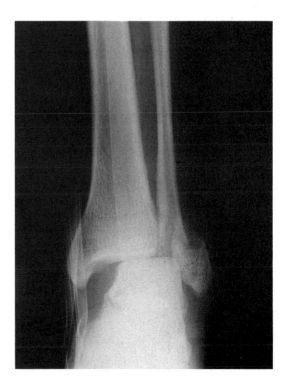

Figure 24.4 – This x-ray should never be seen! Note the gross talar shift in association with a fibular fracture and deltoid ligament rupture. Always reduce the ankle prior to x-ray

4. When applying the backslab, it is helpful if the anterior padding is split to allow application of ice to keep tissue swelling to a minimum prior to surgery.

5. It has been clearly shown that early surgery within 24 hours, if practicable, offers the best results of surgery.

Management based upon classification

Injuries due to rotation, adduction or abduction of the talus within the mortise

These are by far the most common ankle injuries. In injuries of this type, **the level of the fibular fracture gives an indication of the severity of the injury**, with more proximal fractures associated with greater severity (Fig. 24.5). Remember that the fibula may be broken high in the leg, and so not seen on an ankle x-ray!

1.   No fibular fracture

   1.1.   Fracture of the medial malleolus – this pattern is uncommon. If:

   • The fracture is undisplaced, treat in plaster, initially non-weight-bearing, but carefully monitor for subsequent displacement.

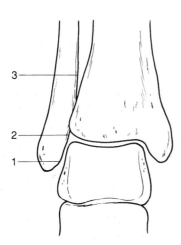

Figure 24.5 – Levels of fibular fracture ; 1. below level of joint, 2. at level of joint, 3. above level of joint. Remember that a high fibular fracture may not be seen on an ankle x-ray!

• The fracture is displaced, refer for closed or (usually) operative reduction.

1.2.   Fracture of the posterior malleolus – this pattern is uncommon (see 3.3).
1.3.   Dislocation of the ankle without fracture – inevitably due to rupture of the medial and lateral ligaments. Needs prompt reduction as there is an incidence of avascular necrosis of the talus following this injury. Immobilize non-weight-bearing for 6–8 weeks.

2.   Fibular fracture below the level of the ankle joint

   2.1.   Fibular fracture with no medial malleolar fracture or deltoid rupture. If:

   • The fibular fracture is undisplaced or minimally displaced, treat in plaster, initially non-weight-bearing, with check x-rays at 1 and 2 weeks. Can then be treated weight-bearing up to 6 weeks.
   • The fibular fracture is significantly displaced (uncommon), refer for consideration of operative reduction.

   2.2.   Fibular fracture with medial malleolar fracture or deltoid rupture. All these fractures have a potential for mortise malalignment. They should be referred – depending upon the policy of the unit, operative reduction may be advised.

3.   Fibular fracture at the level of the ankle joint

   3.1.   Fibular fracture with no medial malleolar fracture or deltoid rupture. There is differing opinion as to how to treat this fracture – most would advocate closely supervised conservative management, although some would advise operative reduction. Refer according to the policy of your unit.
   3.2.   Fibular fracture with medial malleolar fracture or deltoid rupture. These fractures, in most centres, undergo operative reduction.
   3.3.   Fibular fracture with fracture of the posterior malleolus – this usually occurs with medial joint injury in addition. If the

posterior malleolar fragment is less than 30% of the distal tibial surface on the lateral film, it may be treated conservatively. If more than 30%, the fragment requires operative reduction (Fig. 24.6).

4.   Fibular fracture above the level of the ankle joint

All fracture patterns of this type have associated disruption of the syndesomosis. The majority will require open reduction and internal fixation, and should therefore be referred. Some, in addition to the basic fracture fixation, may require a temporary screw ('diastasis screw') to hold the fibula and tibia together in the correct position.

4.1   Associated with fracture of the medial malleolus.
4.2.   Associated with rupture of the deltoid ligament.
4.3.   Associated with fracture of the posterior malleolus.
4.4.   Complex types.

Injuries due to vertical compression forces upon the ankle

These are less common injuries, and are often associated with greater force and disruption of the ankle. The talus is driven superiorly through

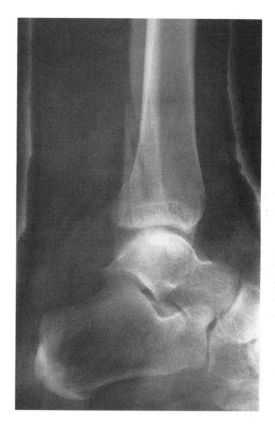

Figure 24.7 – Posterior malleolar fracture in association with a fibular fracture above the level of the ankle joint. Although the fibular fracture requires fixation, the posterior malleolar fragment does not as it represents less than 30% of the distal tibial surface

the distal tibial surface or the inferior tibio-fibular joint, commonly caused by falls from a height or where the ankle is strongly dorsiflexed (Fig. 24.9). **In injuries of this type, the level of the fibular fracture is not helpful in planning treatment.** Many different fracture patterns are possible, and the classic form is termed the **pilon fracture.** These fractures are very difficult to treat and always require admission. Operative treatment is advocated if technically possible, although some require prolonged periods of skeletal traction. The initial management is **protection of the soft tissues** by early reduction of grossly malaligned fractures. If a skeletal traction pin is required, it should be inserted into the calcaneum (assuming there is no fracture in that region).

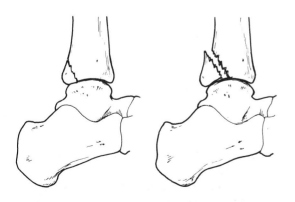

Figure 24.6 – Posterior malleolar fractures. Fractures with less than 30% involvement of the distal tibial surface (left) do not require surgical fixation. Involvement of more than 30% requires stabilization (right).

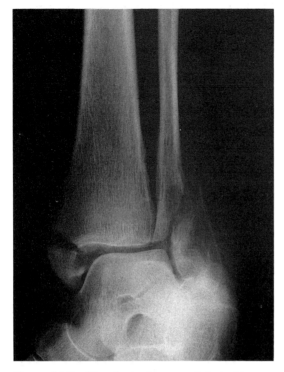

Figure 24.8 – Bimalleolar fracture of the ankle.

Ankle fractures in children

Classification and management

As with any epiphyseal injury, ankle injuries in children can be classified according to the Salter–Harris system, and this gives a basis for their management.

The commonest injury is the Salter–Harris **Type 2** lesion, where a portion of the metaphysis displaces along with the epiphysis (Fig. 24.10):

- If undisplaced, the fracture can be treated in a below-knee plaster non-weight-bearing for 4–6 weeks, initially applying a backslab.
- If displaced, the child should undergo manipulation under anaesthetic (nearly all can be reduced by closed methods), with immobilization for 4–6 weeks.

Type 1 injuries, where the entire distal epiphysis separates from the shaft without a metaphyseal fragment, are rare fractures. The

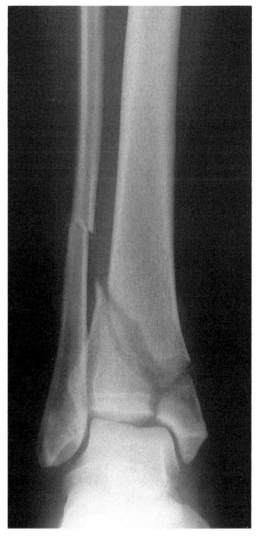

Figure 24.9 – Vertical compression fracture of the ankle.

epiphysis will need to be reduced, possibly with additional percutaneous K wire fixation.

Type 3 injuries, there is a fracture of part of the epiphysis, often with separation. If the displacement is more than 10%, closed reduction and/or open reduction will be required.

Type 4 injuries, a portion of the epiphysis and metaphysis separate. It is important that these fragments are openly reduced.

Type 5 injuries are compression injuries and have a poor prognosis as compared to the other forms. In pure lesions, no reduction or fixation is

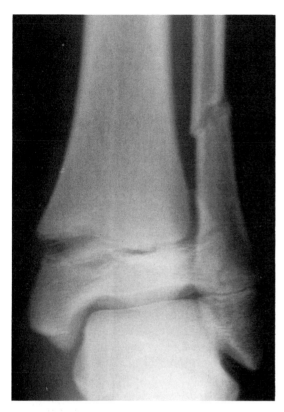

Figure 24.10 – Salter–Harris type 2 fracture of the distal tibial epiphysis

possible. The ankle should be immobilized, non-weight-bearing for at least 6 weeks. Abnormal epiphyseal growth can be anticipated.

Soft tissue injuries around the ankle

There are a number of common clinical soft tissue lesions around the ankle. They may present to the Accident and Emergency Department following an injury or may be due to overuse. Their diagnosis is essentially a clinical one, x-rays only exclude other pathology. It is therefore essential to obtain a history and carry out a thorough clinical examination.

The lateral ligament of the ankle : sprains and tears

Injury to the lateral ligament of the ankle is an exceedingly common disorder seen frequently in the Accident and Emergency setting as a result of an **inversion injury** of the ankle. If a lateral ligament tear is not recognized or inadequately treated, chronic problems can occur (see below). Not all lateral ligament injuries can be treated with a Tubigrip and reassurance that no bone has broken!

Anatomy and biomechanics

The lateral ligament complex consists of three main components (Fig. 24.11):

1. The anterior talo-fibular ligament.
2. The calcaneo-fibular ligament.
3. The posterior talo-fibular ligament.

The three ligaments act as the primary restraint against inversion of the **ankle** (inversion of the **foot** normally occurs at the subtalar joint).

Should the lateral ligament complex be compromised, and left untreated, the result is long-term mechanical instability with repeated giving way of the ankle. A chronic capsulitis and proprioceptive deficiency also ensue, and the ankle is at risk of secondary osteoarthritic change. This can be prevented to some degree by early **recognition** of the problem.

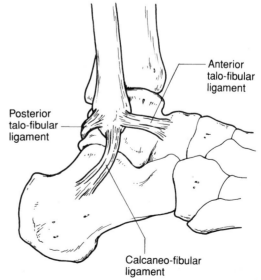

Figure 24.11 – The lateral ligament complex of the ankle

Diagnosis

As stated, the history is most often one of an **inversion injury** of the ankle. Direct injuries (as in sport) to the region are also a cause. The patient with a sprain may be able to walk nearly normally, but a rupture prevents a normal gait in the acute stage.

Examination reveals bruising and swelling over the lateral aspect of the ankle. Sprains usually have diffuse bruising whilst a tear classically has an 'egg-shaped' swelling over the lateral malleolus. There is localized tenderness, with a sprain, maximally over the ligament. The ankle has a decreased range of movement, but paradoxically, a sprain tends to be more painful than a tear. Resisted movement and pain are maximal on inversion with the ankle dorsiflexed.

If a tear is suspected, clinical stress testing can be helpful. Two ligaments of the lateral ligament complex are amenable to stress testing. Local anaesthetic can be introduced into the region if the procedure is too painful.

1. The integrity of the anterior talo-fibular ligament can be established by the **anterior stress test**. One hand holds down the shin whilst the other brings the heel forwards. If pain is elicited a sprain is likely. However, if there is abnormal anterior mobility (compare with the other side), which is often less painful, this is termed the **anterior draw sign**, indicating a rupture of the ligament.
2. The calcaneo-fibular ligament can be similarly examined by the **inversion stress test**.

The place of radiography in inversion injuries of the ankle is controversial, as many unnecessary x-rays can be taken. However, if the patient is efficiently examined, the need for x-rays is reduced. There may be a protocol in your unit. If there is any suspicion of bony tenderness, or tenderness elsewhere in the ankle, an x-ray should be requested. Additionally, if a ligament **rupture** is suggested by the clinical findings, **stress radiography** may be performed. In this test, the stress tests as described above are performed, looking for excessive talar tilt indicative of an unstable ankle. Note however that many normal ankles exhibit talar tilting of up to 10° on stress testing – comparison with the opposite limb is therefore useful.

Management

An ankle sprain, without any evidence of ankle instability, should be treated by **mobilization**, not rested. Early physiotherapy, application of ice, elevation etc. are helpful. A Tubigrip gives no mechanical support, although it can decrease the swelling and increase proprioceptive circuits. The patient can be referred to the General Practitioner or sports clinic if necessary.

A rupture of the lateral ligament of the ankle **must** be recognized acutely. The treatment is controversial. Most centres do not advise surgical repair except in athletes. The most common therapy is immobilization in a below-knee weight-bearing plaster for 4–6 weeks to let the ligament heal. However this is associated with chronic stiffness, and recently cast-braces have been introduced. If you are not sure of the policy of your unit, immobilize in a plaster and refer to the fracture clinic for further assessment.

Differential diagnosis of inversion injuries

Note that in addition to lateral ligament injuries, the following can also occur following an inversion injury of the ankle.

1. Fracture of the base of the fifth metatarsal – this will be missed unless sought clinically as the area is not seen on standard ankle x-rays.
2. Avulsion fracture of the tip of the lateral malleolus – this can be treated as for a ligament tear by a below-knee weight-bearing plaster for 4–6 weeks.
3. Sprain of the calcaneo-cuboid ligament (see Chapter 25).

Other soft tissue injuries of the ankle

Achilles tendinitis

This is seen most commonly in runners and athletes. It may present acutely with posterior ankle pain. There is localized tenderness with pain on dorsiflexion of the foot. Be very careful to distinguish tendinitis from achilles tendon rupture – with a rupture there is usually a history of sudden pain and on examination there is a palpable gap with a positive Simmond's 'squeeze' test (Fig. 24.12, see discussion of the acutely painful lower leg in Chpater 23). Treatment is by conservative measures largely with rest, care with footwear etc. Steroid injections may precipitate a rupture.

Extensor tenosynovitis

This may present acutely following unaccustomed activity. Swelling and tenderness of the extensor tendons on the anterior aspect of the ankle are present. Pain is elicited by plantarflexion of the foot and active resistance of dorsiflexion. Treatment is by conservative means with rest, anti-inflammatories etc. Surgical decompression in chronic cases may be needed.

Peroneal tendinitis

This is a common condition, most often due to overuse. Pain, swelling and tenderness are present over the peroneal tendons on the lateral aspect of the leg and ankle. Pain is elicited by inversion of the foot and by resisted eversion.

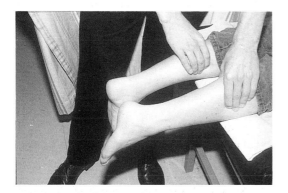

Figure 24.12 – Simmond's test

Treatment is conservative, as with extensor tenosynovitis.

Tendo achilles bursitis

There are a number of bursae around the achilles tendon, the two largest being in front of the tendon and behind it. They can become inflamed following trauma but may do so without injury in certain auto-immune disorders (e.g. reactive arthritis). The condition is diagnosed by the fact that there is a swelling both medial and lateral to the tendon. Treatment is conservative.

Traction osteochondritis of the achilles tendon

An osteochondritis may develop where the tendon inserts into the calcaneum. Pain is localized to that area and is exacerbated by dorsiflexion of the ankle. Treatment is with a heel cushion and physiotherapy etc.

The acutely painful ankle

The patient may present with acute pain in the ankle for the following reasons.

Trauma and soft tissue injuries

See the relevant sections:

- e.g. fractures and dislocations
- e.g. ligament sprains and ruptures
- e.g. achilles tendon rupture
- e.g. tenosynovitis

Acute metabolic and inflammatory conditions

Examples include gout, rheumatoid arthritis, pyrophosphate arthropathy.

Recurrent dislocation of the peroneal tendons

This is a relatively uncommon disorder where the peroneal tendons on the lateral aspect of the ankle have excessive mobility and snap back and forwards over the lateral malleolus. The condition may present acutely, and the snapping may be felt most effectively on repeated eversion and inversion of the ankle. No acute treatment is possible, but surgical repair of the deficient retinaculum lying over the tendons may be needed if the condition does not settle.

Osteochondritis of the talus

This is a condition most common in young adults. It is usually related to trauma in the past, but presents acutely at a later stage. A chondral or osteochondral injury occurs, and the fragment may loosen. The condition may present without trauma as a pure osteochondritis. The patient presents with diffuse ankle pain and may complain of a decreased range of movement, clicking or locking of the ankle. The diagnosis is made on the x-ray, with an osteochondral deficiency in the dome of the talus. A routine orthopaedic referral is indicated.

25
The foot

Fractures of the talus

Anatomy and blood supply of the talus

The talus plays a central role in the function of the hindfoot. Its surfaces form part of three joint complexes (Fig. 25.1):

1. The ankle joint – the dome of the talus articulating with the tibia and fibula.
2. The subtalar joint – articulating with the calcaneum.
3. The talo-navicular joint, part of the mid-tarsal joint.

The talus consists of (Fig. 25.2):

1. The dome.
2. The body with its processes.
3. The neck.
4. The head.

It is worthy of note that the talus has no significant muscular or tendinous attachments. The bone is thus very dependent upon its direct blood supply; if this is lost, **avascular necrosis** is a common sequel. Blood is supplied to the talus in three main groups, into the body, neck and the undersurface. As a result of this arrangement, displaced fractures of the talar neck may interrupt the blood supply to the proximal portion of the body and dome, with subsequent avascular necrosis.

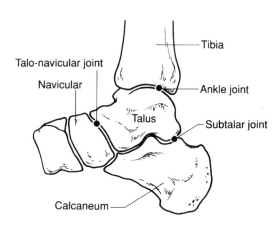

Figure 25.1 – The relationships of the talus

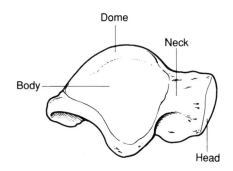

Figure 25.2 – The parts of the talus

Fractures of the dome of the talus

Osteochondral lesions of the dome of the talus (Fig. 25.3) are usually, but not exclusively, due to trauma. They commonly accompany 'ankle sprains', and may not be obvious on the initial x-ray. The lesion can be seen on both the lateral or medial sides of the talus. If the fragment is undisplaced, the fracture is treated conservatively in a non-weight-bearing plaster for 6 weeks. However, displaced fragments are prone to non-union, and many of these require open fixation or excision.

The x-ray appearance of a fragment from the dome of the talus may be seen without recent trauma. The fragment may represent past trauma, or may be a form of osteochondritis tali. Be careful not to interpret such an x-ray as an acute injury.

Fractures of the body and processes of the talus

Fractures of the body of the talus

Fractures of the body of the talus, which are quite uncommon, usually coexist with other

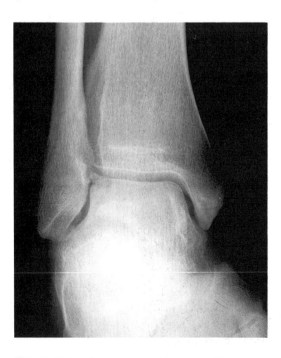

Figure 25.3 – Osteochondral fracture of the dome of the talus

fractures, especially ankle fractures. The main force underlying the injury is compressive, the talus being squashed between the tibia and the calcaneum. The degree of force involved largely dictates the treatment, as some are of such magnitude that the talar bone loss defies surgical reconstruction.

Undisplaced fractures need a period of rest, elevation and restoration of movement, followed by a period of 6–12 weeks in a non-weight-bearing plaster. Displaced fractures, if possible, merit surgical reconstruction. Bone grafting may be necessary. A common sequel is avascular necrosis and collapse of the talus, which may require elective fusion of the ankle and/or subtalar joints.

Fractures of the processes of the talus

There are two processes of the talus, named lateral and posterior. Isolated fractures, which are uncommon, are usually the result of an avulsion injury. Most are combined with other fractures in the region. These fractures can be difficult to visualize on x-rays, but it is important that they are not missed – there is a high non-union rate and persistent pain is a common sequel. Undisplaced fractures should be treated non-weight-bearing for 3 months. If the processes are significantly displaced, accurate open fixation is indicated.

Fractures of the neck of the talus

Talar neck fractures are the most common form of significant talar injury, and are probably the most difficult to treat. The most common mechanism of injury is forced dorsiflexion of the ankle, whereby the anterior tibial margin abuts against the talar neck, e.g. where the pedal of a motor vehicle is forced against the foot. Falls from heights may also produce the fracture, with the foot being dorsiflexed upon landing.

Because of the vascular anatomy in the region, talar neck fractures may result in **avascular necrosis** of the proximal portion of the body.

Classification of talar neck fractures

Hawkins's classification of talar neck fractures is useful in that it allows some form of prognostic indicator and a basis for treatment.

Type 1 Non-displaced vertical fracture of the neck of the talus.

Type 2 Displaced fracture of the talar neck with subluxation or dislocation of the subtalar joint (Fig. 25.4).

Type 3 Displaced fracture of the talar neck with subluxation or dislocation of the subtalar and ankle joints, i.e. the head and body are separated by the tibia.

Type 4 In addition to type 3 pattern, the talar head dislocates from the navicular bone, with which it articulates.

Many talar neck fractures coexist with other injuries, most commonly medial malleolar fractures of the ankle joint.

Management of talar neck fractures

Type 1 fractures

These fractures, with no displacement, must be carefully distinguished from type 2 fractures, and this differentiation should be made by experienced personnel. **The fracture pattern implies that there is no subluxation of the subtalar joint**. The injury should be initially treated in a below-knee backslab, with subsequent immobilization in a below-knee non-weight-bearing plaster for 3 months. As the region is prone to swelling, the patient should be given clear instructions regarding elevation and to return to the department should there be a problem with the circulation. There is a small risk of avascular necrosis of the proximal fragment of the order of 5–10%.

Type 2 fractures

Type 2 fractures are characterized by **subluxation or dislocation of the subtalar joint** – they must be differentiated from type 1 fractures

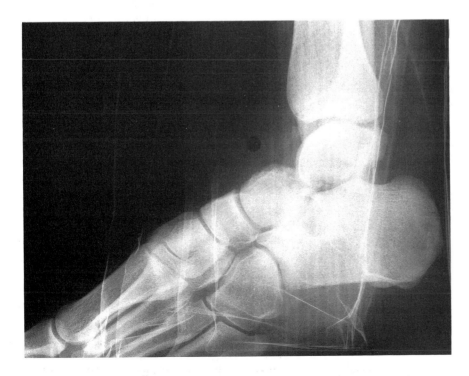

Figure 25.4 – Talar neck fracture

because any displacement must be corrected (see Fig. 25.4). Malunited fractures may result in a permanent limp with a painful gait. These fractures are very prone to swelling, and any displacement should be quickly dealt with to avoid skin necrosis.

As a result of the fracture, the body of the talus assumes a position of plantar flexion, with the distal portion remaining in line with the rest of the foot. If there is any doubt as to whether displacement has occurred, x-rays in both plantar flexion and dorsiflexion may be useful. There is a much higher risk of avascular necrosis of the proximal fragment with this injury, of the order of 50%.

The management of the fracture is a **surgical emergency**, as timely treatment minimizes skin problems and the risk of avascular necrosis. Experienced personnel should be summoned. An attempt at closed fracture reduction is initially made, although commonly open reduction with supplementary K wire fixation is necessary. Although a description of the reduction method is given, it should not be attempted by inexperienced staff. The reduction technique is to apply longitudinal traction and plantarflexion to the foot so as to bring the head of the talus into alignment with the body. Eversion may also help the reduction process. If the reduction is successful, the foot should be immobilized in a plaster slab in full plantarflexion, which is gradually converted to a dorsiflexed position over successive weeks. Immobilization is continued non-weight-bearing for 3 months. Should closed reduction be unsuccessful, immediate conversion to open reduction is necessary.

Type 3 fractures

Type 3 fractures of the talus are highly significant injuries, and again their management constitutes a **surgical emergency**. They are characterized by dislocation of both the subtalar and ankle joints, with the proximal body fragment lying medially in a subcutaneous position. Around one-third of these fractures are open at the time of injury, and a large percentage sustain ischaemic necrosis of the skin over the subcutaneous fragment.

Upon recognition of the injury, experienced personnel should be summoned. Immediate arrangements should be made for reduction in the operating theatre. Closed reduction, the technique of which is outside the scope of this book as it should only be attempted by the orthopaedic surgeon contemplating open surgery, is rarely successful. Open reduction of the fracture is usually necessary. The risk of avascular necrosis approaches 100%.

Type 4 fractures

These are very rare injuries, where, in addition to dislocations at the subtalar and ankle joints, there is a dislocation of the talo-navicular joint. These fractures should be managed as type 3 fractures. They similarly constitute a surgical emergency.

Complications of talar neck fractures

The incidence and severity of complications is proportional to the Hawkins grading. Although prompt appropriate management helps, many talar neck fractures have a poor outcome.

1. Avascular necrosis of the talus, leading to secondary degenerative change.
2. Skin necrosis over the displaced talar fragments – this is minimized by prompt reduction.
3. Infection, usually due to skin necrosis or open injuries.
4. Long-term immobility and stiffness of the subtalar, ankle and mid-tarsal joints.
5. Malunion – this is often due to misdiagnosis, especially of type 2 fractures.

Fractures of the head of the talus

Talar head fractures are, thankfully, very uncommon injuries. The head is compressed against the navicular bone with which it articulates. The result is commonly a very comminuted fracture that defies any form of surgical reconstruction. The incidence of post-traumatic degenerative change is high.

Relatively undisplaced fractures of the head should be immobilized in a non-weight-bearing plaster for 6–12 weeks. Displaced fractures that are not comminuted should be internally fixed, but this is not often possible. Highly comminuted fractures should be treated by early mobilization, non-weight-bearing, so as to prevent a stiff foot.

Dislocations of the talus

The talus commonly dislocates as part of a fracture pattern, and this is described in the section dealing with fractures of the talus. However, talar dislocations may occur as a result of purely ligamentous injury, and these will be described here.

There are two broad patterns of talar dislocation. In both, the mechanism of injury is inversion or eversion of the equinus (plantarflexed) foot. In lesser forces, there is a **subtalar dislocation**, and with greater force there is **total dislocation of the talus**.

Subtalar dislocation of the talus (Fig. 25.5)

This is also termed 'peritalar dislocation'. The talus dislocates at both the talo-calcaneal (i.e. subtalar joint) and the talo-navicular joint, but the ankle joint remains articulated. The injury implies rupture of the lateral ligament of the ankle and the talo-calcaneal ligament. There is often an associated ankle fracture.

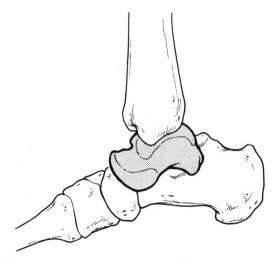

Figure 25.5 – Subtalar dislocation

The dislocation should be promptly reduced so as to protect the skin, which may be under pressure due to the displaced talus. Closed reduction is usually successful, and should be performed under general anaesthetic, but if circumstances dictate, intravenous sedation. Reduction is effected by, with the knee flexed, longitudinal traction, plantarflexion of the foot and correction of any inversion/eversion that may be present. If closed reduction is unsuccessful, urgent open reduction should be performed. The foot should be immobilized, initially in a below-knee backslab and subsequently in a full non-weight-bearing cast for 4–6 weeks.

Subtalar dislocations tend to have a good prognosis if treated appropriately. The main complication is degenerative change at the subtalar joint; the risk of avascular necrosis of the talus is low.

Total dislocation of the talus

This is a rare but very significant injury. The talus is dislocated from all of its three articulations, i.e. the ankle joint as well as the subtalar and talo-navicular joints. All ligamentous attachments of the talus must rupture to allow the talus to dislocate fully. The talus comes to lie in a subcutaneous position, usually laterally in front of the ankle. Many of the injuries are open. The injury almost inevitably results in avascular necrosis of the talus as all its blood supply is disconnected.

The management of total talar dislocation is a **surgical emergency**. Experienced personnel should be summoned. If the injury is open, the wound needs to be urgently debrided. Prompt reduction of the talus is mandatory. General anaesthetic is necessary, and closed reduction is rarely successful. Open reduction usually needs to be supplemented by internal fixation. A below-knee plaster is applied, non-weight-bearing, for 6–12 weeks. The prognosis of the injury is very poor.

Fractures of the calcaneum

Classification

Calcaneal fractures are the most common of all tarsal fractures, and are an important cause of long-term disability. Essex-Lopresti broadly classified calcaneal fractures as follows.

Extra-articular calcaneal fractures

Many extra-articular calcaneal fractures are a result of twisting or sudden muscular force, and are less common (20–30% of all calcaneal fractures).

1. Fractures of the anterior calcaneum.
2. Fractures of the calcaneal tuberosity.
3. Fractures of the sustentaculum tali.
4. Fractures of the body without subtalar joint involvement (Fig. 25.6) (usually due to a fall from a height).

Intra-articular calcaneal fractures

Most intra-articular calcaneal fractures result from falls from a height, and are more common (70–80% of calcaneal fractures).

1. Fractures of the body with subtalar joint involvement (Fig. 25.7).
2. Severely comminuted 'crush' fractures of the body of the calcaneum.

Clinical features of calcaneal fractures

The history of injury often gives a good indication of the type of calcaneal fracture; **any injury involving a fall from a height should have a calcaneal fracture positively excluded**. Note also

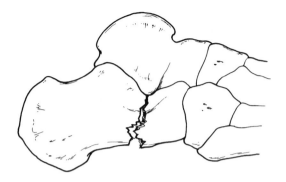

Figure 25.7 – Fracture of the body of the calcaneum with subtalar joint involvement

that any calcaneal fracture caused by falls may be associated with 'crush' fractures of the lumbar spine and fractures of the pelvis, hip, femur and proximal tibia. Remember also that there may be a calcaneal fracture in the other foot!

Calcaneal fractures have a distinctive clinical appearance. The heel appears shorter, flatter and wider, and there is commonly extensive bruising. The patient is rarely able to weight-bear in the presence of a calcaneal fracture.

Radiological evaluation is invaluable. Remember to examine the patient before requesting an x-ray, as ankle views for a suspected 'ankle fracture' may not demonstrate a calcaneal fracture. Standard views are the **lateral** (most useful) and **axial** projections. Oblique x-rays may be useful in unclear cases.

When assessing calcaneal x-rays, the most important fact to establish is **whether there is involvement of the subtalar joint**. If there is subtalar involvement, consideration of surgery is required so as to restore the joint surfaces (although this is not always possible). Radiological assessment also allows definition of **Bohler's angle** (Fig. 25.8). This is the angle between:

(i) a line drawn from the anterior calcaneal process to the posterior calcaneal process;
(ii) a line drawn from the posterior calcaneal process to the calcaneal tuberosity.

The angle between these two lines is normally more than 40° – if less than this, it implies sig-

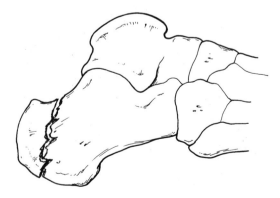

Figure 25.6 – Fracture of the body of the calcaneum posterior to the subtalar joint

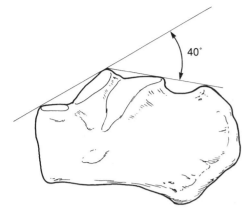

Figure 25.8 – Bohler's angle

nificant compression of the body of the calcaneum.

Extra-articular calcaneal fractures

Fractures of the anterior calcaneum

The anterior calcaneal process articulates with the cuboid joint, forming part of the mid-tarsal joint (with the talo-navicular joint). There are a number of injury patterns.

1. Dislocation of the calcaneo-cuboid joint (see Mid-tarsal Dislocations below).
2. Avulsion fracture of the anterior calcaneum. These relatively common injuries are due to forced adduction of the forefoot, the mid-tarsal ligament pulling off a small area of bone from the calcaneum. The injury should be immobilized in a below-knee backslab, later converted to a below-knee weight-bearing cast for 4–6 weeks. The prognosis is relatively good.
3. Compression fracture of the anterior calcaneal process. This is an uncommon injury where the forefoot is forcefully abducted. There is almost inevitable involvement of the calcaneo-cuboid joint. These fractures, if with significant calcaneo-cuboid incongruency, should undergo open fixation, with bone grafting if necessary to restore bone stock. These fractures tend to fare badly.

Fractures of the calcaneal tuberosity

There are two main forms of tuberosity fractures:

1. Vertical fractures of the tuberosity, without subtalar joint involvement. These fractures tend to do well, although there is initially considerable swelling and discomfort. The fractures are rarely significantly displaced, and should be initially elevated and subsequently mobilized non-weight-bearing for 6 weeks. Plaster immobilization is unnecessary.
2. Horizontal fractures of the tuberosity. These fractures (Fig. 25.9) may compromise the insertion of the achilles tendon. They are caused by either direct injury or by sudden muscular contraction of the gastrocnemius–soleus complex via the achilles tendon. **Undisplaced fractures** may be immobilized in an equinus below-knee backslab, with weight-bearing permitted after 1 week for a further 5 weeks. Check x-rays at weeks 1 and 2 are necessary to ensure that the fracture does not displace. **Displaced ('avulsion') fractures** should be openly reduced to restore correct length to the achilles plantarflexion unit, followed by plaster immobilization for 6 weeks in an equinus plaster.

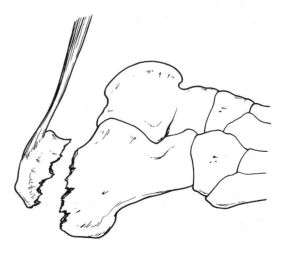

Figure 25.9 – Avulsion fracture of the calcaneal tuberosity

Fractures of the sustentaculum tali

These fractures are best seen on the axial x-ray projection, and are most often minimally displaced. They are due to forced inversion of the forefoot. Undisplaced fractures should be immobilized for 6 weeks in a non-weight-bearing cast. Displaced fractures (rare) require closed and/or open reduction.

Fractures of the body of the calcaneum without subtalar joint involvement

This is a common fracture pattern, in which the fracture line passes posterior to the subtalar joint, thereby sparing it from involvement (see Fig. 25.6). The main cause is a fall from a height. Bohler's angle may be decreased significantly, indicative of a loss of height of the calcaneum. It is imperative to ensure that there is no involvement of the subtalar joint, and CT scanning may be required.

Fractures with minimal displacement are treated conservatively, with initial elevation (they can swell considerably) and non-weight-bearing free of plaster for 6 weeks. Initial compression dressings may decrease swelling and the tendency to form fracture blisters. They have a reasonable prognosis, although prolonged physiotherapy may be required. The treatment of displaced fractures is controversial – operative treatment may allow restoration of heel height, but has a significant number of complications, including stiffness. Conservative treatment can be adopted in many such cases. Even significantly displaced fractures, if without subtalar involvement, have a good prognosis.

Intra-articular calcaneal fractures

Fractures of the body of the calcaneum with subtalar joint involvement

Unfortunately, most fractures of the body of the calcaneum involve the subtalar joint (see Fig. 25.7). The vast majority are caused by falls from a height. There are many fracture patterns and classification systems, none of which is particularly useful in the Accident and Emergency Department. All calcaneal frac-

tures of this type should be referred for further investigation and senior opinion.

The detailed management of the fractures is outside the scope of this book. They require an initial period of elevation at the very least. Most require assessment with CT scanning to evaluate the fracture pattern and the degree of subtalar joint involvement. There is some divergence of opinion as to the advisability of operation to restore the subtalar joint congruity, although most units advocate elevation of the displaced fragments with bone grafting if necessary. The fractures tend to fare badly, with a high incidence of subtalar joint stiffness and secondary degenerative change. The most important contribution to be made in the Accident and Emergency Department is the recognition of the fracture, as early weight-bearing on the fracture can worsen the prognosis considerably.

'Crush' fractures of the body of the calcaneum

Some severely comminuted calcaneal fractures defy description, and fall into this group. The talus is essentially driven through the calcaneal body, resulting in total disorganization of the subtalar and mid-tarsal joints. These injuries are generally not amenable to surgery and do badly. They require initial elevation and prolonged non-weight bearing with early mobilization, and should all be referred.

Tarsal fractures

Isolated fractures of the tarsal bones do occur, but it is important to exclude other injuries, as they commonly exist as part of a larger fracture-dislocation pattern.

Fractures of the navicular bone

There are four main types of navicular fractures:

1. Fractures of the **body** of the navicular These are rarely sole injuries, and coexist with other injuries of the foot. Undisplaced

fractures are treated conservatively in a non-weight-bearing plaster for 6 weeks. Displaced fractures should be referred as they usually require open fixation.

2. Fractures of the **tuberosity** of the navicular (Fig. 25.10) These are avulsion fractures caused by pull-off during eversion by the strong tibialis posterior tendon. Undisplaced fractures can be treated conservatively in a weight-bearing below-knee plaster after initial immobilization in a slab. Significantly displaced fractures should be openly fixed so as to restore the biomechanics of the foot. Do not confuse the accessory navicular bone with a displaced fracture – the accessory bone has rounded edges and is present bilaterally in over two-thirds of cases.

3. **Cortical avulsion fractures** These are the result of eversion or inversion of the foot, resulting in ligamentous pull-off of a portion of the cortex of the navicular. Unless the fragment is large and significantly displaced, the injury is treated conservatively in a plaster.

4. **Stress fractures** of the navicular These are relatively common injuries in sporting populations, and are easily missed. The injury is suspected from the history of medial foot pain without obvious trauma; x-rays do not readily demonstrate the fracture. If the injury is suspected, a bone scan should be

arranged. Treatment is a non-weight-bearing plaster for up to 8–12 weeks. Chronic non-union of a stress fracture can be a difficult problem to manage.

Fractures of the cuboid bone

These are almost exclusively associated with other injury patterns of the foot. Comminuted fractures are not amenable to fixation. Mid-tarsal degenerative change is a common sequel.

Fractures of the cuneiforms

Most isolated cuneiform fractures are caused by direct injury, and the treatment of the overlying soft tissues is important. Most comminuted fractures defy surgical reconstruction. Elevation is an important part of the treatment plan. Immobilization following elevation is often necessary.

Mid-tarsal dislocations

The mid-tarsal region consists of the smaller bones of the tarsus (navicular, cuboid and the three cuneiforms) in association with the mid-tarsal joint, i.e. the calcaneo-cuboid and the talo-navicular. The mid-tarsal joint may be injured by a number of mechanisms, and joint damage is also often associated with fracture of the smaller bones. Therefore great care must be taken when assessing a patient with a tarsal fracture to ensure that there is no accompanying mid-tarsal injury.

Mechanisms of injury

Many mechanisms of injury can produce mid-tarsal injury, i.e. subluxation, dislocation or fracture-dislocation. The detailed mechanisms are outside the scope of this book. However, the common patterns are as a result of forced abduction and adduction of the foot. As a result of associated fractures and ligamentous disruption, many mid-tarsal injuries are unstable (Fig. 25.11).

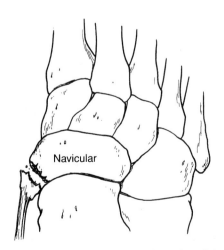

Figure 25.10 – Fracture of the tuberosity of the navicular

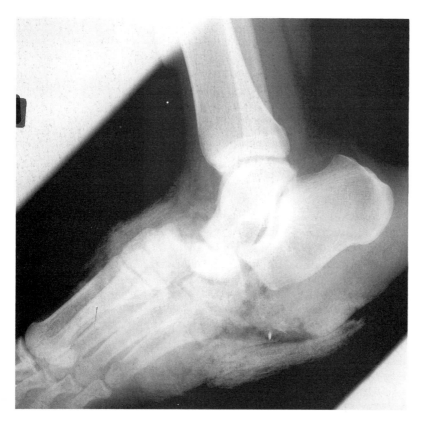

Figure 25.11 – A mid-tarsal dislocation

Management

Most mid-tarsal injuries warrant senior advice as interpretation of x-rays can be difficult. The majority require admission. Dislocations should be promptly reduced, preferably by experienced personnel, and this can be performed in the Accident and Emergency Department under intravenous sedation if necessary. Following reduction, produced by longitudinal traction and correction of deforming forces, the clinical stability of the tarsal region must be established. Further x-rays can then be obtained to assess the integrity of the tarsal bones. Many of the fractures, as they are unstable, require open fixation.

Tarso-metatarsal dislocations

Tarso-metatarsal injuries are not common but are very important to recognize, and are easily missed. Most are the result of high-energy trauma, and can result in long-term complications and morbidity. The tarso-metatarsal joint (Lisfranc's joint) consists of the articulation between proximally the three cuneiforms and the cuboid, and distally five metatarsal bases. Strong ligaments hold the bones together, and it is important to realize that these are damaged as part of any injury in this region. In addition, the local vascular arterial anatomy may be damaged as part of the injury.

Mechanisms of injury

These are many and varied. The most common are:

1. Twisting of the forefoot, often as part of a motor vehicle accident, where the whole forefoot is abducted laterally from the hind foot.

2. Crush injuries, associated with extensive soft tissue damage.

3. Axial compression of the fixed, weight-bearing foot. Note that trivial injury in this way can cause a disruption of the joint.

Clinical features

Tarso-metatarsal injury should be suspected when the above mechanisms have occurred. The clinical features are dependent upon the severity of the injury. 'Sprains' of the joint may occur, and can be confirmed by tenderness in the region and pain on attempted abduction and adduction at the joint. Also remember that a frank dislocation may have spontaneously reduced, and that the injury pattern may be unstable – gross tissue swelling is indicative of this. Dislocation is usually obvious. **Remember to palpate the dorsalis pedis pulse, and promptly reduce the fracture if the distal foot is vascularly compromised.**

Radiographs should be obtained, reduction having taken place initially if deformity is gross. Anterioposterior and lateral x-rays at a minimum are necessary, and oblique views may be helpful. Views of the other foot may be useful in defining the injury. Any fracture should be noted, but in addition, any alteration in the relationship of the bones suggests a ligamentous disruption that may need to be surgically corrected (Fig. 25.12).

Management

Tarso-metatarsal injuries should be assessed by senior personnel. 'Sprains', following exclusion of other injuries and with a normal stability, should be immobilized following a period of elevation in a plaster cast to ensure that all ligaments have healed. All subluxations and dislocations should be admitted, at the very least for elevation and observation of the circulation. Urgent reduction should be performed in the Accident and Emergency Department, preferably by an experienced surgeon. The detailed management following reduction is outside the scope of this book. Many require open fixation of the fracture pattern so as to restore the normal mechanics of the foot.

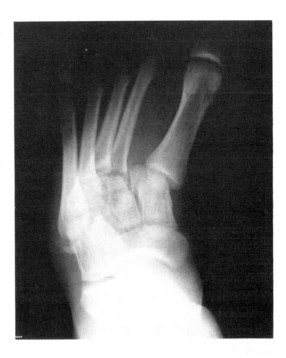

Figure 25.12 – Tarso-metatarsal subluxation

Metatarsal fractures

Metatarsal shaft and neck fractures

Metatarsal fractures are most commonly due to direct blows or crushing mechanisms. The initial treatment must take account of the injury to the overlying soft tissues. The fractures can also result indirectly from twisting injuries, and these result in spiral fractures, especially of the middle three metatarsals. Stress fractures also commonly occur, especially at the region of the fifth metatarsal base and the neck of the second and third metatarsals.

The first metatarsal is a strong bone and integrally involved in the biomechanics of the medial arch of the foot. Most fractures are due to direct trauma, although spiral fractures can occur, especially in athletes and dancers. Direct injuries often have significant soft tissue injury (Fig. 25.13). All open fractures should be admitted and treated in the classic way with antibiotics, wound debridement and fixation if indicated. Many closed fractures may also require admission for elevation, as swelling can be extreme. Displaced shaft fractures usually merit open fixation.

Direct-type fractures of the lesser metatarsals may also be associated with significant soft tissue injury. Consider admission for elevation in multiple fractures. Undisplaced isolated fractures can be treated conservatively, the foot being left free or immobilized in a plaster (care is needed with the latter as swelling may be considerable). Multiple displaced fractures warrant surgical stabilization as the foot may be unstable.

Stress fractures of the metatarsal shafts and necks

These commonly occur in young sporting adults. A history of significant injury may not be obtained, so the fracture must be suspected clinically. The most common site is the neck of the second metatarsal. The fractures tend to do well with conservative treatment, with advice to avoid sport until the fracture has healed. The injury can be treated free or within plaster if especially painful.

Avulsion fractures of the base of the fifth metatarsal

These are very common fractures, seen following an inversion injury of the foot, causing the tendon of peroneus brevis to pull off a portion of the basal bone. **The fracture will be missed unless it is specifically sought, as the patient commonly complains of a painful ankle, and the fifth metatarsal base is not seen on routine ankle x-rays.**

The patient complains of pain following a stumble, specifically an inversion injury. There is a limp, and the patient may not be able to weight-bear. The area around the base of the fifth metatarsal is swollen and bruised, and is tender to palpation. An x-ray may demonstrate a small avulsion fragment, which is usually undisplaced (Fig. 25.14). Distinguish the fracture from a Jones fracture (see below).

The treatment of nearly all of these fractures is conservative. If weight-bearing is not

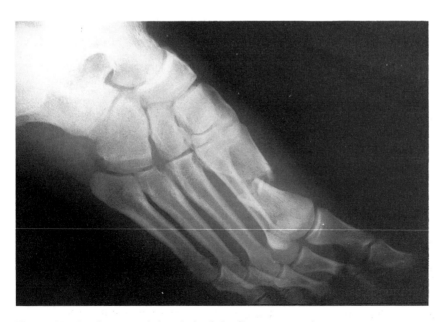

Figure 25.13 – Fracture of the shaft of the first metatarsal

possible, immobilize the foot in a below-knee plaster slab and give the patient some crutches. After a few days, convert the plaster to a fully weight-bearing cast, and leave this on for 2–4 weeks. Less significant injuries can be mobilized immediately with a compression bandage, crutches being needed for 1–2 weeks. Even significantly displaced fractures do not need reduction.

Take care not to confuse an avulsion fragment with small accessory bones around the base of the fifth metatarsal, nor with the epiphyseal line in children (Fig. 25.15) – remember that developmental x-ray features do not hurt when palpated!

Jones fractures – fractures of the basal shaft of the fifth metatarsal

These fractures need to be distinguished from the more common avulsion fractures of the fifth metatarsal base. The fracture is **not** due to an avulsion injury, and is a stress fracture most common in young athletic males. A history of

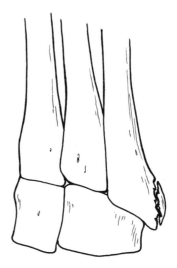

Figure 25.15 – Normal epiphysis at base of fifth metatarsal

definite injury may not be obtained. The characteristic x-ray feature is of a transverse fracture of the basal shaft **distal to the joint line** (Fig. 25.16).

These fractures have a tendency to go on to a painful non-union, and many centres routinely advocate open fixation of the fracture, but the

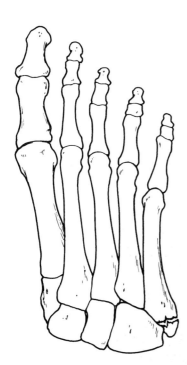

Figure 25.14 – Avulsion fracture of the base of the fifth metatarsal

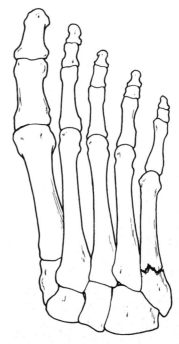

Figure 25.16 – Jones fracture of the fifth metatarsal

minimum treatment is 6 weeks in a non-weight-bearing plaster cast. Refer these patients on to the next available fracture clinic.

Fractures of the metatarsal heads

These are almost always caused by direct blows or crushing injuries, and may be associated with other bone or soft tissue damage. The fractures can be treated conservatively, but elevation etc. is vital as swelling may be considerable. If the displacement is significant, the heads can be reduced by longitudinal traction.

Phalangeal fractures and dislocations

First metatarso-phalangeal joint sprains and dislocations

The first metatarsophalangeal (MTP) joint may be sprained or dislocated. Sprains are the result of hyperextension of the great toe with injury to the dorsal capsule and ligaments. An x-ray may demonstrate an avulsion fracture from the head of the metatarsal. Treatment is conservative but symptoms may be troublesome. 'Neighbour strapping' to the second toe may give some pain relief.

Dislocation of the first MTP joint is uncommon, and results from high-energy trauma. Local skin pressure may be considerable, and the joint should be reduced promptly, if necessary prior to an x-ray. Radiography may demonstrate fracture of a sesamoid in addition. Most reduce with longitudinal traction, under sedation or local anaesthesia. Following reduction, elevation is necessary with later application of a below-knee walking plaster for 4–6 weeks.

Sesamoid fractures

Sesamoid bones may fracture around the first MTP joint for many reasons, including direct trauma, avulsion and stress. Most of the fractures are transverse. The initial treatment is conservative, although later excision of the sesa-

moids may be needed. A walking plaster cast is suitable.

Dislocation of the lesser metatarso-phalangeal joints.

These are very common injuries, usually as a result of lateral or medial forces upon the toe. The injury is clinically obvious, although an x-ray may show an associated fracture. The toe may be reduced under sedation or local anaesthetic 'ring block', and the reduction is effected by longitudinal traction. The process is rarely troublesome. A short period of 'neighbour strapping' may help analgesia.

Fractures of the great toe

Hallux fractures may be caused by a 'stubbing' mechanism, or by direct trauma. There may be intense swelling and a subungual haematoma may develop with distal phalangeal fractures. Elevation is vital and hospitalization may be necessary. Undisplaced fractures may be treated conservatively, but displaced fractures, especially of the proximal phalanx, may warrant open fixation. The treatment of the soft tissues in direct-type injuries is vital, and the fractures are often open. The subungual haematoma, if relieved by trephining, may considerably decrease the pain of the injury.

Lesser toe fractures

These are very common injuries, usually from 'stubbing' or a direct injury. Minimally displaced fractures can be treated with 'neighbour strapping' and elevation etc. Significantly displaced fractures should be reduced under sedation or ring block. Although very painful, recovery is rapid within 2–4 weeks.

Dislocations of the interphalangeal joints of the toes

These are less common than phalangeal fractures, and are easily reduced by longitudinal traction. 'Neighbour strap' the affected digit for a short period. If there is any instability following reduction (due to ligamentous damage), refer the patient for possible K wire fixation.

Soft tissue injuries of the foot

Soft tissue injuries of the foot are common, and can be more devastating than fractures. In many fractures of the foot, treatment of the soft tissues is of more importance, and this requires careful and adequate clinical examination.

The foot is liable to be involved in domestic and industrial accidents, with it being caught in rotatory motors and lawnmowers etc. These are very serious injuries even in the absence of a skeletal injury. Urgent debridement and antibiotic prophylaxis (in many cases including anaerobic cover) is essential.

As with any area of the body, but especially in the foot, **degloving injuries** must be recognized. These injuries are due to shear forces which disconnect the skin and subcutaneous tissue from the underlying structures, thereby compromising their blood supply. Degloving injuries of the sole of the foot are a special problem, and urgent referral to a plastic surgical unit is warranted.

The acutely painful foot

Pain in the foot is an exceedingly common presenting complaint, and a full consideration of all the causes of a painful foot is outside the scope of this book. However, given below are some of the conditions which may cause a patient to present with a painful foot in the emergency setting.

Plantar fasciitis

This is a common problem in the chronic setting, but may also present acutely. It arises from degeneration and inflammation around the plantar fascial attachment to the calcaneum on its medial aspect, causing medial heel and hindfoot pain. The presence of a calcaneal spur has absolutely no relevance to plantar fasciitis, despite numerous referrals for exactly this reason! Clinical signs include tenderness over

the medial calcaneum and pain on dorsiflexion and eversion of the forefoot. Treatment is largely conservative with appropriate lifestyle advice, anti-inflammatories and localized steroid injections in selected cases. Surgical intervention is uncommonly needed in chronic cases.

Stress fractures

Any bone in the foot may be affected by stress fracture, but the most common sites are the proximal fifth metatarsal, second and third metatarsal heads and the navicular bone. There is rarely a history of an isolated injury, and bone scans may be needed if clinically suspected, as x-rays may not demonstrate the fracture. Longer-standing cases may show signs of healing with a periosteal reaction and callus, confirming the diagnosis. Immobilization and referral to a fracture clinic is indicated.

Osteochondritis within the foot

The most common sites for osteochondritis in the foot are:

1. The metatarsal heads (most commonly the second) – **Freiberg's disease**. The aetiology is unclear. The patient complains of continual pain within the forefoot with exacerbation on weight-bearing. The area is very tender to palpation. The x-ray features are characteristic with widening and flattening of the metatarsal head and subsequent degenerative change within the metatarsophalangeal joint. The condition may require surgical excision of the head.
2. The navicular – **Kohler's disease**. This most commonly occurs in young children, with instep pain, and there is osteochondritic change on x-ray. Symptoms universally settle without treatment.

Tarsal coalition

This is a very important condition to recognize, due to initial cartilaginous and subsequent osseous bridging between the tarsal bones. The patient, usually adolescent, complains of an ache on the medial hindfoot. On examination, there is a restricted range of subtalar movement, which is the characteristic feature. An x-ray may demonstrate bony bridging between the bones, but special views are needed to fully visualize the bars. The management is outside the scope of this book, but if the condition is suspected (i.e. by the limitation in subtalar movement), a relatively urgent orthopaedic outpatient referral should be arranged. Prompt excision of a bar before fusion may prevent late pain and degenerative change.

Metatarsalgia

This is a very common chronic disorder in middle age, which may present acutely. Pain is experienced upon weight-bearing in the region of the metatarsal heads, and is probably due to intrinsic musculo-ligamentous insufficiency within the foot. Treatment is rarely curative in the short term and a routine orthopaedic referral may be warranted. Conservative therapy is used in the vast majority of cases. Metatarsalgia should be differentiated from a Morton's neuroma, osteochondritis (Freiberg's disease) and stress fractures.

Morton's neuroma

The plantar digital nerve develops a neuroma just prior to it branching into the toes. It is most commonly seen in the third/fourth toe interspace, and pain is elicited by direct pressure over the area, often with neurological symptoms spreading distally. Surgical excision is curative.

Conditions of the first metatarsophalangeal joint

This area is a common site of disorders. Probably the most common is **gout**, which may especially occur in those on thiazide diuretics or other conditions increasing the serum urate. Acute non-steroidal treatment is indicated, with appropriate investigations to determine the cause. Allopurinol should **not** be used acutely. Bursae as part of a **bunion** may also cause pain and swelling in this region, with local treatment indicated.

The toe nail of the hallux

This is a common site for infective problems, typically the 'ingrowing toe nail'. Initial presentations of infection may be treated with antibiotics, but recurrent infections require wedge resection or other surgical procedure.

Index